W0043244

Precision Anticoagulation Medicine

Hadi Goubran • Gaafar Ragab • Suzy Hassouna
Editors

Precision Anticoagulation Medicine

A Practical Guide

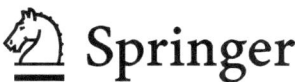 Springer

Editors
Hadi Goubran
Saskatoon Cancer Centre
College of Medicine
University of Saskatchewan
Saskatoon, SK
Canada

Gaafar Ragab
Faculty of Medicine
Cairo University
Giza
Egypt

Suzy Hassouna
College of Human Medicine
Michigan State University
East Lansing, MI
USA

ISBN 978-3-030-25781-1   ISBN 978-3-030-25782-8   (eBook)
https://doi.org/10.1007/978-3-030-25782-8

© Springer Nature Switzerland AG 2020
This work is subject to copyright. All rights are reserved by the Publisher, whether the whole or part of the material is concerned, specifically the rights of translation, reprinting, reuse of illustrations, recitation, broadcasting, reproduction on microfilms or in any other physical way, and transmission or information storage and retrieval, electronic adaptation, computer software, or by similar or dissimilar methodology now known or hereafter developed.
The use of general descriptive names, registered names, trademarks, service marks, etc. in this publication does not imply, even in the absence of a specific statement, that such names are exempt from the relevant protective laws and regulations and therefore free for general use.
The publisher, the authors, and the editors are safe to assume that the advice and information in this book are believed to be true and accurate at the date of publication. Neither the publisher nor the authors or the editors give a warranty, expressed or implied, with respect to the material contained herein or for any errors or omissions that may have been made. The publisher remains neutral with regard to jurisdictional claims in published maps and institutional affiliations.

This Springer imprint is published by the registered company Springer Nature Switzerland AG
The registered company address is: Gewerbestrasse 11, 6330 Cham, Switzerland

This book is dedicated to our beloved families,
Hanaa, Mariam and Farah Goubran
Samia, Ahmed and Sherif Ragab
and the memory of Prof Suzy Hassouna

Preface

Venous thromboembolism and thromboembolic complications of atrial fibrillation are the leading cause of morbidity and mortality across the globe accounting for one in four deaths worldwide in 2010. Its annual incidence rates range from 0.75 to 2.69 per 1000 individuals and increase with age to between 2 and 7 per 1000 among those aged ≥70 years.

For decades, physicians and patients had only two therapeutic options to prevent thrombosis: parenteral unfractionated heparin, one of the oldest medicines currently in use, first discovered in 1916, and the oral warfarin discovered in the late 1930s which necessitated close monitoring with prothrombin time testing.

In the early 1990s, low molecular weight heparins became available as subcutaneous preparations that were offered for both prophylaxis and therapy. The simplicity of their use and dosage fostered a wider use of anticoagulation and allowed for outpatient management of venous thrombosis.

In an effort to address heparin-induced thrombocytopenia, injectable direct antithrombin inhibitors were developed and introduced into our practice algorithms.

In less than two decades later, direct oral anticoagulants with variable therapeutic profiles including direct thrombin inhibitors and anti-factor Xa preparations were offered as therapeutic and prophylactic alternatives to patients with venous thrombosis, for the prevention of thromboembolic complications of atrial fibrillation and as prophylactic tools.

Clinicians are now confronted with an arsenal of anticoagulants and a plethora of clinical trials and guidelines positioning different agents for a given indication and for a particular patient's profile. Many large thrombosis bodies developed apps and therapeutic algorithms to help direct practitioners on how to optimize the use of anticoagulation.

Anticoagulation, therefore, is moving toward a personalized approach where one should choose from the wide palette of anticoagulants, the suitable agent for a given indication in a given profile.

For a clinician in the various medical disciplines today to make an evidence-based anticoagulation decision, a road map is needed to navigate through the different agents, indications, and intrinsic patients' characteristics.

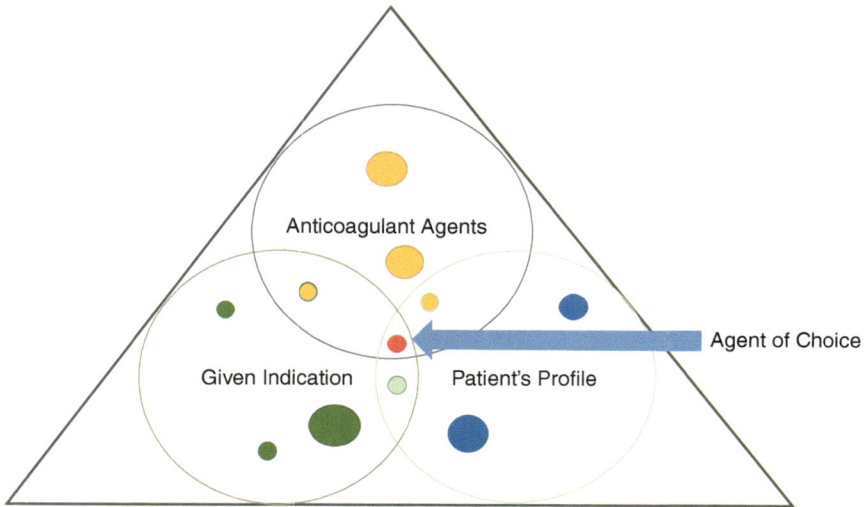

In this book, and with the contribution of a large group of clinicians from different disciplines and different parts of the world, we tried to draw an anticoagulation guide map based on the different therapeutic options available, the approved or accepted indications supported by clinical evidence, and patients' profiles.

This book is not meant at all to replace any local, regional, or national guideline as many institutions, scientific bodies, and nations have developed their own specific guidelines that should be followed rigorously. It is meant only to integrate most of the available resources in a comprehensive format.

The first chapter of this book attempted at reviewing the commonly available anticoagulants with simple prescription tools to help their administration and monitoring. The following chapters address the anticoagulation based on patients and diseases including anticoagulation in the general population, in cardiac patients, in the pediatric population, in the context of cancer, or in pregnancy and lactation.

Anticoagulation in rheumatic patients and in patients with the antiphospholipid syndrome as well as anticoagulation in renal patients was also addressed separately.

Thromboprophylaxis in surgical and medical patients is also given their due consideration.

The last two chapters describe the indications and methods to bridge anticoagulation in the context of procedures and surgical interventions as well as the tool to reverse their action in case of bleeding.

A better understanding of coagulation and the underlying pathophysiology of thrombosis in the different clinical contexts calls for the development of newer targeting anticoagulants. The field is therefore in rapid evolution moving steadily toward a more precise, personalized approach.

It is sad that Dr. Hassouna, our coeditor, passed away peacefully on October 2018 during the early preparation of this book. She was Professor of Medicine, Division of Thrombosis, Elsa D. and Carl E. Rehberg Hematology Research Professor, and Director, Special Coagulation Center at Michigan State University (MSU). In her proliferative career, she contributed tremendously to the understanding of blood coagulation, particularly the vitamin K-dependent factors and also, therefore, natural anticoagulants like protein C. In 1989, she was the first in the world to publish a second biochemical cause in protein C associated with thrombosis by documenting resistance to inactivation of both activated factor V and factor VIII by activated protein C. She will always be remembered as a delightful personality and an outstanding researcher and medical educator.

In a famous quote, Dr. Samuel Johnson said: "knowledge is of two kinds. We know a subject ourselves or we know where we can find information upon it." In the ever-expanding horizons of thrombosis and anticoagulation, we do not claim to have the knowledge, but we can modestly hope to offer our reader a tool to navigate and our fellow physicians an instrument that helps in decision-making.

Saskatoon, SK, Canada   Hadi Goubran
Giza, Egypt   Gaafar Ragab

Contents

Contributors

Ahmed Abdulgawad, MB.BCh, MSc, MD, MD (Hematology) MRCP Hematology Department, Faculty of Medicine, Cairo University, Giza, Egypt

Hamdy M. A. Ahmed, MB.BCh, MSc, MD Division of Clinical Immunology and Rheumatology, University of Alabama at Birmingham, Birmingham, USA

Rheumatology and Clinical Immunology, Faculty Of Medicine Cairo University, Giza, Egypt

Jérôme Avouac, MD, PhD Université Paris Descartes, Service de Rhumatologie, Hôpital Cochin, Paris, France

Rashad S. Barsoum, MB.BCh, MD, FRCP, FRCP Edin The Cairo Kidney Center, Cairo, Egypt

Department of Internal Medicine and Nephrology, Kasr-El-Aini Medical School, Cairo University, Cairo, Egypt

Mark Bosch, MD, FRCPC Saskatoon Cancer Centre, College of Medicine, University of Saskatchewan, Saskatoon, SK, Canada

Kelsey Brose, MD, FRCPC Saskatoon Cancer Centre, College of Medicine, University of Saskatchewan, Saskatoon, SK, Canada

Veronica Codullo, MD, PhD Université Paris Descartes, Service de Rhumatologie, Hôpital Cochin, Paris, France

Cherine El-Dabh, MD Cleveland Clinic and Lerner School of Medicine, Abu Dhabi, UAE

Mohamed Elemary, MB.BCh. MSc, MD Saskatoon Cancer Centre, College of Medicine, University of Saskatchewan, Saskatoon, SK, Canada

Hadi Goubran, MB.BCh, MSc, MD, FACP, FRCP Edin (UK) Saskatoon Cancer Centre, College of Medicine, University of Saskatchewan, Saskatoon, SK, Canada

Hany Guirguis, MB.BCh, MSc, FRCP Edin, FRCPC Scarborough Health Network, Toronto, ON, Canada

Haissam Haddad, BSc,MD,FRCPC,FACC,FAAC,FRCP Edin Department of Medicine, Division of Cardiology, University of Saskatchewan, Saskatoon, SK, Canada

Tony Haddad, MD Department of Medicine, College of Medicine, University of Saskatchewan, Saskatoon, SK, Canada

Caroline Hart, MD, FRCPC Saskatoon Cancer Centre, College of Medicine, University of Saskatchewan, Saskatoon, SK, Canada

Mohamed Tharwat Hegazy, MB.BCh, MSc, MD Internal Medicine Department, Rheumatology and Clinical Immunology Unit, Faculty of Medicine, Cairo University, Cairo, Egypt

Iman Fathy Iskander, MB.BCh, MSc, MD Pediatrics & Neonatology, College of Medicine, Cairo University, Giza, Egypt

Ahmed Maher Kaddah, MB.BCh, MSc, MD Pediatrics and Pediatric Hematology, College of Medicine, Cairo University, Giza, Egypt

Mervat Mattar, MB.BCh, MSc, MD Internal Medicine and Hematology, Cairo University, Giza, Egypt

Otto Moodley, MD, FRCPC Saskatoon Cancer Centre, College of Medicine, University of Saskatchewan, Saskatoon, SK, Canada

Joshua Nero, MD, FRCPC Section of Gastroenterology, Department of Internal Medicine, Max Rady College of Medicine, University of Manitoba, Winnipeg, MB, Canada

Udoka Okpalauwaekwe, MD, FRCPC Division of Cardiology, College of Medicine, University of Saskatchewan, Saskatoon, SK, Canada

Ibraheem Othman, MB.BCh, MSc, MD Alain Blair Cancer Centre and College of Medicine, University of Saskatchewan, Regina, SK, Canada

Derek Pearson, MD, FRCPC Saskatoon Cancer Centre, College of Medicine, University of Saskatchewan, Saskatoon, SK, Canada

Gaafar Ragab, MB.BCh, MSc, MD Internal Medicine Department, Rheumatology and Clinical Immunology Unit, Giza, Egypt

Waleed Sabry, MB.BCh, MSc, MD Saskatoon Cancer Centre and Division of Oncology, College of Medicine, University of Saskatchewan, Saskatoon, SK, Canada

Nishant Sharma, MD, FRCPC Division of Cardiology, College of Medicine, University of Saskatchewan, Saskatoon, SK, Canada

Jay S. Shavadia, MD, FRCPC Division of Cardiology, College of Medicine, University of Saskatchewan, Saskatoon, SK, Canada

Tamer Shehab, MB.BCh, MRCP (UK) The Cairo Kidney Center, Cairo, Egypt

Department of Nephrology, Sahel Teaching Hospital, Ministry of Health, Cairo, Egypt

Julie Stakiw, MD, FRCPC Saskatoon Cancer Centre, College of Medicine, University of Saskatchewan, Saskatoon, SK, Canada

Vinita Sundaram, MB.BCh. MD Saskatoon Cancer Centre, Saskatoon, SK, Canada

Hanaa Wanas, PhD The Cairo Kidney Center, Cairo, Egypt

Department of Pharmacology, Kasr-El-Aini Medical School, Cairo University, Cairo, Egypt

Alex Zhai, MD, FRCPC Division of Cardiology, Department of Medicine, University of Saskatchewan, Saskatoon, SK, Canada

Chapter 1
Coagulation and Anticoagulants

Hadi Goubran, Mark Bosch, and Julie Stakiw

Abbreviations

ACCP	American College of Chest Physicians
AF	Atrial fibrillation
APC	Activated protein C
aPTT	Activated Partial thromboplastin time
AT	Antithrombin
AUC	Area under the curve
BID	Twice daily
C4BP	C4b-binding protein
CAD	Coronary artery disease
Cmax	Maximum (or peak) serum concentration
CrCl	Creatinine clearance
CYP	Cytochrome
DOACs	Direct oral anticoagulants
DVT	Deep venous thrombosis
ECT	Eccrine time
HIT	Heparin-induced thrombocytopenia
HMK	High-molecular-weight kininogen
LMWH	Low-molecular-weight heparin
MI	Myocardial infarction
NOACs	Non-vitamin K antagonist oral anticoagulants

H. Goubran (✉) · M. Bosch · J. Stakiw
Saskatoon Cancer Centre, College of Medicine, University of Saskatchewan,
Saskatoon, SK, Canada
e-mail: hadi.goubranmessiha@saskcancer.ca; Mark.bosch@saskcancer.ca;
Julie.stakiw@saskcancer.ca

© Springer Nature Switzerland AG 2020
H. Goubran et al. (eds.), *Precision Anticoagulation Medicine*,
https://doi.org/10.1007/978-3-030-25782-8_1

1

PAD	Peripheral artery disease
PCI	Percutaneous coronary intervention
PE	Pulmonary embolization
P-gp	Permeability glycoprotein
PK	Pre-kallikrein
SC	Subcutaneous
STEMI	ST segment elevation myocardial infarction
TAFI	Tissue factor pathway inhibitor
TF	Tissue factor
THR	Total hip replacement
TKR	Total knee replacement
TT	Thrombin time
UFH	Unfractionated Heparin
VKA	Vitamin K antagonist
VKORC1	Vitamin K epoxide reductase
VTE	Venous thromboembolism

Introduction

The coagulation process that leads to hemostasis involves numerous reactions that culminate into the conversion of soluble fibrinogen to insoluble strands of fibrin which entraps platelets to forms a stable thrombus.

The Coagulation Cascade

Classically the coagulation cascade has been described as a dual model pathway with the intrinsic and extrinsic pathways merging into a common pathway that, following the activation of factor X, leads to the generation of thrombin which then converts fibrinogen into fibrin [1]. This model reflects to the screening coagulation laboratory tests, prothrombin time (PT) and activated partial thromboplastin time (aPTT), which correspond to the extrinsic and intrinsic pathways respectively. Factor XII, high-molecular-weight kininogen (HMK), or Pre-Kallekrein (PK) deficiency, on the other hand, does not cause a clinical bleeding tendency.

The "extrinsic" and "intrinsic" pathways are interdependent in vivo as it was recognized that the factor VIIa/tissue factor (TF) complex can activate factor IX as well as factor X [2]. Figure 1.1 illustrates the coagulation cascade. Thrombin is capable of directly activating factor XI on the charged surface of activated platelets [3, 4]. Factor XII, HMK, and PK might therefore not be required for hemostasis. This led to a concept of hemostasis in which TF is the primary physiologic activator [5].

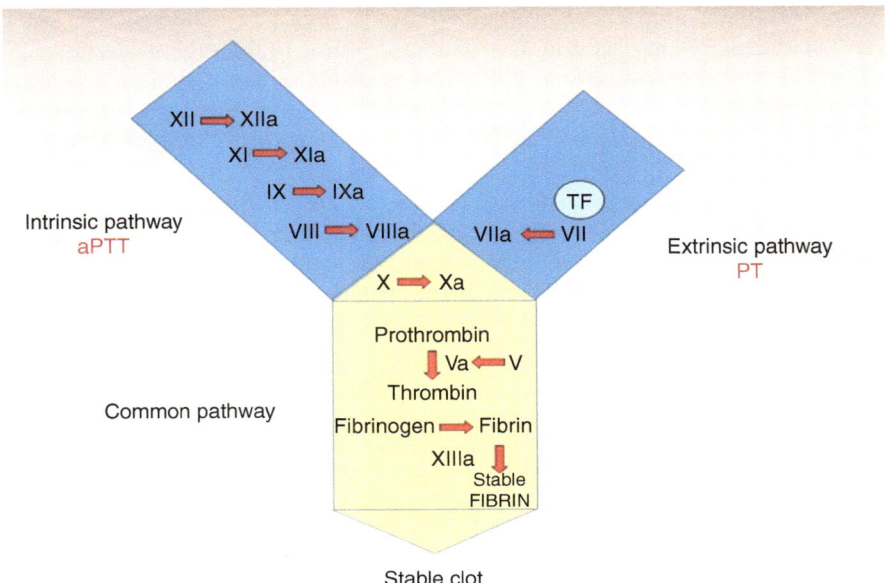

Fig. 1.1 The coagulation cascade with its intrinsic and extrinsic pathway leading to a common pathway and the formation of a stable fibrin clot

Cell-Based Model of Hemostasis

Another model of hemostasis, the cell-based model, highlights the important interactions between cells directly involved in hemostasis and coagulation factors and views hemostasis as occurring in three overlapping phases. It represents a more accurate description of the interaction between cellular activity and coagulation proteins that leads to thrombus formation and hemostasis [6].

The initiation phase of coagulation is triggered when a break in the vessel wall allows plasma to come into contact with TF-bearing extravascular cells [7]. Cancer cells or microparticles can also express TF [8, 9]. Factor VII in plasma tightly binds to cellular TF rapidly activating coagulation [7]. If the procoagulant stimulus is sufficiently strong, adequate amounts of factors Xa, IXa, and thrombin are formed, successfully igniting the coagulation process [5].

Amplification of the coagulant response occurs at the platelet surface where the procoagulant stimulus is amplified as platelets become activated and accumulate activated cofactors on their surfaces. Activated factor X causes a burst of thrombin production. Microparticles are irregularly shaped vesicles that are smaller than platelets (<1 μm in diameter) [9]. They arise from the plasma membrane of blood-borne cells during cell activation, exposure to shear stress, or apoptosis [10]. P-selectin, a cell adhesion molecule, is also expressed on the endothelium and activated platelets [11]. Both microparticles and P-selectin promote thrombosis during the amplification phase of coagulation [11].

Finally, in the propagation phase, the active proteases combine with their cofactors on the platelet surface and large-scale generation of thrombin takes place [5]. Thrombin converts the soluble fibrinogen to insoluble fibrin strands, leading to thrombus formation.

Thrombin also activates factor XIII, which stabilizes the thrombus by cross-linking fibrin. The resulting fibrin mesh is strong enough to trap and hold cellular components of the thrombus (platelets and/or red blood cells) [1].

Factor Xa plays a central role in both the original extrinsic/intrinsic model, as well as the cell-based model of hemostasis with its three phases. One molecule of factor Xa catalyzes the formation of approximately 1000 thrombin molecules [12]. Figure 1.2 illustrates the cell-based model of hemostasis.

Natural Anticoagulants, Predisposing Factors, and Exposing Factors of Clot Formation

Natural anticoagulants are circulating proteins that tend to modulate, limit, and balance thrombin production.

Encoded by the *PROS1* gene, protein S is a vitamin K-dependent plasma glycoprotein synthesized by the liver that exists in the circulation in a free form or a complex one, bound to complement C4b-binding protein (C4BP) [13]. It functions as a cofactor to protein C in the inactivation of Factors Va and VIIIa. Only the free form has cofactor activity [14]. *PROS1* gene mutations result in quantitative or qualitative protein S deficiency with increased thrombotic risks [15].

Protein C, encoded by the *PROC* gene found on chromosome 2 [16], is also a vitamin K-dependent zymogen. Its activated form plays an important role in regulating anticoagulation, inflammation and apoptosis, and endothelial function [17]. When activated by protein S, activated protein C (APC) performs these operations primarily by proteolytically inactivating proteins factor Va and factor VIIIa. APC is classified as a serine protease as it contains a residue of serine in its active site [18]. Deficiency or resistance to the action of protein C will result in an enhanced thrombotic risk [19]. Resistance to activated protein C occurs in congenital and acquired states [20]. The factor V Leiden mutation, caused by a single nucleotide substitution resulting in an R506Q missense mutation, results in factor V resistance to APC inactivation and is the most common heritable cause of venous thrombosis [20].

Antithrombin (AT), a glycoprotein produced by the liver, contains three disulfide bonds and a total of four possible glycosylation sites [20]. Its activity is increased many folds by heparins, which enhance its binding to factors IIa and Xa [21]. Whereas unfractionated heparin binds IIa and Xa in a 1:1 ratio, low-molecular-weight heparins have more affinity to Xa [22]. Deficiencies of antithrombin result in thrombophilia and increased clotting risks.

Other natural anticoagulants include heparin cofactor II and tissue factor pathway inhibitor.

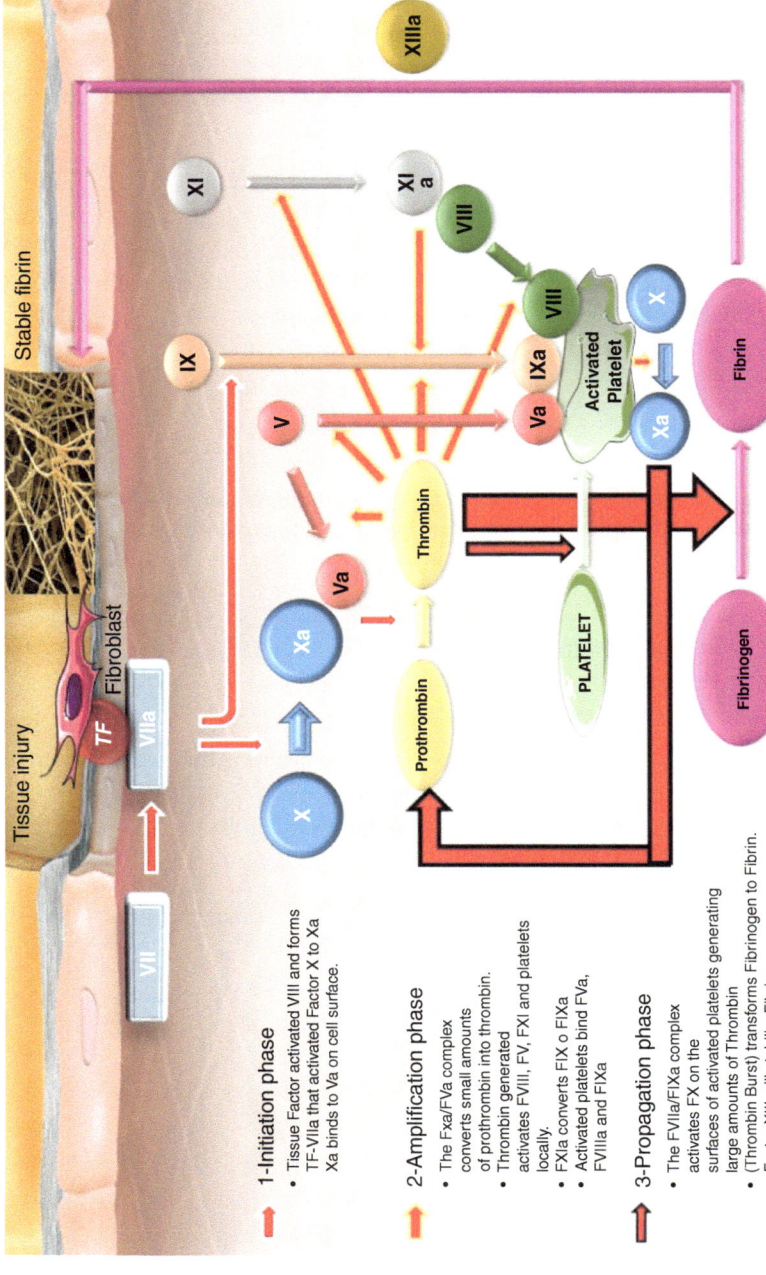

Fig. 1.2 The cell-based model of hemostasis in three phases: initiation, amplification, and propagation. The result is the formation of a stable clot

Disturbance of the hemostatic balance between coagulation factors and natural anticoagulants will favor clot formation. As an example, an imbalance can also occur in the presence of excess coagulation factors associated with the prothrombin 20210 G/A mutation, associated with elevated levels of factor II in plasma, which causes a significantly increased risk of developing venous thrombosis. It is the second most important genetic risk factor for venous thrombosis in Caucasian populations [23, 24].

The genetic predisposition therefore can lead to unprovoked clots or paves the way for thrombosis to develop when the patient is exposed to a second hit that includes hormonal therapy [25], immobilization [26], hospitalization [27], trauma [28], surgery [29], and the development of cancer [30]. If such triggers are strong enough, a provoked thrombosis can develop even in individuals with no genetic predisposition.

Anticoagulants

For decades, clinicians had only two anticoagulant tools: heparin and warfarin. With a better understanding of the coagulation cascade and advancements in basic science, a full arsenal of anticoagulants are now available and should be used with precision, tailored to meet the need of individual patients in a personalized manner. The choice is based on the indications for anticoagulation, the bleeding risks, and the presence of comorbidities including renal or hepatic disease and the convenience of administration.

Anticoagulants include:

- Indirect thrombin inhibitors which encompass heparin, low-molecular-weight heparins, pentasaccharide, and heparinoids
- Vitamin K antagonists, namely, warfarin and related molecules
- Parenteral direct thrombin inhibitors
- Non-vitamin K antagonist oral anticoagulants (NOACs) also known as direct oral anticoagulants (DOACs) which include dabigatran, the direct thrombin inhibitor, or a series of direct anti-factor Xa molecules

The doses of anticoagulants mentioned in this chapter reflect manufacturers' recommendations. Figure 1.3 illustrates the site of action of the different anticoagulants on the coagulation cascade.

Injectable Indirect Thrombin/Anti-Xa Inhibitors

Indirect thrombin inhibitors act through binding AT and enhancing its inactivation of factor Xa and thrombin. Unfractionated heparin inhibits both thrombin as well as factor Xa. Low-molecular-weight heparins, on the other hand, act predominantly on

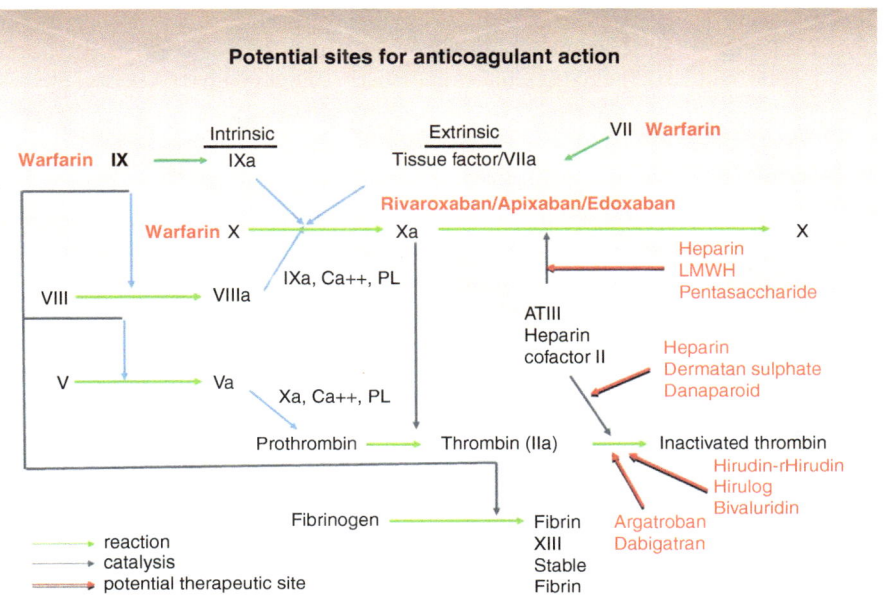

Fig. 1.3 Site of action of the different anticoagulant agents on the coagulation cascade

factor Xa and to a lesser extent on IIa. The synthetic pentasaccharide fondaparinux is an indirect factor Xa inhibitor.

Unfractionated Heparin (UFH)

Historic Background

Heparin is one of the oldest drugs, which nevertheless remains in widespread clinical use as an inhibitor of blood coagulation [31]. It was discovered around 1922 by Howell (Baltimore) and was further developed by the teams of Best (Toronto) and Jorpes (Stockholm). It was not until 1971 onward when Kakkar (London) propagated its routine use for the prevention of postoperative thrombosis [32, 33].

Heparin is a sulfated mucopolysaccharide derived from bovine or porcine lungs or intestine and contains glucuronic acid and N-acetyl glucosamine residues. It binds endothelial cell surface and antithrombin enhancing its neutralizing activity of factors IIa, IXa, and Xa. It also interacts with platelet factor 4.

Indications

With the advent of low-molecular-weight heparins and other novel anticoagulants, the use of UFH is currently limited to cardiovascular indications and for the management and prevention of venous thromboembolism (VTE) in the presence of renal impairment.

Formulation

1000, 5000, and 10,000, (20,000) units/ml (heparin sodium with 0.01 benzyl alcohol)

Route and Dose

Therapeutic

(i). Continuous infusion by an infusion pump after an initial bolus of 80–100 units/ kg (max 10,000 units). A continuous infusion given at a rate of 15–22 units/kg per hour is required to maintain therapeutic levels. Dose adjustment is made based on monitoring anti-Xa and aPTT. The infusion can be given either as a high or a low intensity based on indications (VTE vs. cardiovascular) with a gradual or a rapid approach based on bleeding risks.

(ii). Subcutaneous UFH (deep subcutaneous to avoid hematoma formation) can be given either by an unmonitored dose regimen with an initial dose of 333 units/ kg followed by 250 Units/kg q 12 h. A monitored approach is used when an immediate effect is needed with a loading dose of 5000 units by IV followed by 250 units/kg Sc. q 12 h with testing at 6 h.

Prophylactic

Heparin is given at a dose of 5000 international units subcutaneously every 8–12 h with no monitoring.

Monitoring

Heparin assay/aPTT,   hemoglobin,   and   signs   of   bleeding   should   be monitored.

Platelet count should be performed at baseline and every 2–3 days on days 4–14 of therapy.

(i). Continuous infusion: Therapeutic range for treatment of VTE is at 0.3–0.7 units per milliliter (anti-Xa Units) corresponding to a PTT of 1.5–2.5 times baseline values. Standard monograms help adjust the dose of heparin [34].

(a) High intensity/rapid nomogram (VTE) using aPTT and anti-Xa for control

ATPP (sec)	UFH bolus	Hold Infusion	Rate Change	Repeat aPTT
Less than 45	Repeat x1	0	Inc 450 U/h	6 h
45–59	Repeat ½	0	Inc 300 U/h	6 h
60–69	0	0	Inc 150 U/h	6
70–90	**0**	**0**	**NO CHANGE**	**Next A.M.**
100–109	0	0	Dec 150 U/h	6 h
110–125	0	30 min	Dec 300 U/h	6 h
>125	0	60 min	Dec 450 U/h	6 h

Anti-Xa(IU/ml)	UFH bolus	Hold Infusion	Rate Change	Repeat aPTT
<0.1	Repeat 40 U/kg	0	Inc 3 U/kg/h	6 h
0.1–0.19	Repeat 20 U/kg	0	Inc 2 U/kg/h	6 h
0.2–0.029	0	0	Inc 1 U/kg/h	6
0.3–0.7	**0**	**0**	**NO CHANGE**	**Next A.M.**
0.71–0.8	0	0	Dec 1 U/kg/h	6 h
0.81–1.7	0	60 min	Dec 2 U/kg/h	6 h
>1.7	0	90 min	Dec 3 U/kg/h	6 h

(b) Low intensity, gradual (cardiovascular indications/high bleeding risks)) using aPTT and anti-Xa for control

ATPP (sec)	UFH bolus	Hold Infusion	Rate Change	Repeat aPTT
Less than 45	Repeat x1 or 0	0	Inc 200 U/h	6 h
45–59	0	0	Inc 100 U/h	6 h
60–84	**0**	**0**	**N change**	**Next a.m**
85–94	0	0	Dec 100 U/h	6 h
95–110	0	60 min	Dec 200 U/h	6 h
>110	0	120 min	Dec 300 U/h	6 h

Anti-Xa(IU/ml)	UFH bolus	Hold Infusion	Rate Change	Repeat aPTT
<0.1	Repeat 20 U/kg	0	Inc 2 U/kg/h	6 h
0.1–0.29	0	0	Inc 1 U/kg/h	6
0.3–0.7	**0**	**0**	**N change**	**Next a.m.**
0.71–0.8	0	0	Dec 1 U/kg/h	6 h
0.81–1.7	0	60 min	Dec 2 U/kg/h	6 h
>1.7	0	90 min	Dec 3 U/kg/h	6 h

(ii). SC monitored UFH, the aPTT, or anti-Xa should be measured 6 h after the administered doses maintaining APTT at 2–2.5 times baseline values. The following nomogram highlights the approach for dose adjustment.

Anti-Xa (IU/ml)	Intervention
<0.15	Inc 48 U/kg/12 h
0.15–0.29	Inc 24 U/kg/12 h
0.3–0.7	**No change**
0.17–1.0	Dec 24 U/kg/12 h
>1	Dec 48 U/kg/12 h

Side Effects

A. Bleeding: minimized by careful patient selection, close control of dosage, and proper monitoring.
B. Osteoporosis and mineral deficiencies have been described with prolonged heparin use.
C. Heparin induced thrombocytopenia [HIT] [35] occurs in 1–4% of patients treated for a minimum of 7 days (see Chap. 2).

Contraindications

UFH is contraindicated in HIT, hypersensitivity to the medication and in the presence of active or recent bleeding or bleeding diathesis and in the presence of significant thrombocytopenia.

Reversal

Discontinuation often results in avoiding excessive anticoagulation. If reversal is needed, protamine sulfate may be given at a dose of 1 milligram for every 100 units of UFH. The rate of the infusion should not exceed 50 milligrams per 10 min. (see Chap. 13).

Low-Molecular-Weight Heparins [LMWHs]

In contrast to UFH, LMWHs inhibit activated factor X and to a lesser extent factor IIa. Numerous studies have demonstrated that they are as efficacious as UFH for the treatment and prevention of venous thromboembolism. LMWHs are administered subcutaneously and do not require monitoring if given in the therapeutic dose and in the presence of adequate kidney functions with predictable pharmacokinetics [36].

LMWHs are frequently used for perioperative prophylaxis and prophylaxis in medical patients. In addition, LMWHs can be used as initial anticoagulants, given for 7–10 days prior to bridging to warfarin or as extended anticoagulants in cancer patients. They also have many cardiovascular indications [37].

Epidural or spinal hematomas may occur in patients undergoing anticoagulation with LMWHs or heparinoids who receive neuraxial (epidural or spinal) anesthesia or spinal puncture [38].

Figure 1.4 illustrates the different LMWH and their corresponding therapeutic and prophylactic doses with the percentage of renal and hepatic elimination.

Low-molecular-weight heparins are not interchangeable as they differ with respect to their pharmacological properties and their capacity to inhibit factor Xa vs. factor IIa varies greatly. They increase the release and activity of tissue factor pathway inhibitor (TFPI) from endothelial cells under both static conditions and arterial shear stress [47].

	Plasma ½ life	Prophylactic dose	Therapeutic dose	Elimination	Form
Bemiparin (Badyket®, Heparox, Hepdren, Ivorat) [39]	5–6 h	**Surgical** **Orthopedic** **Medical** 2500–3500 IU/SC q 24 h	<50Kg 5000 IU/SC q 24 h 50-70Kg 7500 IU/SC q 24 h 70-100Kg 10,000 IU/SC q 24	**Renal/Hepatic**	Bemiparin **PFS** 2500 IU 0.2ml 3500 IU 0.2ml 5000 IU 0.2ml 7500 IU 0.3ml 10,000 IU 0.4ml
Certoparin [40]	1.5 h	**Surgical** 3000 IU/SC q 24 h ×7–10 days	–	**Renal**	**PFS** 3000 IU/0.3 mL
Dalteparin (Fragmin®) [41]	3–5 h	**Surgical** 2500 IU pre 2500 IU/SC **Orthopedic** 2500 IU pre or immediate post-op 5000 IU/24 h **Medical** 5000 IU/SC q 24 h	**VTE/Cancer** 200 units IU/kg SC qDay **UA/MI** 120 IU/kg SC q12h for 5–8 days (concurrent with aspirin 75–165 mg qDay) Not to exceed 10,000 units/dose or 18,000 units/day	CrCl <30 mL/min: monitor anti-Xa level to determine appropriate dose	**PFS** 2500 IU/0.2 ml 5000 IU/0.2 ml 7500 IU/0.3 ml **Vial** 10,000 IU/ml 25,000 IU/ml
Enoxaparin (Clexane-Lovenox) [42]	4.5 h	**Surgical/Ortho** 40 mg/SCq24h (world except USA) 30 mg/SC q12 h (USA) **Medical** 40 mg/SC q 24 h	**VTE** 1 mg/kg/SC q12h Or 1.5 mg/kg/Sc q 24 h **UA/MI** 1 mg/kg/SC q 12 h in (concurrent with aspirin therapy (100–325 mg qDay) **STEMI** 30 mg IV bolus once plus 1 mg/kg/ SC once followed by 1 mg/kg/SC q 12 h (maximum 100 mg for the first two doses only, followed by 1 mg/kg for the remaining doses)	CrCl <50 mL/min: monitor anti-Xa level to determine appropriate dose	**PFS** 40 mg/0.4 ml 60 mg/0.6 ml 80 mg/0.8 ml 100 mg/ml 30 mg/0.3 ml 120 mg/0.8 ml 150 mg/ml

Fig. 1.4 Commonly used LMWH, their half-lives, indications, elimination, and formulations

	Plasma ½ life	Prophylactic dose	Therapeutic dose	Elimination	Form
Nadroparin (Fraxiparine) [43]	3.5 h	**Surgical/Medical** 2850 IU/SC q 24 h **Orthopedic** High risk 38 IU/kg/SC q 24 × 3 days then 57 IU/kg/SC q 24 h. **Dialysis** 65 IU/kg for extracorporeal system	**VTE** 171 U/kg q 24 h or 86 IU/kg/q 12 h (0.1 ml/10 kg/q 12 h)	25–33% dose reduction if CrCl 30–50 D/C if CrCl<50 ml/min.	**PFS** 2850 IU/0.3 ml 3800 IU/0.4 ml 5700 IU/0.6 ml 7600 IU/0.8 ml
Parnaparin (Fluxum) [44]	6 h	**Surgical** 3200 IU/SC 2 h pre-op, then 3200 u/SC q 24 h × 7 **Orthopedic** 4250 IU/SC 12 h pre-op, then 4250 IU/SC 12 h post-op and then q 24 h × 10 days.	**VTE** 6400 IU/SC/q 24 h	Mainly renal	**PFS** 3200 IU/0.3 ml 4250 IU/0.4 ml 6400 IU/0.6 ml
Reviparin (Clivarine) [45]	1.5 h	**Surgical** 1750 SC 12 h pre-op then every 24 **Orthopedic** 4200 IU/SC 12 h prior then q 24	**VTE** 175 IU/SC q 12 h **PTCI** 7000 IU/IV then 10,500 IU/IV infusion/24 h	monitor anti-Xa If CrCl 30–50 ml/min D/C < 50 ml/min	**PFS** 1750 IU/0.25 ml 4200 IU/0.6 ml **Vial** 7000 IU/ ml 10,500 IU/1.5 ml
Tinzaparin (Innohep-Logiparin) [46]	3–4 h	**Surgical** 3500 IU/SC q 24 h **Orthopedic** Hip 50 IU/kg/SC q 24 h **Knee** 75 IU/kg SC q 24 h	**VTE** 175 IU/kg/SC 24 h	monitor anti-Xa if CrCl<30 ml/min	**PFS** 2500 IU/0.25 ml 3500 IU/0.35 ml 4500 IU/0.45 ml 8000 IU/0.4 ml 10,000 IU/0.5 ml 12,000 IU/0.6 ml 14,000 IU/0.7 ml 16,000 IU/0.8 ml 18,000 IU/0.9 ml **Vial** 10,000 IU/ml 20,000 IU/ml

Fig. 1.4 (continued)

LMWHs are usually administered by deep SC injection into the skin fold of the abdominal wall, held between thumb and forefinger and alternating between right and left, anterior and posterior areas.For IV administration, they may be administered in IV line with 0.9% NaCl or D5W.

Indications and Dosage [39–46]

1. Deep Vein Thrombosis (Prophylaxis)
   LMWHs are used to prevent the occurrence of pulmonary embolism in patients at risk for thromboembolic complications who are undergoing abdominal surgery and hip or knee replacement surgery, as well as in medical patients with severely restricted mobility during acute illness.

   (a) *Abdominal surgery (For extended prophylaxis following cancer surgery* (please refer to Chap. 10).
   - *Bemiparin*: 2500–3500 IU SC q 24 h.
   - *Certoparin*: 3000 IU/SC q 24 h ×7–10 days.
   - *Dalteparin*: 2500 IU preoperative then 2500 IU/SC q24 h × 7–10 days.
   - *Enoxaparin*: 40 mg SC qDay; initiate 2 h preoperatively × 7–10 days.
   - With renal impairment: Prophylaxis in abdominal surgery, 30 mg SC qDay.
   - *Nadroparin*: 2850 IU/SC q 24 high risk, 38 IU/Kg/SC q 24 × 3 days, and then 57 IU/Kg/SC q 24 h.
   - *Parnaparin*: 3200 IU/SC 2 h pre-op and then 3200 u/SC q 24 h × 7.
   - *Reviparin*: 1750 SC 12 h pre-op and then every 24.
   - *Tinzaparin*: 3500 IU/SC q 24 h.
   (b) *Knee or hip replacement surgery*
   - *Bemiparin*: 2500–3500 IU SC q 24 h.
   - Dalteparin: 2500 IU preoperative or immediate postoperative and then 5000 IU/SC q24.
   - Enoxaparin:
     30 mg SC q12h; initiate therapy 12–24 h postoperatively and continue for 10 days or up to 35 days postoperatively or until the risk of DVT has been significantly reduced or patient is on anticoagulant therapy.
     For hip replacement surgery, consider administering 40 mg SC qDay, initiated 9–15 h preoperatively, and continue for 10 days or up to 35 days postoperatively or until the risk of DVT has been significantly reduced or the patient is on anticoagulant therapy.
     With renal impairment: coadministered with warfarin, maximum 1 mg/kg SC qDay.
   - *Nadroparin*: High risk, 38 IU/Kg/SC q 24 × 3 days and then 57 IU/Kg/SC q 24 h.
   - *Parnaparin*: 4250 IU/SC 12 h pre-op, then 4250 IU/SC 12 h post-op, and then q 24 h × 10 days.
   - *Reviparin*: 4200 IU/SC 12 h prior then q 24.
   - *Tinzaparin*: Hip 50 IU/Kg/SC q 24 h. Knee75 IU/Kg SC q 24 h.

(c) *Medical patients with restricted mobility* (please refer to Chap. 11)
  - *Bemiparin*: 2500–3500 IU SC q 24 h.
  - *Cetroparin*: 3000 IU SC q 24 h.
  - *Dalterparin*: 5000 IU SC q 24 h.
  - *Enoxaparin*:
    40 mg SC qDay; continue until risk of DVT has been significantly (6–11 days) reduced or patient is on anticoagulant therapy. Reduced to30 mg SC qDay if CrCl<30 ml/min.
  - *Nadroparin*: 2850 IU SC q 24 h.
  - *Tinzaparin*: 4500 IU SC q 24 h.

2. Initial out-patient and in-patient treatment of DVT and PE Continue enoxaparin for a minimum of 5 days and until a therapeutic oral anticoagulant effect has been achieved (INR 2.0–3.0):
   - Treatment could be continued in the context of cancer-associated thrombosis and in pregnancy.
   - LMWHs are also used during bridging of warfarin in the perioperative or peri-interventional process.
     - *Dalteparin*: 200 units IU/kg SC qDay - In cancer patients, treatment intensity may be reduced based on the results of the CLOT trial (200 IU per kilogram once daily for 1 month, followed by a daily dose of approximately 150 IU per kilogram for 5 months).
     - *Enoxaparin*:
       Acute DVT with or without PE, when administered in conjunction with warfarin sodium
       1 mg/kg SC q12h, OR 1.5 mg/kg SC qDay (administer at same time each day)
       With renal impairment:1 mg/kg SC qDay
     - *Nadroparin*: Patients weighing 40–100 kg, subcutaneous, 171 anti-factor Xa IU per kg of body weight once a day or 86 anti-factor Xa IU per kg of body weight (0.1 ml/10 kg) two times a day in patients who have an increased risk of bleeding
     - *Parnaparin*: 6400 IU/SC/ q 24 h
     - *Reviparin*: 175 IU/SC q 12 h
     - *Tinzaparin*: 175 IU/Kg/SC q 24 h

3. Unstable angina and non-Q-wave myocardial infarction
   Prophylaxis of ischemic complications of unstable angina and non-Q-wave myocardial infarction, when concurrently administered with aspirin:
   - *Dalteparin*: 120 IU/kg SC q12h for 5–8 days (concurrent with aspirin 75–165 mg qDay).
     Not to exceed 10,000 units/dose or 18,000 units/day.
   - *Enoxaparin*: 1 mg/kg SC q12h regimen includes aspirin (100–325 mg/day PO), 1 mg/kg SC qDay if CrCl<30 ml/min.
   - *Nadroparin*: Angina, unstable (treatment), and myocardial infarction, non-Q-wave subcutaneous, initially 86 anti-factor Xa international units (IU) per kg of body weight followed by 86 anti-factor Xa IU per kg of body weight every 12 h for 6 days.

4. Acute ST-segment elevation myocardial infarction (STEMI)
   - *Enoxaparin*:
     Reduces the rate of the combined endpoint of recurrent myocardial infarction or death in patients with acute STEMI receiving thrombolysis and being managed medically or with percutaneous coronary intervention (PCI).
     All patients should receive aspirin as soon as they are identified as having STEMI and should be maintained on 75–325 mg PO qDay unless contraindicated.
     <75 years: Loading dose, 30 mg IV bolus once plus 1 mg/kg SC once; not to exceed 100 mg cumulative loading dose. Maintenance: 1 mg/kg SC q12h.
     If Cr Cl <30 ml/min: 30 mg IV single bolus plus 1 mg/kg SC and then 1 mg/kg SC qDay.
     >75 years: No IV bolus 0.75 mg/kg SC q12h not to exceed 75 mg/dose for first 2 doses only, followed by 0.75 mg/kg for remaining doses.
     If CrCl<30 ml/min: No initial bolus; maintain at 1 mg/kg SC qDay.

5. Concomitant use with percutaneous coronary interventions (PCI)
   - *Enoxaparin*:
     If the last enoxaparin dose was given <8 h before balloon inflation, no additional dosing is needed.
     If the last enoxaparin dose was given 8–12 h before balloon inflation, an IV bolus of 0.3 mg/kg should be administered.
     If PCI occurs >12 h after the last SC dose, use established anticoagulation therapy (full-dose unfractionated heparin or LMWH).
     For the patient who has not received prior anticoagulant therapy: 0.5–0.75 mg/kg bolus dose.
   - *Reviparin*: 7000 IU/IV then 10,500 IU/IV Infusion/24 h

Warning and Precautions

- Spinal or epidural hematomas, which may result in long-term or permanent paralysis, can occur with the use of anticoagulants and neuraxial (spinal/epidural) anesthesia or spinal puncture. The risk of these events may be higher with postoperative use of indwelling epidural catheters or concomitant use of other drugs affecting hemostasis such as NSAIDs [38, 48].
- Low body weight (<45 kg for women or < 57 kg for men): Increased exposure has been observed with prophylactic (non-weight adjusted) dosage; carefully monitor for signs/symptoms of bleeding [49].

Monitoring

No monitoring is needed during the routine use of LMWH. In extreme body weights, pregnancy and in patients with renal impairment, measurement of anti-Xa activity may guide therapy.

The therapeutic anti-Xa level for LMWH is 0.5–1.0 IU/mL 4 h after a daily dose, whereas a reasonable anti-Xa target range for deep venous thromboses prophylaxis might be 0.2–0.5 IU/mL [50, 51].

Bridging

LMWHs are used during reversal; the timing of their administration in relation to surgery and procedures is highlighted in Chap. 12.

Reversal

Incomplete reversal with protamine – 1 mg of protamine may reverse 1 mg of enoxaparin.(see Chap. 13).

Other glycosaminoglycans include dextran and pentosane, the use of which is limited to extracorporeal circulation and experimental laboratory use.

Pentasaccharide

Avidly binds antithrombin with recycling to bind new molecules configured to inhibit factor Xa (Fig. 1.5). Figure 1.6 illustrates the characteristics of pentasaccharides.

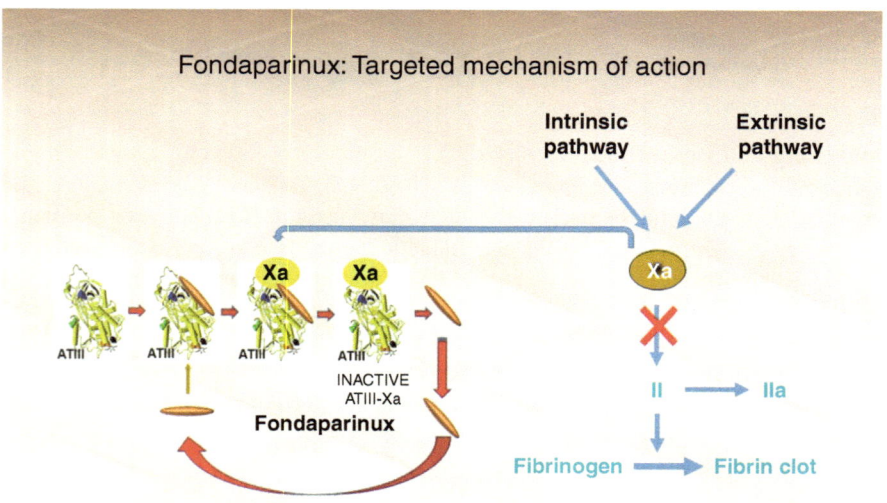

Fig. 1.5 Fondaparinux interacts with antithrombin which is configured to bind and inhibit factor Xa preventing the conversion of prothrombin to thrombin and hence fibrin formation. (Illustration based on Olson ST et al., 1992 [53])

	Plasma ½ life	Prophylaxis	Therapeutic	Elimination	Formulation
Fondaparinux (Arixtra®) [52–54]	15 h	**Orthopedic/ Surgery Medical** 2.5 mg/SC/q 24 h (1.5 mg/SC/q 24 h) **Acute Coronary Syndrome** 2.5 mg/SC/q 24 h	**VTE /(HIT)** <50 kg: 5 mg SC q 24 h 50–100 kg: 7.5 mg SC q 24 h >100 kg: 10 mg SC q 24 h	**Renal** D/C if CrC;<30 mL/min	**PFS** 2.5 mg/0.5 mL 5 mg/0.4 mL 7.5 mg/0.6 mL 10 mg/0.8 mL
Idraparinux (Investigational)	95.1 h	2.5 mg SC q week	–	2.5 mg SC q 1st week then 1.5 mg SC q week if CrCl<30 ml/min	2.5 mg vial

Fig. 1.6 Pentasaccharides, their half-lives, indications, elimination, and formulation

Fondaparinux

Formulation 2.5 mg, 5 mg, 7.5 mg and 10 mg for subcutaneous injection.

Indication and Dose

Deep Vein Thrombosis Prophylaxis Following Hip Fracture, Hip Replacement, and Knee Replacement Surgery

- For patients undergoing hip fracture, hip replacement, or knee replacement surgery, the recommended dose of fondaparinux is 2.5 mg administered by subcutaneous injection once daily after hemostasis has been established.
- Administer the initial dose no earlier than 6–8 h after surgery. Administration of fondaparinux earlier than 6 h after surgery increases the risk of major bleeding.
- The usual duration of therapy is 5–9 days; up to 11 days of therapy was administered in clinical trials.
- In patients undergoing hip fracture surgery, an extended prophylaxis course of up to 24 additional days is recommended. In patients undergoing hip fracture surgery, a total of 32 days (perioperative and extended prophylaxis) was reported in clinical trials.

Deep Vein Thrombosis Prophylaxis Following Abdominal Surgery

- In patients undergoing abdominal surgery, the recommended dose of fondaparinux is 2.5 mg administered by subcutaneous injection once daily after hemostasis has been established. Administer the initial dose no earlier than 6–8 h after surgery.

Administration of fondaparinux earlier than 6 h after surgery increases the risk of major bleeding.

- The usual duration of administration is 5–9 days, and up to 10 days of fondaparinux was administered in clinical trials.

Deep Vein Thrombosis Prophylaxis in Medical Patients

- 2.5 mg SC q 24 h. (Doses of 1.5 mg SC q 24 h suggested for elderly and renal impairment [55, 56].

Deep Vein Thrombosis and Pulmonary Embolism Treatment, Including HIT

In patients with acute symptomatic DVT and in patients with acute symptomatic PE, the recommended dose of fondaparinux is:

- 5 mg (body weight < 50 kg)
- 7.5 mg (body weight 50–100 kg)
- 10 mg (body weight > 100 kg) by subcutaneous injection once daily

Initiate concomitant treatment with warfarin sodium as soon as possible, usually within 72 h. Continue treatment with fondaparinux for at least 5 days and until a therapeutic oral anticoagulant effect is established (INR 2–3).

The usual duration of administration of fondaparinux is 5–9 days;

Acute Coronary Syndrome

Fondaparinux at a dose of 2.5 mg is similar to enoxaparin in reducing the risk of ischemic events at 9 days, but it substantially reduces major bleeding and improves long term mortality and morbidity [54].

Off-label use Heparin-induced thrombocytopenia in full therapeutic dose [52]

Warnings and Precautions

1. *Neuraxial Anesthesia and Postoperative Indwelling Epidural Catheter Use:*
   Spinal or epidural hematomas, which may result in long-term or permanent paralysis, can occur with the use of anticoagulants and neuraxial (spinal/epidural) anesthesia or spinal puncture. The risk of these events may be higher with postoperative use of indwelling epidural catheters or concomitant use of other drugs affecting hemostasis such as NSAIDs [38].
2. *Renal impairment*: Fondaparinux increases the risk of bleeding in patients with impaired renal function due to reduced clearance.
3. *Body weight less than 50 kg*: As the risk of bleeding is increased, it is contraindicated if CrCl < 30 ml/min and is associated with increased bleeding risks when between 30 and 50 ml/min.
4. *Thrombocytopenia*: Risk of bleeding is increased significantly.
5. *Pregnancy, lactation, and pediatric population*: Not tested.

Bridging

Refer to indication and dosage.

Reversal of Anticoagulation

There is no reversal of fondaparinux. Dialysis eliminates 20% of the agent (see Chap. 13).

Fondaparinux molecules leave the configured antithrombin to interact with another molecule in a reverberating manner [53].

Vitamin K Antagonists [VKAs] and Warfarin

VKAs are a group of substances that reduce blood clotting by reducing the action of vitamin K through the inhibition of vitamin K epoxide reductase (VKORC1). This results in recycling of the inactive vitamin K epoxide back to the active reduced form of vitamin K. VKAs, therefore, block the γ-carboxylation of prothrombin; factor VII, IX, and X residues; as well as proteins C and S. They also affect protein Z. Anticoagulation is therefore dependent on the half-life of the coagulation factor/natural anticoagulant involved. The short half-life of protein C and factor VIIa can subsequently lead to a transient hypercoagulable state observed with the initiation of VKAs and explains the need to start patients with VTE on a heparin until a full depletion of the procoagulant factors is reached in 5–7 days [57].

Mutations of the gene coding for (VKORC1) can give rise to warfarin resistance.

VKAs include coumarins (4-hydroxycoumarins) which include warfarin, acenocoumarol, phenprocoumon, and dicoumarol as well as indandiones which include phenindione.

Warfarin

Historic Background

Warfarin is the most widely used anticoagulant in the world. It was estimated that in 2006 at least 1% of the population and 8% of the people over 80 years of age were using the medication [58].

In the late 1920s, it was noticed that previously healthy cattle in the Canadian Prairies and northern USA, grazing on sweet clover hay, began dying of internal bleeding with no obvious precipitating cause. Such damp hay was infected by molds and contained a hemorrhagic substance. Roderick, a local veterinarian, demonstrated that the acquired coagulation disorder was caused by what he called a "plasma prothrombin defect" [59]. The toxic agent was identified at the University of Wisconsin as bishydroxycoumarin [60] and its structurally similar agent warfarin (Wisconsin Alumni Research Foundation – adding ARIN from coumarin) was promoted as rodenticide [59].

Bioavailability and Half-Life

Warfarin is a racemic mixture of R and S isomers; it is usually administered as sodium salt with 100% bioavailability and a half-life of 36 h. Warfarin and its derivatives have a small therapeutic window.

Formulation

Warfarin is available as warfarin sodium in the following strength: 1, 2, 2.5, 3, 4, 5, 6, and 10 mg tablets.

Dose and Administration

Treatment is usually initiated with a loading dose of 5–10 mg and adjustments are made based on the prothrombin time (expressed in INR) at about 1 week. An average maintenance dose of 5–7 mg orally daily targeting an INR of 2–3 is used for the treatment and prophylaxis of VTE and atrial fibrillation. A target INR of 2.5–3.5 is used for patients with artificial valves and those who need more intense anticoagulation.

Since the medication is dependent on VKORC1 and is metabolized through P450 CYP2C9 [61], inherited polymorphism may have a significant impact on the dose of the medication. This led to the consideration of patient-specific genotype for the adjustment of warfarin therapy [62]. Wells and coworkers also highlighted the role of CYP4F2 [63].

It is usually recommended to administer the drug at bed-time to be ingested with water and away from food to avoid drug-food interactions. Hepatic disease and thyroid dysfunction may also significantly affect the action of warfarin.

The following nomogram could guide the adjustment of INR for patients on warfarin [64].

Target 2.0–3.0 and No Bleeding

Measured INR	Dosage adjustment	Next INR
<1.5	Consider extra dose, increase weekly dose by 10–20%	4–7 days
1.5–1.9	Increase weekly dose by 5–10%	7–14 days
2.0–3.0	**No change**	**See follow-up algorithm (below)**
3.1–3.5	Decrease weekly dose by 5–10%	7–14 days
3.6–4.0	Decrease weekly dose by 10–20%	7–14 days
4.1–4.9	Hold 0–2 day(s) and decrease weekly dose by 20%	4–7 days

Target INR 2.5–3.5 and No Bleeding

Measured INR	Dosage adjustment	Next INR
<1.5	Consider extra dose, increase weekly dose by 10–20%	4–7 days
1.5–2.4	Increase weekly dose by 5–10%	7–14 days
2.5–3.5	**No change**	**See follow-up algorithm (below)**
3.6–4.0	Decrease weekly dose by 5–10%	7–14 days
4.1–4.5	Consider holding 1 dose, Decrease weekly dose by 10%	7–14 days
4.6–4.9	Hold 0–2 day(s) and decrease weekly dose by 10–20%	4–7 days

Follow-Up Algorithm

Number of consecutive INRs in range	Repeat INR
1	4–7 days
2	14 days
3	21 days
4	28 days

For Target 2–3

- If INR 1.8–1.9, consider no dosage change, and repeat INR in 7–14 days.
- *If INR 2.0–2.1, or 2.8–3.0, consider repeating INR in 14 days regardless of number of consecutive in range INRs.
- If INR 3.1–3.2, consider no dose change, and repeat INR in 7–14 days.

For Target 2.5–3.5

- If recent mechanical heart valve within 6–8 weeks, consider bridging therapy with therapeutic dose low-molecular-weight heparin.
- If INR 2.3–2.4, consider no dose change, and repeat INR in 7–14 days.
- If INR 2.5–2.6 or 3.3–3.4, consider repeating INR in 14 days, regardless of number of consecutive in-range INRs.
- If INR 3.6–3.7, consider no dose change, and repeat INR in 7–14 days.

Warfarin Resistance

Two types of warfarin resistance have been described:

(a) "Functional" resistance is defined as progression or recurrence of thrombosis despite being on therapeutic range of anticoagulation from the laboratory perspective and is often seen in patients with cancer mandating the switch to alternate anticoagulation [65].
(b) "True" warfarin resistance is rare (< 0.1%) and is defined as warfarin requirements greater than 70 mg per week to maintain the international normalized ratio (INR) in the target therapeutic range [66].

It is usually related to VKORC1 or CYP3C9 mutations or resulting from a gross drug-drug interaction and necessitates the consideration of alternate anticoagulant.

Warfarin Interactions

Food, Food Supplement, and Herbal Interactions

VKAs interact with food containing vitamin K (reducing its actions) [67, 68]; therefore, the intake of foods rich in vitamin K (an average consumption of ½ cup/day) should be about the same each day. If patients want to consume more, the daily amount needs to be consistent.

Examples of food servings rich in vitamin K are illustrated in Fig. 1.7:

Other Interactions

Alcoholic beverages: Alcohol can affect warfarin dose and should be avoided.

Dietary supplements and herbal medications: Many dietary supplements (arnica, bilberry, butchers broom, cat's claw, St John's wort, feverfew, Dong quai, garlic, ginger, ginkgo, and others) can alter the INR/PT. The safest policy for individuals on warfarin is to avoid all dietary supplements. This includes any vitamin/mineral supplements that list vitamin K on the label. If they are taken regularly on a daily basis, they pose less of a problem than if taken off and on.

Vitamin E supplements: Vitamin E intake above 1000 International Units (IU) per day may increase the risk of excess bleeding. Research suggests that doses up to 800 IU may be safe for individuals on warfarin, but the evidence is not conclusive [69, 70].

Drug Interactions [69–73]

CYP450 isozymes involved in the metabolism of warfarin include CYP2C9, 2C19, 2C8, 2C18, 1A2, and 3A4. The more potent warfarin S-enantiomer (60% of the overall anticoagulation response) is metabolized by CYP2C9, while the R-enantiomer is metabolized by CYP1A2 and 3A4.

- Inhibitors of CYP2C9, 1A2, and/or 3A4 have the potential to increase the effect (increase INR) of warfarin by increasing the exposure of warfarin.
- Inducers of CYP2C9, 1A2, and/or 3A4 have the potential to decrease the effect (decrease NR) of warfarin by decreasing the exposure of warfarin.

Coumarins may also affect the action of other drugs. Hypoglycemic agents (chlorpropamide and tolbutamide) and anticonvulsants (phenytoin and phenobarbital) may accumulate in the body as a result of interference with either their metabolism or excretion.

Food serving	Size	Vitamin K (mcg/serving size)
Broccoli, cooked	1 cup	220
Brussels sprouts, cooked	1 cup	219
Collard, cooked	½ cup	418
Parsley, raw	¼ cup	246
Swiss chard, cooked	½ cup	287
Turnip greens, cooked	½ cup	265

Fig. 1.7 Illustrates the content of vitamin K in common food servings [67, 68]

It has been reported that concomitant administration of warfarin and ticlopidine may be associated with cholestatic hepatitis. Figure 1.8 - Established or Potential Drug-Drug Interactions with VKA.

A detailed list of drug interactions could be reviewed in references [70–73].

Contraindications

1. As with all anticoagulants, VKAs are contraindicated with active bleeding or in patients with increased risk of bleeding, e.g., low platelets, severe liver disease, and uncontrolled hypertension. For patients undergoing surgery or invasive procedures, a bridging approach should be considered (Discussed in detail Chap. 12).

Name	Effect	Clinical comment
Nonsteroidal anti-inflammatory drugs (NSAIDs)	May affect prothrombin time May inhibit platelet aggregation May increase risk of gastrointestinal bleeding, peptic ulceration and/or perforation May increase bleeding risk	Close monitoring of patients receiving nonsteroidal anti-inflammatory agents (NSAIDs) is recommended to be certain that no change in anticoagulation dosage is required. Bleeding risk is increased when these drugs are used concomitantly with warfarin. Adjust dosage accordingly or discontinue if necessary. Consult the labeling of all concurrently used drugs to obtain further information about interactions with warfarin or adverse reactions pertaining to bleeding.
Anticoagulants Platelet anti-aggregants Thrombolytics Serotonin reuptake inhibitors	May increase bleeding risk	Bleeding risk is increased when these drugs are used concomitantly with warfarin. Closely monitor patients receiving any such class of drug with warfarin. Adjust dosage accordingly or discontinue if necessary.
Antibiotics and antifungals	May change international normalized ratio (INR)	There have been reports of changes in INR in patients taking warfarin and antibiotics or antifungals, but clinical pharmacokinetic studies have not shown consistent effects of these agents on plasma concentrations of warfarin. Coadministration with warfarin should be avoided or closely monitor INR when starting or stopping any antibiotic or antifungal in patients taking warfarin.

Fig. 1.8 Established and potential drug group interactions with VKA and their effect on INR

2. Warfarin should not be given to people with heparin-induced thrombocytopenia until platelet count has improved or normalized [70].
3. Warfarin is usually best avoided in people with protein C or protein S deficiency without proper bridging as these thrombophilic conditions increase the risk of skin necrosis, which is a rare but serious side effect associated with warfarin [74].
4. Pregnancy: Warfarin is contraindicated in pregnancy as it passes the placental barrier and may cause fetal bleeding. It is commonly associated with poor outcome and is also teratogenic, resulting in a constellation of abnormalities known as fetal warfarin syndrome (FWS). The incidence of birth defects appears to be around 5%, although higher figures (up to 30%) have been reported in some studies [54]. Depending on when exposure occurs during pregnancy, two distinct combinations of congenital abnormalities can arise [75]. It should be definitely avoided in the first trimester.

Warfarin administration in the second and third trimesters is much less commonly associated with birth defects and, when they do occur, is considerably different from FWS.

According to the American College of Chest Physicians (ACCP), warfarin may be used in lactating women who wish to breast-feed [56]. Data does not suggest that warfarin crosses into the breast milk [75].

Adverse Events

1. Bleeding: The risk of severe bleeding is typically at 1–3% per year [76]. Bleeding can occur from many sources with intracranial bleeds and gastrointestinal ones being the most serious [77].

    Risk of bleeding is increased if the INR is out of the therapeutic range [78]. This risk increases greatly once the INR exceeds 4.5 [79].

    The risks of bleeding are increased further when warfarin is combined with antiplatelet drugs such as clopidogrel, aspirin, or nonsteroidal anti-inflammatory drugs [80].

    The bleeding risk prediction can be calculated using one of the following scoring systems:
    - HAS-BLED SCORE [81]: With a maximum score of 9

	Condition	
H	Hypertension (systolic blood pressure > 160 mmHg)	1
A	Abnormal renal function (defined as the presence of chronic dialysis or renal transplantation or serum creatinine 200 µmol/L (>~2.3 mg/dL))	1
	Abnormal liver function (defined as chronic hepatic disease (e.g., cirrhosis) or biochemical evidence of significant hepatic derangement (e.g., bilirubin >2x upper limit of normal, in association with AST/ALT/ALP >3x upper limit normal)	1
S	Stroke (previous history of stroke)	1
B	Bleeding (major bleeding history (anemia or predisposition to bleeding))	1
L	Labile INRs (refers to unstable/high INRs or poor time in therapeutic range (e.g., <60%))	1
E	Elderly (age >/= 65)	1
D	Drug therapy (concomitant therapy such as antiplatelet agents, NSAIDs)	1
	Alcohol intake (consuming 8 or more alcoholic drinks per week)	1
	Total	9

- The scoring system translates into percentage of bleeding/Year:

HAS-BLED score	Bleeds % per Year
0	1.13
1	1.02
2	1.88
3	3.74
4	8.70
5	12.50
Any score	1.56

HEMORR2HAGES is another scoring system used to stratify the risk of bleeding in patients on warfarin. The ATRIA score uses a weighted additive scale of clinical findings for better bleeding risk stratification [82].

2. Warfarin necrosis is a rare but serious and often life-threatening complication resulting from treatment with warfarin and commonly occurs shortly after commencing treatment in patients with a deficiency of protein C. As warfarin initially decreases protein C levels faster than the coagulation factors, it can paradoxically induce a transient hypercoagulable state leading to massive thrombosis with skin necrosis and gangrene of limbs. Its natural counterpart, purpura fulminans, occurs in children who are homozygous for certain protein C mutations [83].
3. Calcification: Several studies have alluded to vascular calcification as a complication of prolonged warfarin use [84].
4. Osteoporosis is a controversial side effect. A retrospective study on 14,564 Medicare patients receiving warfarin for more than 1 year, showed that its use was linked with an increased risk of osteoporosis-related fracture in men. There was no association in women. The mechanism entails interaction with bone proteins [85].
5. Purple toe syndrome is another rare complication occurring during the first few weeks of warfarin therapy and is thought to result from cholesterol embolization of the blood vessels in the skin of the toes or plantar surface of the foot. It may require discontinuation of the therapy [86].

Bridging of Anticoagulation See Chap. 12.

Overdose and Reversal See Chap. 13.

Injectable Direct Thrombin Inhibitors

Hirudo medicinalis, the medicinal leeches, were used extensively in the eighteenth and nineteenth centuries to treat a wide variety of diseases. It was not until the twentieth century that the anticoagulation properties of an extract from the salivary glands of leeches were characterized as hirudin [87]. Hirudins are formed of amino-acid sequence that binds to thrombin in a 1:1 ratio in a non-covalent manner.

A group of other molecules was thereafter developed binding thrombin in a 1:1 ratio with covalent bonding [88].

Hirudins

Recombinant hirudins are formed of 65-amino acid sequence that binds in an irreversible manner to the active binding site (exocite) of thrombin, neutralizing its function [88]. They act also on fibrin-bound thrombin within thrombi. Figure 1.9 illustrates the binding of hirudin to thrombin.

  (i). Lepuridine: Initially approved for the management of HIT [89–92].
 (ii). Deserudine: A different formulation approved for thromboprophylaxis in the orthopedic context [93, 94].

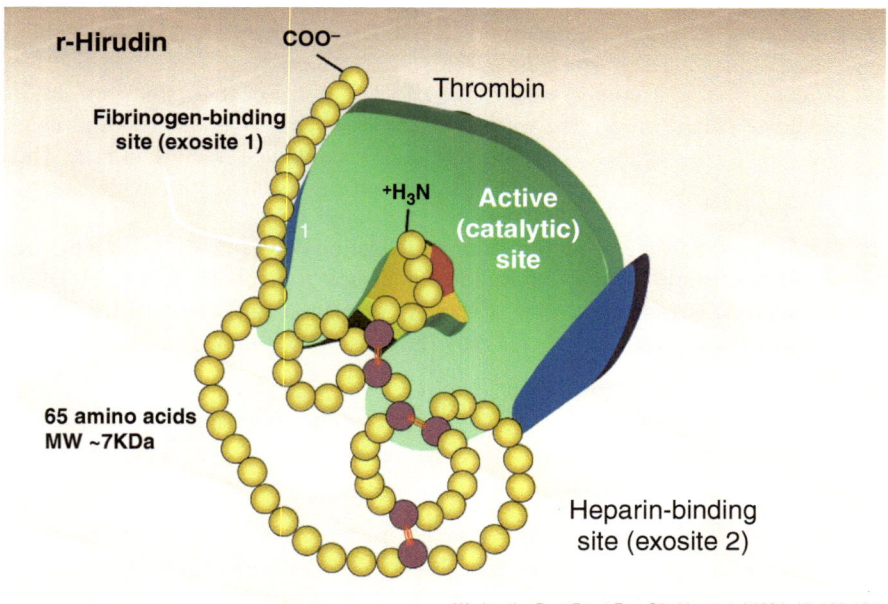

Warkentin. *Best Pract Res Clin Haematol 2004; 17: 105-125*

Fig. 1.9 Mechanism of action of r-Hirudin, blocking exosite 1 of thrombin and inhibiting its action in an irreversible manner. (From Warkentin [101]. Used with Permission [101]) (iii). rb-Hirudin variant: A third formulation available primarily for thromboprophylaxis but also for HIT management. It is also marketed as a gel or cream for topical treatment. Figure 1.10 illustrates the different injectable direct thrombin inhibitors and their characteristics.

Bivaluridin

Formulation   250 mg vial of lyophilized powder to be dissolved in 5 ml of distilled water and added to 5% D/W.

Indications
Bivalirudin (Angiomax) is a bivalent transient direct thrombin inhibitor with short half-life (25 min) and a clearance of 20% renal and 80% metabolic. It is indicated in [102]:
- Patients undergoing PCI with provisional use of glycoprotein IIb/IIIa inhibitor (GPI)
- With, or at risk of, HIT or heparin-induced thrombocytopenia and thrombosis syndrome (HITTS), undergoing PCI
- With unstable angina undergoing percutaneous transluminal coronary angioplasty (PTCA)

Dose [102]
- IV bolus dose of 0.75 mg/kg, followed immediately by an infusion of 1.75 mg/kg/h for the procedure duration. Activated clotting time should be performed at 5 min from bolus and an additional bolus of 0.3 mg/kg should be given if needed.
- Infusion may be continued for up to 4 h post-procedure.
- In patients with STEMI, continuation of therapy at a rate of 1.75 mg/kg/h following PCI/PTCA for up to 4 h post-procedure should be considered.
- After 4 h, an additional IV infusion of bivaluridin may be initiated at a rate of 0.2 mg/kg/h (low-rate infusion), for up to 20 h, if needed.

Renal Adjustment   Bolus given at regular dose, infusion rate adjusted accordingly [102]:
- CrCl 30–59 mL/min – 1.75 mg/kg/h
- CrCl <30 mL/min – 1 mg/kg/h
- Dialysis patients – 0.25 mg/kg/h

Argatroban [103–106]

Form   Vial 125 mL glass vial contains 125 mg of argatroban (1 mg/mL); 250 mg in 2.5 ml (100 mg/ml)

Hirudin	HIT IV use	Prophylaxis SC	Monitoring	Renal Adjustment	Form
Lepirudin (Refludan) [95]	0.4 mg/kg body weight (up to 110 kg) slowly intravenously (e.g., over 15–20 seconds) as a bolus dose, followed by 0.15 mg/kg body weight (up to 110 kg)/h as a continuous intravenous infusion [95][a] Bridging to warfarin[b]	N/A	Infusion rate adjusted according to the aPTT ratio. (at 4 h) Therapeutic window is 1.5–2.5. If above 2.5, stop infusion for 2 h. Restart, with 50% dose reduction and assess in 4 h. If below 1.5, increment dose by 20% and recheck in 4 h. Rates of 0.21 mg/kg/h should not be exceeded Allergic reactions[c]	D/C CrCl<50 ml/min	Vial 50 mg
Desirudin (Ipravask Revasc)	N/A	15 mg SC q 12 h	No monitoring	CrCl 31–60 mL/min 5 mg SC q 12 h CrCl <31 mL/min 1.7 mg SC q 12 h	Lyophilized powder 15 mg
rb-varian Hirudin (Thrombexx) [96]	Same as leperudin	15 mg SC q 12 h	No monitoring	Only if used IV	Amp 15 mg

[a]In practice [97, 98]
  Patients with normal renal function: 0.1 mg/kg × h
  Mild-to-moderate renal impairment: 0.01 mg/kg × h
  Severe renal impairment: 0.005 mg/kg × h
[b]Converting to oral anticoagulant therapy [99, 100]
  Warfarin initiated only after substantial recovery from HIT has occurred with lepirudin therapy
  Reduce dosage gradually until the aPTT ratio is just above 1.5, then initiate therapy with warfarin avoiding loading dose and with modest doses
  Overlap lepirudin and warfarin therapy for a minimum of 4–5 days until the target INR is reached
[c]Allergic reaction can occur and 40% of patient develop antibodies to lepirudin

Fig. 1.10 The various injectable direct thrombin inhibitors, indications, monitoring, and formulations

Indications

Argatroban is a synthetic, small-molecule, univalent direct thrombin inhibitor derived from L-arginine. It is approved for the use in HIT with or without thrombosis and in coronary angioplasties in patients with HIT. It interferes with INR rendering bridging problematic [103–106].

Dose

For adult patients without hepatic impairment, the dose is 2 µg/kg/min, administered as a continuous infusion.

Monitoring

Argatroban is monitored using the aPTT attaining steady-state levels within 2.5 h or with dosage adjustment.

Check aPTT 2 h after initiation of therapy to confirm that the patient has attained the desired therapeutic range (1.5–3).

Dosage adjustment Dose can be adjusted as clinically indicated (not to exceed 10 µg/kg/min), until the steady-state aPTT is 1.5–3.0 times the initial baseline value (not to exceed 100 seconds) – The following nomogram can be used to titrate the drug [104].

aPTT(Sec)	Hold infusion	Rate Change	Next test
<36	0	Inc 1 mcg/kg/min	3 h
37–44	0	Inc 0.5 mcg/kg/min	3 h
45–90	**0**	**No change**	**Next morning**
91–120	0	Dec 0.5 mcg/kg/min	3 h
121–149	60 min	Dec 1 mcg/kg/mi	3 h
>150	Stop	Hold till aPTT<90 Then resume at ½ rate	Q 2 h until aPTT<90

Renal and Hepatic adjustment No renal adjustment of the dose is needed. For patients with moderate hepatic impairment, an initial dose of 0.5 µg/kg/min is recommended, whereas the initial dose can be reduced up to 0.05 µg/kg/min in severe liver disease.

Transition to Warfarin [106]

- Warfarin initiated only after substantial recovery from HIT has occurred with argatroban therapy.
- If dose <2mcg/Kg/min D/C when INR is >4 on combined therapy and remeasure INR in 4–6 h.
- Restart argatroban if INR below range and repeat until desired INR is achieved.
- If dose is >2mcg/Kg/min, decrease rate to 2mcg/Kg/min and measure INR at 4–6 h and proceed accordingly.

A formula was developed to calculate INR attributable to warfarin when argatroban is given at 2mcg/Kg/min.

Warfarin INR = 0.19 + 0.57 (INR warfarin + argatroban).

NOACs/DOACs

Non-vitamin K antagonist oral anticoagulants (NOACs) are now widely used in patients with non-valvular atrial fibrillation (AF) and for the prevention and treatment of VTE. The term "DOAC" (direct oral anticoagulant) is also used to describe these medicines.

They share the common advantages of the lack of need for laboratory monitoring as they are given in fixed doses, regardless of the patient's weight.

Contraindications

1. NOAC treatment is contraindicated, notably, in patients with a mechanical heart valve (77, 78).
2. Concomitant treatment with any other anticoagulant, including:

   - UFH, except at doses used to maintain a patent central venous or arterial catheter
   - LMWH, such as enoxaparin and dalteparin
   - Heparin derivatives, such as fondaparinux, and oral anticoagulants
   - Hepatic disease (including Child-Pugh class B and C) associated with coagulopathy, having clinically relevant bleeding risk

   Their use has not been studied in the following conditions:

- Cerebral venous sinus thrombosis.
- Portal and splenic vein thrombosis.
- Non-lower limb DVT.
- NOACs are not suitable for use in patients with hemodynamically significant valvular heart disease.
- Pregnancy and lactation.
- The safety of NOACs has not been established in children less than 18 years of age, although recent studies supported their use.

NOACs Include

Oral Direct Thrombin Inhibitor: Dabigatran

Formulation 75, 110, and 150 mg capsules of dabigatran etexilate (Pradaxa, Pradax)

Indications

Dabigatran is an oral direct thrombin inhibitor formulated as dabigatran etexilate mesylate and indicated in the following conditions:

1. Thromboprophylaxis after orthopedic surgery [107]
2. Stroke prevention in atrial fibrillation [108]
3. Treatment of DVT and PE (excluding cancer-associated thrombosis) [109]

Dose

1. *Thromboprophylaxis after orthopedic surgery*:

   - Start with 110 mg 1–4 h after surgery and increase to 220 mg once daily (OD) starting the day after surgery; the 220 mg OD dose is continued for at least 14 days and up to 35 days.

2. *Atrial Fibrillation*:

   - Patients aged 80 years and older, or over 75 years old, with one risk factor for bleeding should be treated with a dose of 110 mg BID. All other patients should receive 150 mg BID . The manufacturer suggests that for patients with creatinine clearance (CrCl) >30 mL/min, the recommended dose of dabigatran is 150 mg taken orally, twice daily, with or without food. For patients with severe renal impairment (CrCl 15–30 mL/min), the recommended dose is 75 mg twice daily with no recommendations for patients with a CrCl <15 mL/min or on dialysis cannot be provided [108].

3. *Treatment of DVT and PE*:

   - Dabigatran 150 mg BID is started after 5–10 days of initial treatment with a parenteral anticoagulant. There is no recommended dose adjustment in patients with moderate renal impairment (CrCl 30–50 mL/min). The reduced dose of 110 mg has never been evaluated in a VTE treatment clinical trial [109].

In patients with moderate renal impairment (CrCl 30–50 mL/min), concomitant use of the P-gp inhibitor dronedarone or systemic ketoconazole can be expected to increase dabigatran effect in a similar way to that observed in severe renal impairment.

Contraindications [110]

- Active pathological bleeding
- History of a serious hypersensitivity reaction to dabigatran
- Valvular heart disease
- Pregnancy and lactation
- Child-Pugh C

Risk of Bleeding

Dabigatran increases the risk of bleeding and can cause significant and sometimes fatal bleeding. Risk factors for bleeding include the use of drugs that increase the risk of bleeding in general (e.g., antiplatelet agents, heparin, fibrinolytic therapy, and chronic use of NSAIDs) and labor and delivery. Discontinue the medication in patients with active pathological bleeding.

In the RE-LY (Randomized Evaluation of Long-term Anticoagulant Therapy) study, a life-threatening bleed (bleeding that met one or more of the following criteria: fatal, symptomatic intracranial, reduction in hemoglobin of at least 5 grams per deciliter, transfusion of at least 4 units of blood, associated with hypotension requiring the use of intravenous inotropic agents, or necessitating surgical intervention) occurred at an annualized rate of 1.5% and 1.8% for dabigatran 150 mg and warfarin, respectively [108].

The risk of major bleeds was similar with dabigatran 150 mg and warfarin across major subgroups defined by baseline characteristics, with the exception of age, where there was a trend toward a higher incidence of major bleeding on dabigatran (hazard ratio 1.2, 95% CI, 1.0 to 1.4) for patients ≥75 years of age.

There was a higher rate of major gastrointestinal bleeds in patients receiving dabigatran 150 mg than in patients receiving warfarin (1.6% vs. 1.1%, respectively, with a hazard ratio vs. warfarin of 1.5, 95% CI, 1.2 to 1.9), and a higher rate of any gastrointestinal bleeds (6.1% vs. 4.0%, respectively).

Drug Interactions [110]

P-glycoprotein 1 (permeability glycoprotein, abbreviated as P-gp or Pgp) is a cell membrane protein that pumps many foreign substances out of cells. Its inducers or inhibitors affect dabigatran action significantly. Figure 1.11 illustrates the different P-gp inducers and inhibitors affecting dabigatran.

P-gp Inducers
Rifampin   Decreased its AUC and Cmax by 66% and 67%, respectively
P-gp Inhibitors
Dronedarone   Increased its AUC and Cmax by 99% and 73%, respectively

Ketoconazole
  Increased its AUC and Cmax by 138% and 135%, respectively
Multiple doses
  Increased its AUC and Cmax by 153% and 149%, respectively

Verapamil   Increased – Variable dependent on formulation
Amiodarone   Increased its AUC and Cmax by 58% and 50%, respectively. The increase in exposure was mitigated by a 65% increase in the renal clearance of dabigatran in the presence of amiodarone. The increase in renal clearance may persist after amiodarone is discontinued because of amiodarone's long half-life
Quinidine   Increased its AUC and Cmax by 53% and 56%, respectively
Clarithromycin   Coadministered clarithromycin had no impact on the exposure to dabigatran

Fig. 1.11 P-gp inducers and inhibitors and their effect on dabigatran

Other Drugs

Clopidogrel: When dabigatran etexilate was given concomitantly with a loading dose of 300 mg or 600 mg clopidogrel, the dabigatran AUC and Cmax increased by approximately 30% and 40%, respectively. The concomitant administration of dabigatran etexilate and clopidogrel resulted in no further prolongation of capillary bleeding times compared to clopidogrel monotherapy.

Enoxaparin: Enoxaparin 40 mg given subcutaneously for 3 days with the last dose given 24 h before a single dose of dabigatran had no impact on the exposure to dabigatran or the coagulation measures aPTT, ECT, or TT.

Diclofenac, ranitidine, and digoxin: None of these drugs alter exposure to dabigatran.

The concomitant use of proton pump inhibitors, H2 antagonists, diclofenac and digoxin did not appreciably change the trough concentration of dabigatran.

Impact of Dabigatran on Other Drugs

In clinical studies exploring CYP3A4, CYP2C9, P-gp, and other pathways, dabigatran did not meaningfully alter the pharmacokinetics of amiodarone, atorvastatin, clarithromycin, diclofenac, clopidogrel, digoxin, pantoprazole, or ranitidine.

Conversion to Warfarin [110]

When converting from Dabigatran to warfarin, adjust the starting time of warfarin based on creatinine clearance as follows:

- For CrCl ≥50 mL/min, start warfarin 3 days before discontinuing Dabigatran.
- For CrCl 30–50 mL/min, start warfarin 2 days before discontinuing Dabigatran.
- For CrCl 15–30 mL/min, start warfarin 1 day before discontinuing Dabigatran.
- For CrCl <15 mL/min, no recommendations can be made.

Converting from or to Parenteral Anticoagulants

For patients currently receiving a parenteral anticoagulant, start dabigatran 0–2 h before the next scheduled dose of the parenteral drug or at the time of discontinuation of a continuously administered parenteral drug.

For patients currently taking dabigatran, wait for 12 h (CrCl ≥30 mL/min) or 24 h (CrCl <30 mL/min) after the last dose before initiating treatment with a parenteral anticoagulant.

Bridging of anticoagulation Please refer to Chap. 12.

Reversal of anticoagulation Idarucizumab, a monoclonal antibody fragment, was developed to reverse the anticoagulant effect of dabigatran [111] under the commercial name of Praxbind. It is indicated in patients treated with dabigatran (Pradaxa) when reversal of the anticoagulant effects is needed for emergency surgery or urgent

Generic	Commercial	Formulation	Renal
Apixaban	Eliquis®	2.5, 5 mg	Discontinue/not indicated if Cr Cl < 15 ml/min Reduce dose for stroke if Cr Cl <30 ml/min.
Betrixaban	Bevyxxa®	40, 80 mg	Contraindicated if CrCl<30 ml/min
Edoxaban	Lixiana®	15, 30, 60 mg	Contraindicated if CrCl<30 ml/min.
Rivaroxaban	Xarelto®	2.5, 10, 15, 20 mg Tablets	Discontinue/not indicated if Cr Cl < 15 ml/min Reduce dose for stroke to 15 mg if Cr Cl 30–49 ml/min.

Fig. 1.12 The different factor Xa inhibitors, their commercial name, formulation, and renal adjustment

procedures, or in the event of life-threatening or uncontrolled bleeding. The dose is 5 g IV, provided as two separate vials each containing 2.5 g/50 mL – for details on reversal, please refer to Chap. 13.

Oral Direct Factor Xa Inhibitors

These molecules are indicated in the prevention of stroke and systemic embolism in patients with AF with one or more risk factors, in the prevention of VTE following hip and knee replacement and the treatment of new and secondary prevention of DVT and PE. Figure 1.12 illustrates the different factor Xa inhibitors.

Apixaban [112]

Formulation

Tablets, 2.5 mg and 5 mg

Indications

Apixaban is indicated for:

1. Prevention of VTE in adult patients who have undergone elective knee or hip replacement surgery
2. Prevention of stroke and systemic embolism in patients with AF (atrial fibrillation)
3. Treatment of venous thromboembolic events (DVT, PE) and prevention of recurrent DVT and PE
4. Treatment of VTE in the context of cancer

Contraindications [112]

- Clinically significant active bleeding or in patients with spontaneous or acquired hemostatic impairment
- Hepatic disease associated with coagulopathy

- Concomitant systemic treatment with strong inhibitors of both CYP 3A4 and P-gp such as azole-antimycotics, e.g., ketoconazole, itraconazole, voriconazole, or posaconazole, and HIV protease inhibitors, e.g., ritonavir (Inhibitors of both CYP 3A4 and P-gp)
- Concomitant treatment with any other anticoagulant, including UH, except at doses used to maintain a patent central catheters, LMWH, fondaparinux, and other oral anticoagulants, such as warfarin, dabigatran, and rivaroxaban, except under circumstances of switching therapy to or from apixaban
- Hypersensitivity to apixaban or to any ingredients of the formulation

Dose

1. *Prevention of VTE following elective hip or knee replacement surgery* [113].
   - The recommended dose of apixaban is 2.5 mg twice daily.
   - The initial dose should be taken 12–24 h after surgery, and after hemostasis has been obtained.
   - In patients undergoing hip replacement surgery, the recommended duration of treatment is 32–38 days.
   - In patients undergoing knee replacement surgery, the recommended duration of treatment is 10–14 days.

2. *Stroke prevention in patients with AF* [114, 115]
   - The recommended dose of apixaban is 5 mg taken orally twice daily.
   - In patients fulfilling at least two (2) of the following characteristics, a reduced dose of apixaban 2.5 mg twice daily is recommended:
     - Age $\geq$ 80 years, body weight $\leq$ 60 kg
     - Serum creatinine $\geq$ 133 micromole/L (1.5 mg/dL)

3. *Treatment of DVT and PE and prevention of recurrent DVT and PE and CAT* [116–118].
   - The recommended dose of apixaban for the treatment of acute DVT or PE is 10 mg taken orally twice daily for 7 days, followed by 5 mg taken orally twice daily.
   - The duration of therapy should be individualized.
     - Short duration of therapy (at least 3 months) should be offered to provoked VTEs
     - Extended duration should be based on permanent risk factors or idiopathic DVT or PE.
   - If additional anticoagulation is required after the minimum of 6 months of treatment for DVT or PE, the recommended dose for the continued prevention of recurrent DVT and PE is 2.5 mg taken orally twice daily.

NB: Acute Coronary Syndrome In the PPRAISE-2 trial, the addition of apixaban, at a dose of 5 mg twice daily, to antiplatelet therapy in high-risk patients after an acute coronary syndrome increased the number of major bleeding events without a significant reduction in recurrent ischemic events [119].

Precautions in Special Populations [112]

Renal Impairment

1. *Prevention of VTE following elective hip or knee replacement surgery, treatment of DVT and PE, and prevention of recurrent DVT and PE*

    *   No dose adjustment is necessary in patients with mild or moderate renal impairment (eCrCl ≥30 mL/min).
    *   Limited clinical data in patients with severe renal impairment (eCrCl 15–29 mL/min) indicate that apixaban plasma concentrations are increased. Therefore, apixaban is to be used with caution in these patients because of potentially higher bleeding risk.
    *   There is very limited clinical experience in patients with creatinine clearance <15 ml/min, and there are no data in patients undergoing dialysis; therefore, apixaban is not recommended in these situations.

2. *Stroke prevention in patients with AF*

    *   No dose adjustment is necessary in patients with mild or moderate renal impairment, or in those with eCrCL 25–30 mL/min, unless the criteria for dose reduction are met: Patients with serum creatinine ≥133 micromol/L (1.5 mg/dL) who are also ≥80 years or whose body weight ≤ 60 kg should receive a dose of apixaban 2.5 mg twice daily.
    *   In patients with eCrCL 15–24 mL/min, no dosing recommendation can be made as clinical data are very limited.
    *   Because there are no data in patients with creatinine clearance <15 ml/min, or in those undergoing dialysis, apixaban is not recommended in these patients.

Hepatic Impairment

Apixaban is contraindicated in patients with hepatic disease associated with coagulopathy and clinically relevant bleeding risk and should be used with caution in patients with mild or moderate hepatic impairment (Child Pugh A or B).

Patients with elevated liver enzymes (ALT/AST > 2 × ULN, or total bilirubin ≥1.5 × ULN) were excluded in clinical trials. Therefore, apixaban should be used with caution in these patients.

Concomitant Use of Antiplatelet Agents

The concomitant use of apixaban with antiplatelet agents increases the risk of bleeding. If concomitant antiplatelet therapy is contemplated for indications related to coronary artery disease, a careful assessment of the potential risks of bleeding should be made against potential benefits.

Drug Interactions [112]

- Concomitant systemic treatment with strong inhibitors of both CYP 3A4 and P-gp such as azole-antimycotics, e.g., ketoconazole, itraconazole, voriconazole, or posaconazole, and HIV protease inhibitors, e.g., ritonavir (Inhibitors of both CYP 3A4 and P-gp).
- Clarithromycin (500 mg, twice daily), an inhibitor of P-gp and a strong inhibitor of CYP3A4, led to a 1.6-fold and 1.3-fold increase in mean apixaban AUC and Cmax respectively but requires no dosage adjustment for apixaban. It should, however, be used with caution.
- Coadministration of apixaban with rifampin, a strong inducer of both CYP 3A4 and P-gp, led to an approximate 54% and 42% decrease in mean apixaban AUC and Cmax, respectively. Combined use with strong inducers of both CYP 3A4 and P-gp should generally be avoided, since efficacy of apixaban may be compromised.

Switching from to and from Other Anticoagulation Agents

Switching from or to Parenteral Anticoagulants

In general, switching treatment from parenteral anticoagulants to apixaban (or vice versa) can be done at the next scheduled dose.

Switching from VKA to Apixaban

When switching patients from a VKA, such as warfarin, to apixaban, discontinue warfarin or other VKA therapy, and start apixaban when the international normalized ratio (INR) is below 2.0.

Switching from Apixaban to VKA

As with any short-acting anticoagulant, there is a potential for inadequate anticoagulation when transitioning from apixaban to a VKA. It is important to maintain an adequate level of anticoagulation when transitioning patients from one anticoagulant to another.

Apixaban should be continued concurrently with the VKA until the INR is ≥2.0.

- For the first 2 days of the conversion period, the VKA can be given in the usual starting doses without INR testing.
- Thereafter, while on concomitant therapy, the INR should be tested just prior to the next dose of apixaban, as appropriate.
- The medication can be discontinued once the INR is >2.0.
- Once discontinued, INR testing may be done at least 12 h after the last dose and should then reliably reflect the anticoagulant effect of the VKA.

Anticoagulation Bridging (See Chap. 12)

Reversal of anticoagulation The U.S. FDA has approved Andexxa, the first factor Xa inhibitor antidote indicated for patients treated with rivaroxaban and apixaban, when reversal of anticoagulation is needed due to life-threatening or uncontrolled bleeding. It is a recombinant, virally inactivated factor Xa that markedly reduced anti-factor Xa activity, and 82% of patients had excellent or good hemostatic efficacy at 12 h [120] (see Chap. 13).

Betrixaban [121]

Formulation

Capsules of 40mg and 80 mg

Indications

- Prophylaxis of VTE in adult patients hospitalized for an acute medical illness who are at risk for thromboembolic complications due to moderate or severe restricted mobility and other risk factors for VTE [121].

Dose

- The recommended dose is an initial single dose of 160 mg.
- Followed by 80 mg once daily. Daily oral doses should be given at the same time of day with food.
- The recommended duration of treatment is 35–42 days.

Precautions

A. *Severe renal impairment (CrCl ≥ 15 to < 30 mL/min)*:
   - The recommended dose of betrixaban is an initial single dose of 80 mg followed by 40 mg once daily.
B. *Use with P-gp inhibitors*:
   - For patients receiving or starting concomitant P-gp inhibitors, the recommended dose is an initial single dose of 80 mg followed by 40 mg once daily.
C. *Spinal/epidural anesthesia or puncture when neuraxial anesthesia (spinal/epidural anesthesia) or spinal/epidural puncture is employed* [121]:
   - Patients treated with antithrombotic agents for the prevention of thromboembolic complications are at risk of developing an epidural or spinal hematoma which can result in long-term or permanent paralysis.
   - Do not remove an epidural catheter earlier than 72 h after the last administration of Betrixaban. Do not administer the next dose earlier than 5 h after the removal of the catheter. If traumatic puncture occurs, delay the administration for 72 h.

D. *Coadminstration of antiplatelets or thrombolytic therapy and/or NSAIDs*:
  • Coadministration of anticoagulants, antiplatelet drugs, and thrombolytics may increase the risk of bleeding.
E. *Missed dose*:
  • If a dose is not taken at the scheduled time, the dose should be taken as soon as possible on the same day and should not be doubled to make up for the missed dose.
F. *Pregnancy, lactation, and pediatric population*:
  • No data available.

Side Effects and Bleeding Risks

The most common adverse reactions with Betrixaban were bleeding (> 5%) with major bleeding occurring in less than 1% of patients.

In the APEX trial, overall 54% vs. 52% of patients receiving betrixaban experienced at least one adverse reaction vs. enoxaparin. The frequency of patients reporting serious adverse reactions was similar between the two arms [122].

Bleeding Reversal

Overdose of betrixaban increases the risk of bleeding and a specific reversal agent is not available. There is no experience with hemodialysis in individuals receiving betrixaban. Protamine sulfate, vitamin K, and tranexamic acid are not expected to reverse the anticoagulant activity of betrixaban.

Edoxaban [123]

Formulation

15, 30, and 60 mg tablets

Indications

• Non-valvular atrial fibrillation (NVAF) to prevent stroke and systemic embolism (excluding mechanical heart valves, rheumatic mitral stenosis, or moderate/severe non-rheumatic mitral stenosis) [124]
• Acute VTE treatment (DVT and PE) must be preceded by 5–10 days of the parenteral anticoagulant) (not recommended in hemodynamically unstable acute PE or those requiring thrombectomy or thrombolysis) [125]
• Cancer-associated thrombosis (CAT) [126]
• VTE prevention [Published data but not on product monograph] [127]

As it accumulates in hepatic and/or renal dysfunction, its use mandates stable creatinine clearance (CrCl) greater than 30 mL/min and stable liver function.

Contraindications [123, 126]

- Mechanical heart valves.
- Patients at high risk for bleeding.
- Pregnant/breastfeeding as safety and dosing have not been studied.
- Significant liver disease with coagulopathy and clinically relevant bleeding risk.
- CrCL >95 mL/min: Do not use; increased risk of ischemic stroke compared with warfarin in NVAF trial.
- CAT with GIT or urothelial malignancy with high bleeding risks.

Dose

Figure 1.13 illustrates the indications and dosage of edoxaban and the minimal creatinine clearance permitted with its use [123].

Precautions [123]

- Decline in anticoagulant effect after a missed dose.
- Very limited data with extremes of weight (under 50 kg, over 120 kg or BMI > 40) [108].
- Has not been tested in children below 18 years of age.
- Patients with ALT or AST greater than 2 × ULN or total bilirubin greater than 1.5 × ULN were excluded in clinical trials.
- CrCL >95 mL/min: Do not use; increased risk of ischemic stroke compared with warfarin in NVAF trial.
- CrCl should be determined at baseline and then annually with more frequent monitoring in patients older than 75 years old, with renal dysfunction (CrCl <60 mL/min), or when there is a decline in renal functions.

Drug Interactions: [120]

- Concomitant use of strong P-gp inhibitors (cyclosporine, dronedarone, erythromycin, quinidine, ketoconazole) requires a dose reduction to 30 mg daily.

Stroke prevention in non-valvular atrial fibrillation	60 mg once daily if CrCl >50 mL/min
	30 mg once daily if one or more of the following:
	    CrCl30-50 mL/min
	    Body weight ≤ 60Kg
	    Concomitant P-gp inhibitor
	    (excluding amiodarone or verapamil)
		CrCl < 30 mL/min, not recommended

Hip and knee replacement	Not approved in Canada Published data suggest 30 mg	**CrCl < 30 mL/min,** not recommended
Acute DVT/PE treatment	Parenteral anticoagulant × 5–10 days, then edoxaban as per AF dosing	**CrCl < 30 mL/min,** not recommended
Cancer-associated thrombosis	Parenteral anticoagulant × 5–10 days, then edoxaban as per AF dosing	**CrCl < 30 mL/min,** not recommended

Fig. 1.13 Indications and dosage of edoxaban and the minimal creatinine clearance permitted with its use

- P-gp inducers (rifampin, phenytoin, carbamazepine, phenobarbital, St John's wort) and HIV protease inhibitors may significantly affect drug metabolism, and therefore, its use should be avoided.
- Combination therapy with antiplatelets increases bleeding risk.

Switching Between Agents [123]

From Warfarin to Edoxaban
Discontinue warfarin and start edoxaban when INR 2.5 or less. From non-warfarin anticoagulant (oral or parenteral, e.g., LMWH, rivaroxaban, dabigatran, apixaban) to edoxaban: Start edoxaban at the time the next scheduled dose of the non-warfarin anticoagulant was to be administered.
For unfractionated heparin infusions, stop the infusion and start edoxaban 4 h later

From Edoxaban to Warfarin
- Start warfarin and administer edoxaban at half the prescribed dose (either 30 mg or 15 mg for those on a reduced dose for one or more of the following: CrCl 15-50 mL/min; <60Kg; use with P-gp inhibitor except amiodarone or verapamil). Once INR is 2 or greater, discontinue edoxaban. Note: Edoxaban can affect INR; therefore, when starting warfarin, INR may be unreliable. If possible, checking INR just prior to next edoxaban dose may better reflect the anticoagulant effect of warfarin.

From edoxaban to non-warfarin anticoagulants (oral or parenteral) (e.g., LMWH, apixaban, rivaroxaban, dabigatran):
- Discontinue edoxaban and give first dose of non-warfarin anticoagulant at the time the next dose of edoxaban is due.

Bridging Anticoagulation (Please refer to Chap. 12)

Anticoagulation around invasive procedures [128] (e.g., surgery, elective day procedures, major dental procedures):

- As with warfarin, very low-risk bleed procedures (such as dental extraction) do not require withholding edoxaban.
- Due to the onset/offset time of edoxaban, peri-procedural use of LMWH is not required.

Renal function (CrCl mL/min)	Last intake of drug prior to procedure	
	Low bleeding risk	High bleeding risk
30 or more	At least 24 h	At least 48 h

Reversal: Management of Bleeding Episodes with Edoxaban (For anticoagulation reversal, please refer to Chap. 13)

- Vitamin K, protamine, tranexamic acid, plasma, and/or idarucizumab will not reverse drug effects.
- In the event of major hemorrhagic complications, discontinue edoxaban and refer patient for urgent assessment and locally developed management strategies.
- Limited evidence demonstrates prothrombin complex concentrates (e.g., Octaplex®/Beriplex®) are able to reverse the anticoagulant effect, but the effect of these agents on bleeding outcomes is limited [123].
- Specific antidotes are not yet available in Canada, but Andexxa seems to be a promising option [120].

Rivaroxaban [129]

Formulation

It is supplied as 2.5 mg, 10mg, 15 mg, and 20 mg film-coated tablets.

Indications

Rivaroxaban (10 mg, 15 mg, 20 mg) is indicated for:

1. Prevention of VTE in patients who have undergone THR or total knee replacement (TKR) surgery.
2. Treatment of venous thromboembolic events (DVT, PE) and prevention of recurrent DVT and PE. It is not recommended as an alternative to unfractionated heparin in patients with pulmonary embolus who are hemodynamically unstable, or who may receive thrombolysis or pulmonary embolectomy.
3. Management of cancer-associated thrombosis.
4. Prevention of stroke and systemic embolism in patients with AF, in whom anticoagulation is appropriate.

Rivaroxaban film-coated tablet (2.5 mg), in combination with 75–100 mg acetylsalicylic acid (ASA), is indicated for the prevention of stroke, myocardial infarction and cardiovascular death, and for the prevention of acute limb ischemia and mortality in patients with coronary artery disease (CAD) with or without peripheral artery disease (PAD).

Dose

1. *Recommended dose and dosage adjustment prevention of VTE after THR and TKR:*
   - *One 10 mg tablet* once daily. Rivaroxaban 10 mg may be taken with or without food.
   - The initial dose should be taken within 6–10 h after surgery, provided that hemostasis has been established. If hemostasis is not established, treatment should be delayed.

- The duration of administration depends on the type of surgery:
  - After elective THR surgery, patients should be administered rivaroxaban for 35 days.
  - After elective TKR surgery, patients should be administered rivaroxaban for 14 days.

2. *Treatment of VTE and Prevention of recurrent DVT and PE*

- The recommended dose for the initial treatment of acute DVT or PE *is 15 mg twice daily (one tablet in the morning and one in the evening) for the first 3 weeks* followed by *20 mg once daily for the continued treatment* and prevention of recurrent DVT and PE.
- Short duration of therapy (at least 3 months) should be considered in patients with DVT or PE provoked by major transient risk factors (e.g., recent major surgery or trauma). The duration of therapy should be individualized after careful assessment of the treatment benefit against the risk for bleeding following completion of at least 6 months treatment for DVT or PE.
- The recommended dose for prevention of recurrent DVT and PE is *20 mg or 10 mg once daily* based on an individual assessment of the risk of recurrent DVT and PE against the risk for bleeding.

The recommended maximum daily dose is 30 mg during the first 3 weeks of treatment and 20 mg thereafter [129].

3. *Cancer-associated thrombosis* is treated similarly; however, major bleeding in clinical trials was higher in gastrointestinal (13.1%) and urothelial (7.9%) cancers, and it would seem unreasonable to use DOACs to manage CAT in such cancers [130].

4. *Prevention of stroke and systemic embolism in patients with AF*:

- The recommended dose is one 20 mg tablet of rivaroxaban taken once daily with food.
- For patients with moderate renal impairment (CrCl 30–49 mL/min), the recommended dose is 15 mg once daily with food [129].

5. *Prevention of stroke, MI, cardiovascular death, acute limb ischemia, and mortality in patients with CAD with or without PAD*:

- The recommended vascular protection regimen for patients with CAD with or without PAD is *one tablet of 2.5 mg rivaroxaban twice daily,* in combination with a once daily dose of 75–100 mg ASA.
- Tablets may be taken with or without food.
- In patients with CAD with or without PAD, treatment should be continued long term provided the benefit outweighs the risk.
- It is not indicated in combination with dual antiplatelet therapy

Factors increasing rivaroxaban plasma levels	Severe renal impairment (CrCl <30 mL/min) Concomitant systemic treatment with strong inhibitors of both CYP 3A4 and P-gp
Pharmacodynamic interactions	NSAID platelet aggregation inhibitors, including ASA, clopidogrel, prasugrel, ticagrelor, selective serotonin reuptake inhibitors (SSRI), and serotonin norepinephrine reuptake inhibitors (SNRIs)
Diseases/procedures with bleeding risks	Congenital or acquired coagulation disorders; thrombocytopenia or functional platelet defects; uncontrolled severe arterial hypertension; active ulcerative gastrointestinal disease; recent gastrointestinal bleeding, vascular retinopathy, such as hypertensive or diabetic; recent intracranial hemorrhage; intraspinal or intracerebral vascular abnormalities; recent brain, spinal, or ophthalmological surgery; bronchiectasis or history of pulmonary bleeding
Others	Age > 75 years

Fig. 1.14 Factors affecting rivaroxaban levels [129]

Precautions and Bleeding Risks

The bleeding risks associated with the use of rivaroxaban are increased in the following conditions. Figure 1.14 illustrates the factors affecting rivaroxaban levels.

Rivaroxaban should be used with caution in patients with moderate renal impairment having a creatinine clearance close to the severe renal impairment category (CrCl <30 mL/min), or in those with a potential to have deterioration of renal function to severe impairment during therapy. In patients with severe renal impairment (CrCl 15 < 30 mL/min), rivaroxaban plasma levels may be significantly elevated compared to healthy volunteers (1.6-fold on average). This may lead to an increased bleeding risk. Due to limited clinical data, rivaroxaban must be used with caution in these patients. No clinical data are available for patients with CrCl <15 mL/min and therefore its use is not recommended. Patients who develop acute renal failure while on rivaroxaban should discontinue such treatment [129].

Switching from One Anticoagulant to Another

Adequate level of anticoagulation should be maintained when transitioning patients from one anticoagulant to another.

Switching from Parenteral Anticoagulants to Rivaroxaban

Rivaroxaban can be started when the infusion of full-dose intravenous heparin is stopped or 0–2 h before the next scheduled injection of full-dose subcutaneous LMWH or fondaparinux. In patients receiving prophylactic heparin, LMWH, or fondaparinux, it can be started 6 or more hours after the last prophylactic dose.

Switching from Rivaroxaban to Parenteral Anticoagulants

Discontinue rivaroxaban and give the first dose of parenteral anticoagulant at the time that the next rivaroxaban dose was scheduled to be taken.

Switching from Vitamin K Antagonists (VKAs) to Rivaroxaban

Stop the VKA and determine the INR. If the INR is ≤2.5, start rivaroxaban at the usual dose. If the INR is >2.5, delay the start until the INR is ≤2.5.

Switching from Rivaroxaban to a VKA

• Rivaroxaban should be continued concurrently with the VKA until the INR is ≥2.0. For the first 2 days of the conversion period, the VKA can be given in the usual starting doses without INR testing.
• Thereafter, while on concomitant warfarin therapy, the INR should be tested just prior to the next dose of rivaroxaban, as appropriate. Rivaroxaban can be discontinued once the INR is >2.0.
• Once it is discontinued, INR testing may be done at least 24 h after the last dose reflecting the anticoagulant effect of the VKA.

Anticoagulation Bridging: See Chap. 12

Reversal of anticoagulation The US FDA has approved Andexxa, the first factor Xa inhibitor antidote indicated for patients treated with rivaroxaban and apixaban, when reversal of anticoagulation is needed due to life-threatening or uncontrolled bleeding. It is a recombinant, virally inactivated factor Xa. Details about reversal are discussed in Chap. 13.

Choice of Anticoagulants

A decade ago, the choice of anticoagulants was limited to heparins and its derivatives, VKA as well as injectable direct thrombin inhibitors that were used only in the context of HIT and to a much lesser extent in thromboprophylaxis.

Over the last decade, novel oral anticoagulants have offered a wider palette of anticoagulation that should be tailored with precision to meet the needs of specific patients.

The choice is therefore made based on the current evidence, taking into account the reason for anticoagulation and the patient's comorbidities and preferences.

Figure 1.15 illustrates the suggested choice of anticoagulants based on the thrombosis etiology and risk and the patient's comorbidities and characteristics [*(N) Chapter number where topic is discussed in detail. Agents between brackets = use with caution].

	GENERAL[2]	PEDIATRICS[4]	PREGNANCY[5]	IMMUNE/APS[7,8]	HEPATIC[2]	RENAL[9]
VTE provoked	UH/LMWH VKA/DOACs	UH/LMWH/ VKA (NOACs)	UH/LMWH	UH/LMWH VKA (DOACs)	UH/LMWH (VKA/DOACs)	UH/(LMWH) VKA (DOACs)
VTE unprovoked	*UH/LMWH VKA/DOACs*	UH/LMWH/ VKA (NOACs)	UH/LMWH	UH/LMWH VKA (DOACs)	UH/LMWH (VKA/DOACs)	UH VKA (DOACs)
PE with hemodynamic instability	UH/LMWH VKA/	UH/LMWH/ VKA	UH/LMWH	UH/LMWH VKA	UH/LMWH VKA	UH VKA
HIT	DTI/Fondaparinux	DTI /Fondaparinux	(DTI/ Fondaparinux)	DTI/ Fondaparinux	DTI/ Fondaparinux	Argatroban
Odd site thrombosis	UH/LMWH VKA/	UH/LMWH/ VKA	UH/LMWH	UH/LMWH VKA	UH/LMWH (VKA)	UH VKA
Cancer-associated thrombosis[6]	UH/LMWH Edoxaban Rivaroxaban (Apixaban)	UH/LMWH/	UH/LMWH	UH/LMWH VKA	UH/LMWH Edoxaban Rivaroxaban (Apixaban)	UH (DOACs)
Atrial fibrillation[3]	UH/LMWH/VKA/ DOACs	UH/LMWH/ VKA	UH/LMWH	UH/LMWH VKA (DOACs)	UH/LMWH (VKA/DOACs)	UH (DOACs)
Mechanical valve[3]	UH/VKA	UH/VKA	UH/LMWH	UH/LMWH VKA	UH/LMWH (VKA)	UH VKA
Valvular heart disease/HF[3]	UH/LMWH VKA	UH/LMWH/ VKA	UH/LMWH	UH/LMWH VKA	UH/LMWH (VKA)	UH VKA
Thromboprophylaxis medical patients[11]	UH/LMWH Betrixaban	–	UH/LMWH	UH/LMWH	UH/LMWH	UH
Thromboprophylaxis surgical patients[10]	UH/LMWH	UH/LMWH	UH/LMWH	UH/LMWH	UH/LMWH	UH
Thromboprophylaxis orthopedic patients[10]	UH/LMWH DOACs-rHirudin	UH/LMWH	UH/LMWH	UH/LMWH	UH/LMWH (DOACs)	UH (DOACs)
Unstable angina/ Non-STEMI[3]	UH/Dalteparin Enoxaparin Dalteparin Fondaparinux Bivaluridin	–	UH/Dalteparin Enoxaparin Dalteparin	UH/Dalteparin Enoxaparin Dalteparin Fondaparinux Bivaluridin	UH/Dalteparin Enoxaparin Dalteparin Fondaparinux Bivaluridin	UH/Dalteparin Enoxaparin Dalteparin Bivaluridin
STEMI[3]	UH/Enoxaparin	–	UH/Enoxaparin	UH/Enoxaparin	UH/Enoxaparin	UH/Enoxaparin
With PCI[3]	UH/Enoxaparin Reviparin	–	UH/Enoxaparin Reviparin	UH/Enoxaparin Reviparin	UH/Enoxaparin Reviparin	UH/Enoxaparin Reviparin

Fig. 1.15 Suggested choice of anticoagulants based on the thrombosis etiology and risk and the patient's comorbidities and characteristics. [(N) Chapter number where the topic is discussed in detail. Agents between brackets = use with caution/no enough evidence]

References

1. Colman RW, Clowes AW, George JN, et al. Overview of hemostasis. In: Colman RW, Clowes AW, George JN, et al., editors. Hemostasis and thrombosis: basic principles and clinical practice. 5th ed. Philadelphia: Lippincott, Williams & Wilkins; 2006. p. 1–16.
2. Osterud B, Rapaport SI. Activation of factor IX by the reaction product of tissue factor and factor VII: additional pathway for initiating blood coagulation. Proc Natl Acad Sci U S A. 1977;74:5260–4.
3. Oliver J, Monroe D, Roberts H, Hoffman M. Thrombin activates factor XI on activated platelets in the absence of factor XII. Arterioscler Thromb Vascular Biol. 1999;19:170–7.
4. Baglia FA, Walsh PN. Prothrombin is a cofactor for the binding of factor XI to the platelet surface and for platelet-mediated factor XI activation by thrombin. Biochemistry. 1998;37:2271–80.
5. Hoffman M, Monroe D. A cell-based model of hemostasis. Thromb Haemost. 2001;85:958–65.
6. Hoffman M, Monroe DM. Coagulation 2006: a modern view of hemostasis. Hematol Oncol Clin North Am. 2007;21:1–11.
7. Wildgoose P, Kisiel W. Activation of human factor VII by factors IXa and Xa on human bladder carcinoma cells. Blood. 1989;73:1888–95.
8. Goubran HA, Burnouf T, Radosevich M, El-Ekiaby M. The platelet-cancer loop. Eur J Intern Med. 2013;24:393–400.

9. Burnouf T, Chou ML, Goubran H, Cognasse F, Garaud O, Seghatchian J. An overview of the role of microparticles/microvesicles in blood components: are they clinically beneficial or harmful? Transfus Apher Sci. 2015;53(2):137–45.
10. Davizon P, Lopez JA. Microparticles and thrombotic disease. Curr Opin Hematol. 2009;16:334–41.
11. Furie B, Furie BC. Mechanisms of thrombus formation. N Engl J Med. 2008;359:938–49.
12. Mann KG, Brummel K, Butenas S. What is all that thrombin for? J Thromb Haemost. 2003;1:1504–14.
13. Long GL, Marshall A, Gardner JC, Naylor SL. Genes for human vitamin K-dependent plasma proteins C and S are located on chromosomes 2 and 3, respectively. Somat Cell Mol Genet. 1988;14(1):93–8.
14. Castoldi E, Hackeng TM. Regulation of coagulation by protein S. Curr Opin Hematol. 2008;15(5):529–36.
15. García de Frutos P, Fuentes-Prior P, Hurtado B, Sala N. Molecular basis of protein S deficiency. Thromb Haemostasis. 2007;98(3):543–56.
16. Foster DC, Yoshitake S, Davie EW. The nucleotide sequence of the gene for human protein C. Proc Natl Acad Sci U S A. 1985;82(14):4673–7.
17. Mosnier LO, Zlokovic BV, Griffin JH. The cytoprotective protein C pathway. Blood. 2007;109(8):3161–72.
18. Nicolaes GA, Dahlbäck B. Congenital and acquired activated protein C resistance. Semin Vasc Med. 2003;3(1):33–46.
19. Chrobák L, Dulícek P. Resistance to activated protein C as pathogenic factor of venous thromboembolism. Acta Medica. 1996;39(2):55–62.
20. Bjork I, Olson JE. Antithrombin, a bloody important serpin (in Chemistry and Biology of Serpins): Plenum Press; 1997. p. 17–33. ISBN 0-306-45698-2.
21. Amiral J, Seghatchian J. Revisiting antithrombin in health and disease, congenital deficiencies and genetic variants, and laboratory studies on α and β forms. Transfus Apher Sci. 2018;57(2):291–7.
22. Ofosu FA. Mechanisms for the anticoagulant effect of heparin and related polysaccharides. Nouv Rev Fr Hematol. 1988;30(3):155–60.
23. Vicente V, González-Conejero R, Rivera J, Corral J. The prothrombin gene variant 20210A in venous and arterial thromboembolism. Haematologica. 1999;84(4):356–62.
24. Seligsohn U, Lubetsky A. Genetic susceptibility to venous thrombosis. N Engl J Med. 2001;344:1222–31.
25. Suchon P, Al Frouh F, Ibrahim M, Sarlon G, Venton G, Alessi MC, Trégouët DA, Morange PE. Genetic risk factors for venous thrombosis in women using combined oral contraceptives: update of the PILGRIM study. Clin Genet. 2017;91(1):131–6.
26. Nemeth B, van Adrichem RA, van Hylckama VA, Bucciarelli P, Martinelli I, Baglin T, Rosendaal FR, Cessie S, Cannegieter SC. Venous thrombosis risk after cast immobilization of the lower extremity: derivation and validation of a clinical prediction score, L-TRiP(cast), in three population-based case-control studies. PLoS Med. 2015;12(11):e1001899; discussion e1001899.
27. Dentali F, Di Micco G, Giorgi Pierfranceschi M, Gussoni G, Barillari G, Amitrano M, Fontanella A, Lodigiani C, Guida A, Visonà A, Monreal M, Di Micco P. Rate and duration of hospitalization for deep vein thrombosis and pulmonary embolism in real-world clinical practice. Ann Med. 2015;47(7):546–54.
28. Ruskin KJ. Deep vein thrombosis and venous thromboembolism in trauma. Curr Opin Anaesthesiol. 2018;31(2):215–8.
29. Sue-Ling HM, Johnston D, McMahon MJ, Philips PR, Davies JA. Pre-operative identification of patients at high risk of deep venous thrombosis after elective major abdominal surgery. Lancet. 1986;1(8491):1173–6.
30. Abdol Razak NB, Jones G, Bhandari M, Berndt MC, Metharom P. Cancer-associated thrombosis: an overview of mechanisms, risk factors, and treatment. Cancers (Basel). 2018;10(10)

31. Aláez-Versón CR, Lantero E, Fernàndez-Busquets X. Heparin: new life for an old drug. Nanomedicine (Lond). 2017;12(14):1727–44.
32. Hemker HC. A century of heparin: past, present and future. J Thromb Haemost. 2016;14(12):2329–38.
33. Torri G, Naggi A. Heparin centenary - an ever-young life-saving drug. Int J Cardiol. 2016;212(Suppl 1):S1–4.
34. Cruickshank MK, Levine MN, Hirsh J, Roberts R, Siguenza M. A standard heparin nomogram for the management of heparin therapy. Arch Intern Med. 1991;151(2):333–7.
35. Warkentin TE. Heparin-induced thrombocytopenia. Curr Opin Crit Care. 2015;21(6): 576–85.
36. Hirsh J, Ofosu F, Buchanan M. Rationale behind the development of low molecular weight heparin derivatives. Semin Thromb Hemost. 1985;11(1):13–6.
37. Gray E, Mulloy B, Barrowcliffe TW. Heparin and low-molecular-weight heparin. Thromb Haemost. 2008;99(5):807–18.
38. Leffert LR, Dubois HM, Butwick AJ, Carvalho B, Houle TT, Landau R. Neuraxial anesthesia in obstetric patients receiving thromboprophylaxis with unfractionated or low-molecular-weight heparin: a systematic review of spinal epidural hematoma. Anesth Analg. 2017;125(1):223–31.
39. Planès A. Review of bemiparin sodium--a new second-generation low molecular weight heparin and its applications in venous thromboembolism. Expert Opin Pharmacother. 2003;4(9):1551–61.
40. Donadini MP, Ageno W, Guasti L, Squizzato A. Certoparin for the treatment and prevention of thrombosis: pharmacological profile and results from clinical studies. Expert Opin Drug Metab Toxicol. 2013;9(7):901–9.
41. Pr FRAGMIN Monograph. Dalteparin sodium injection solution anticoagulant/antithrombotic agent © Pfizer Canada Inc. 2018 date of initial approval: September 30, 1994. Date of Revision:October 18, 2018.
42. PRODUCT MONOGRAPH PrLOVENOX®(Enoxaparin sodium solution for injection, manufacturer's standard) ATC Code: B01AB05 Anticoagulant/Antithrombotic Agent sanofi-aventis Canada Inc. 2905 Place Louis-R.-Renaud Laval, Quebec H7V 0A3. Date of Approval: September 11, 2018.
43. PRODUCT MONOGRAPH PrFRAXIPARINE® nadroparin calcium injection (9,500 anti-Xa IU/mL) 0.2 mL, 0.3 mL, 0.4 mL, 0.6 mL and 1.0 mL prefilled syringe. Aspen Pharmacare Canada Inc 111 Queen Street East, Suite 450, Toronto, Ontario, M5C 1S2 Submission Control No: 195973. Date of Revision: July 11, 2017.
44. Bugamelli S, Zangheri E, Montebugnoli M, Guerra L. Clinical use of parnaparin in major and minor orthopedic surgery: a review. Vasc Health Risk Manag. 2008;4(5):983–90.
45. Del Bono R, Martini G, Volpi R. Update on low molecular weight heparins at the beginning of third millennium. Focus on reviparin. Eur Rev Med Pharmacol Sci. 2011;15(8): 950–9.
46. PRODUCT MONOGRAPH Prinnohep® tinzaparin sodium Sterile solution for SC injection. Anticoagulant/Antithrombotic LEO Pharma Inc Thornhill, ON L3T 7W8 www.leo-pharma.com/canada. Date of Revision: Date of Approval: May 26, 2017.
47. Nenci GG. Low molecular weight heparins: are they interchangeable? No. J Thromb Haemost. 2003;1(1):12–3.
48. Dolenska S. Neuraxial blocks and LMWH thromboprophylaxis. Hosp Med. 1998;59(12):940–3.
49. Barba R, Marco J, Martín-Alvarez H, Rondon P, Fernández-Capitan C, Garcia-Bragado F, Monreal M, RIETE investigators. The influence of extreme body weight on clinical outcome of patients with venous thromboembolism: findings from a prospective registry (RIETE). J Thromb Haemost. 2005;3(5):856–62.
50. Babin JL, Traylor KL, Witt DM. Laboratory monitoring of low-molecular-weight heparin and fondaparinux. Semin Thromb Hemost. 2017;43(3):261–9.

51. Pannucci CJ, Prazak AM, Scheefer M. Utility of anti-factor Xa monitoring in surgical patients receiving prophylactic doses of enoxaparin for venous thromboembolism prophylaxis. Am J Surg. 2017;213(6):1143–52.
52. PRODUCT MONOGRAPH PrARIXTRA® fondaparinux sodium injection 2.5 mg/0.5 mL 5.0 mg/0.4 mL 7.5 mg/0.6 mL 10.0 mg/0.8 mL ATC Classification: B01AX05 Synthetic Antithrombotic Aspen Pharma Trading Limited 3016 Lake Drive Citywest Business Campus Dublin 24 Ireland Date of Preparation: 12 March 2015.
53. Olson ST, Björk I, Sheffer R, Craig PA, Shore JD, Choay J. Role of the antithrombin-binding pentasaccharide in heparin acceleration of antithrombin-proteinase reactions. Resolution of the antithrombin conformational change contribution to heparin rate enhancement. J Biol Chem. 1992;267(18):12528–38.
54. Fifth Organization to Assess Strategies in Acute Ischemic Syndromes Investigators, Yusuf S, Mehta SR, Chrolavicius S, Afzal R, Pogue J, Granger CB, Budaj A, Peters RJ, Bassand JP, Wallentin L, Joyner C, Fox KA. Comparison of fondaparinux and enoxaparin in acute coronary syndromes. N Engl J Med. 2006;354(14):1464–76.
55. Silvestri F, Pasca S, Labombarda A, Barbi A, Desideri M, Guidi P, Rogato A, Zaramella M, Bergamo M, Ageno W, Barillari G. Safety of fondaparinux in the prevention of venous thromboembolism in elderly medical patients: results of a single-center, retrospective study. Minerva Med. 2014;105(3):221–8.
56. Ageno W, Riva N, Noris P, Di Nisio M, La Regina M, Arioli D, Ria L, Monzani V, Cuppini S, Lupia E, Giorgi Pierfranceschi M, Dentali F, FONDAIR study group. Safety and efficacy of low-dose fondaparinux (1.5 mg) for the prevention of venous thromboembolism in acutely ill medical patients with renal impairment: the FONDAIR study. J Thromb Haemost. 2012;10(11):2291–7.
57. Ufer M. Comparative pharmacokinetics of vitamin K antagonists: warfarin, phenprocoumon and acenocoumarol. Clin Pharmacokinet. 2005;44(12):1227–46.
58. Pirmohamed M. Warfarin: almost 60 years old and still causing problems. Br J Clin Pharmacol. 2006;62:509–11.
59. Roderick LM. The pathology of sweet clover disease in cattle. J Am Veterinary Med Assoc. 1929;74:314–25.
60. Link, The discovery of dicumarol and its sequels. Circulation. 1959;19(1):97–107.
61. Beinema M, et al. Pharmacogenetic differences between warfarin, acenocoumarol and phenprocoumon. Thromb Haemost. 2008;100(6):1052–7.
62. Gandara E, Wells PS. Will there be a role for genotyping in warfarin therapy? Curr Opin Hematol. 2010;17(5):439–43.
63. Wells PS, et al. A regression model to predict warfarin dose from clinical variables and polymorphisms in CYP2C9, CYP4F2, and VKORC1: derivation in a sample with predominantly a history of venous thromboembolism. Thromb Res. 2010;125(6):e259–64.
64. http://med.umich.edu/cvc/prof/anticoag/dose.htm
65. Watzka M, et al. Thirteen novel VKORC1 mutations associated with oral anticoagulant resistance: insights into improved patient diagnosis and treatment. J Thromb Haemost. 2011;9(1):109–18.
66. Sinxadi P, Blockman M. Warfarin resistance. Cardiovasc J Afr. 2008;19(4):215–7.
67. https://www.cc.nih.gov/ccc/patient_education/drug_nutrient/coumadin1.pdf
68. Stenton S, Bungard T, Akman B. Interactions between warfarin and herbal products, minerals, and vitamins: a pharmacist's guide. Can J Hosp Pharm. 2001;54:186–92.
69. Important Drug and Food Information from the National Institutes of Health Clinical Center Drug-Nutrient Interaction Task Force. Important information to know when you are taking: Warfarin (Coumadin) and Vitamin K. https://www.cc.nih.gov/ccc/patient_education/drug_nutrient/coumadin1.pdf
70. Coumadin, Product Monograph, Bristol-Myers Squibb Canada, March, 2017.
71. Bungard T, Yakiwchuk E. Drug interactions involving warfarin: practice tool and practical management tips. CPJ/RPC. 2011;144(1):21–30.

72. Brayfield A. Martindale: The Complete Drug Reference. London: Pharmaceutical Press; 2017.
73. Nutescu E, Chuatrisorn I, Hellenbart E. Drug and dietary interactions of warfarin and novel oral anticoagulants: an update. J Thromb Thrombolysis. 2011;31(3):326–43.
74. Bolognia JL, Jorizzo JL, Rapini RP. Dermatology. 2nd ed. St. Louis: Mosby/Elsevier; 2008. p. 331–40.
75. Loftus CM. Fetal toxicity of common neurosurgical drugs. Neurosurgical aspects of pregnancy. Park Ridge: American Association of Neurological Surgeons; 1995. p. 11–3.
76. Bates SM, Greer IA, Middeldorp S, Veenstra DL, Prabulos AM, Vandvik PO. VTE, thrombophilia, antithrombotic therapy, and pregnancy: antithrombotic therapy and prevention of thrombosis, 9th ed: American College of Chest Physicians Evidence-Based Clinical Practice Guidelines. Chest. 2012;141(2 Suppl):e691S–736S.
77. Holbrook A, Schulman S, Witt DM, Vandvik PO, Fish J, Kovacs MJ, Svensson PJ, Veenstra DL, Crowther M, Guyatt GH. Evidence-based management of anticoagulant therapy: antithrombotic therapy and prevention of thrombosis, 9th ed: American College of Chest Physicians Evidence-Based Clinical Practice Guidelines. Chest. 2012;141(2 Suppl):e152S–84S.
78. Garcia D, Crowther MA, Ageno W. Practical management of coagulopathy associated with w1arfarin. BMJ. 2010;340:c1813. https://doi.org/10.1136/bmj.c1813. PMID 20404060.
79. Brown DG, Wilkerson EC, Love WE. A review of traditional and novel oral anticoagulant and antiplatelet therapy for dermatologists and dermatologic surgeons. J Am Acad Dermatol. 2015;72(3):524–34.
80. Delaney JA, Opatrny L, Brophy JM, Suissa S. Drug drug interactions between antithrombotic medications and the risk of gastrointestinal bleeding. CMAJ. 2007;177(4):347–51.
81. Lip GY. Implications of the CHA(2)DS(2)-VASc and HAS-BLED scores for thromboprophylaxis in atrial fibrillation. Am J Med. 2011;124(2):111–4.
82. Fang MC, Go AS, Chang Y, Borowsky LH, Pomernacki NK, Udaltsova N, Singer DE. A new risk scheme to predict warfarin-associated hemorrhage: the ATRIA (Anticoagulation and Risk Factors in Atrial Fibrillation) Study. J Am Coll Cardiol. 2011;58(4):395–401.
83. Chan YC, Valenti D, Mansfield AO, Stansby G. Warfarin induced skin necrosis. Br J Surg. 2000;87(3):266–72.3.
84. Goldhaber S, Poterucha T. Warfarin and vascular calcification. Am J Med. 2016;129(6):635. e1–4.
85. Risk of osteoporotic fracture in elderly patients taking warfarin: results from the National Registry of Atrial Fibrillation 2. Arch Inter Med. 166(2):241–6.
86. Talmadge DB, Spyropoulos AC. Purple toes syndrome associated with warfarin therapy in a patient with antiphospholipid syndrome. Pharmacotherapy. 2003;23(5):674–7.
87. Markwardt F. Studies on the mechanism of the anticoagulant effect of hirudin. Naunyn Schmiedebergs Arch Exp Pathol Pharmakol. 1956;229(4):389–99. German.
88. Dodt J, Seemüller U, Maschler R, Fritz H. The complete covalent structure of hirudin. Localization of the disulfide bonds. Biol Chem Hoppe Seyler. 1985;366(4):379–85.
89. Greinacher A, Volpel H, Janssens U, et al. Recombinant hirudin (lepirudin) provides safe and effective anticoagulation in patients with heparin-induced thrombocytopenia. Circulation. 1999;99:73–80.
90. Greinacher A, Janssens U, Berg G, et al. Lepirudin (recombinant hirudin) for parenteral anticoagulation in patients with heparin-induced thrombocytopenia. Circulation. 1999;100:587–93.
91. Greinacher A, Eichler P, Lubenow N, et al. Heparin-induced thrombocytopenia with thromboembolic complications: meta-analysis of 2 prospective trials to assess the value of parenteral treatment with lepirudin and its therapeutic aPTT range. Blood. 2000;96:846–51.
92. Lubenow N, Eichler P, Lietz T, Greinacher A, Hit Investigators Group. Lepirudin in patients with heparin-induced thrombocytopenia - results of the third prospective study (HAT-3) and a combined analysis of HAT-1, HAT-2, and HAT-3. J Thromb Haemost. 2005;3(11):2428–36.
93. Eriksson BI, Ekman S, Lindbratt S, Baur M, Bach D, Torholm C, Kälebo P, Close P. Prevention of thromboembolism with use of recombinant hirudin. Results of a double-blind, multicenter

trial comparing the efficacy of desirudin (Revasc) with that of unfractionated heparin in patients having a total hip replacement. J Bone Joint Surg Am. 1997;79(3):326–33.

94. Eriksson BI, Wille-Jørgensen P, Kälebo P, Mouret P, Rosencher N, Bösch P, Baur M, Ekman S, Bach D, Lindbratt S, Close P. A comparison of recombinant hirudin with a low-molecular-weight heparin to prevent thromboembolic complications after total hip replacement. N Engl J Med. 1997;337(19):1329–35.

95. PRODUCT MONOGRAPH PrREFLUDAN® lepirudin [rDNA] lyophilized powder (MFR) for intravenous injection 50 mg vial Antithrombotic Bayer Inc. Date of Approval: May 29th, 2007.

96. Goubran HA, Hanna AAZ, Sholkamy S. Efficacy and safety of a novel Hansenula polymorpha-derived recombinant RB-variant Hirudin for thromboprophylaxis in orthopaedic patients, ISTH Geneva, 2007. J Thrombosis Haemostasis. 2007;5(Suppl.2):667.

97. Selleng K, Warkentin TE, Greinacher A. Heparin-induced thrombocytopenia in intensive care patients. Crit Care Med. 2007;35(4):1165–76.

98. Warkentin TE, Greinacher A, Koster A, Lincoff AM. Treatment and prevention of heparin-induced thrombocytopenia: American College of Chest Physicians Evidence-Based Clinical Practice Guidelines (8th Edition). Chest. 2008;133(6 Suppl):340S–80S.

99. Berlex Laboratories. Refludan (lepirudin) injection prescribing information. Montville; 2004.

100. Messmore HL, Jeske WP, Wehmacher WH, et al. Benefit-risk assessment of treatments for heparin-induced thrombocytopenia. Drug Safety. 2003;26:625–41. [PubMed 12814331].

101. Warkentin TE. Bivalent direct thrombin inhibitors: hirudin and bivalirudin. Best Pract Res Clin Haematol. 2004;17(1):105–23.

102. PRODUCT MONOGRAPH PrANGIOMAX® Bivalirudin for Injection 250 mg/vial Professed Standard Direct Thrombin Inhibitor Intravenous Injection Sandoz Canada Inc. 145 Jules-Léger Street Boucherville, Québec J4B 7K8 Date of Revision: September 28, 2016.

103. UNC Health care guideline – John MacKay and Debbie Montague, UNC, 06/11.

104. Ansara AJ, Arif S, Warhurst RD. Weight based argatroban dosing nomogram for treatment of heparin-induced thrombocytopenia. Ann Pharmacother. 2009;43:9–18.

105. Argatroban package inserst, GlaxopsmithKline September, 2009.

106. Argatroban, Product Monograph, Pfizer Canada, revision June 25, 2013.

107. Eriksson BI, Dahl OE, Rosencher N, Kurth AA, van Dijk CN, Frostick SP, Kälebo P, Christiansen AV, Hantel S, Hettiarachchi R, Schnee J, Büller HR, RE-MODEL Study Group. Oral dabigatran etexilate vs. subcutaneous enoxaparin for the prevention of venous thromboembolism after total knee replacement: the RE-MODEL randomized trial. J Thromb Haemost. 2007;5(11):2178–85.

108. Wallentin L, Yusuf S, Ezekowitz MD, Alings M, Flather M, Franzosi MG, Pais P, Dans A, Eikelboom J, Oldgren J, Pogue J, Reilly PA, Yang S, Connolly SJ, RE-LY investigators. Efficacy and safety of dabigatran compared with warfarin at different levels of international normalised ratio control for stroke prevention in atrial fibrillation: an analysis of the RE-LY trial. Lancet. 2010;376(9745):975–83.

109. Schulman S, Kearon C, Kakkar AK, Mismetti P, Schellong S, Eriksson H, Baanstra D, Schnee J, Goldhaber SZ, RE-COVER Study Group. Dabigatran versus warfarin in the treatment of acute venous thromboembolism. N Engl J Med. 2009;361(24):2342–52.

110. PRODUCT MONOGRAPH Pr PRADAXA® Dabigatran Etexilate Capsules Capsules 75 mg, 110 mg and 150 mg Dabigatran Etexilate, (as Dabigatran Etexilate Mesilate) Anticoagulant Boehringer Ingelheim Canada Ltd. 5180 South Service Road Burlington, ON L7L 5H4 BICL 0266 17, 18 and 19 Date of Revision: February 7, 2019.

111. Pollack CV Jr, Reilly PA, van Ryn J, Eikelboom JW, Glund S, Bernstein RA, Dubiel R, Huisman MV, Hylek EM, Kam CW, Kamphuisen PW, Kreuzer J, Levy JH, Royle G, Sellke FW, Stangier J, Steiner T, Verhamme P, Wang B, Young L, Weitz JI. Idarucizumab for dabigatran reversal - full cohort analysis. N Engl J Med. 2017;377(5):431–44.

112. PRODUCT MONOGRAPH PrELIQUIS® apixaban tablets 2.5 mg and 5 mg Anticoagulant Pfizer Canada Inc. 17,300 Trans-Canada Highway Kirkland, Quebec H9J 2M5 Bristol-Myers

Squibb Canada Co. Montreal, Canada H4S 0A4 www.bmscanada.ca. Date of Preparation: 23 October 2018.

113. Lassen MR, et al. For the ADVANCE-3 investigators. Apixaban versus enoxaparin for thrombophylaxis after hip replacement. New Engl J Med. 2010;363:2487–98.

114. Granger CB, Alexander JH, McMurray JJ, Lopes RD, Hylek EM, Hanna M, et al. ARISTOTLE Committees and Investigators. Apixaban versus warfarin in patients with atrial fibrillation. N Engl J Med. 2011;365(11):981–992.

115. Connolly SJ, Eikelboom J, Joyner C, Diener HC, Hart R, Golitsyn S, et al. AVERROES Steering Committee and Investigators. Apixaban in patients with atrial fibrillation. N Engl J Med. 2011;364(9):806–817.

116. Agnelli G, Buller HR, Cohen A, et al. Oral apixaban for the treatment of acute venous thromboembolism. N Engl J Med. 2013;369:799–808.

117. Agnelli G, Buller HR, Cohen A, et al. Apixaban for extended treatment of venous thromboembolism. N Engl J Med. 2013;368:699–708.

118. McBane RD, Wysokinski WE, Le-Rademacher J, Ashrani AA, Tafur AJ, Gundabolu K, Perez-Botero J, Perepu U, Anderson DM, Kuzma C, Leon Ferre R, Henkin S, Lenz C, Loprinzi C. Apixaban, dalteparin, in active cancer associated venous thromboembolism, the ADAM VTE Trial. Abstract 421. St Diego: American Society of Hematology; 2018.

119. Alexander JH, Lopes RD, James S, Kilaru R, He Y, Mohan P, Bhatt DL, et al. APPRAISE-2 Investigators. Apixaban with antiplatelet therapy after acute coronary syndrome. N Engl J Med 2011;365(8):699–708.

120. Connolly SJ, Crowther M, Eikelboom JW, Gibson CM, Curnutte JT et al. ANNEXA-4 Investigators. Full Study Report of Andexanet Alfa for Bleeding Associated with Factor Xa Inhibitors. N Engl J Med. 2019. https://doi.org/10.1056/NEJMoa1814051.

121. HIGHLIGHTS OF PRESCRIBING INFORMATION These highlights do not include all the information needed to use BEVYXXA safely and effectively. FDA, 2017.

122. Nafee T, Gibson CM, Yee MK, Alkhalfan F, Chi G, Travis R, et al. Betrixaban for first-line venous thromboembolism prevention in acute medically ill patients with risk factors for venous thromboembolism. Expert Rev Cardiovasc Ther. 2018;16(11):845–55.

123. Lixiana product monograph. (Servier Canada Inc), July 26, 2017.

124. Giugliano RP, Ruff CT, Braunwald E, Murphy SA, Wiviott SD, Halperin JL, Waldo AL, Ezekowitz MD, Weitz JI, Špinar J, Ruzyllo W, Ruda M, Koretsune Y, Betcher J, Shi M, Grip LT, Patel SP, Patel I, Hanyok JJ, Mercuri M. Antman EM; ENGAGE AF-TIMI 48 Investigators. Edoxaban versus warfarin in patients with atrial fibrillation. N Engl J Med. 2013;369(22):2093–104.

125. Hokusai-VTE Investigators, Büller HR, Décousus H, Grosso MA, Mercuri M, Middeldorp S, Prins MH, Raskob GE, Schellong SM, Schwocho L, Segers A, Shi M, Verhamme P, Wells P. Edoxaban versus warfarin for the treatment of symptomatic venous thromboembolism. N Engl J Med. 2013;369(15):1406–15.

126. Raskob GE, van Es N, Verhamme P, Carrier M, Di Nisio M, Garcia D, Grosso MA, Kakkar AK, Kovacs MJ, Mercuri MF, Meyer G, Segers A, Shi M, Wang TF, Yeo E, Zhang G, Zwicker JI, Weitz JI, Büller HR, Hokusai VTE Cancer Investigators. Edoxaban for the treatment of cancer-associated venous thromboembolism. N Engl J Med. 2018;378(7):615–24.

127. AlHajri L, Jabbari S, AlEmad H, AlMahri K, AlMahri M, AlKitbi N. The efficacy and safety of edoxaban for VTE prophylaxis post-orthopedic surgery: a systematic review. J Cardiovasc Pharmacol Ther. 2017;22(3):230–8.

128. Steffel J, Potpara TS. Challenges in clinical decision-making on concomitant drug therapies in patients with atrial fibrillation taking oral anticoagulants. Eur Heart J. 2018;40:1569. https://doi.org/10.1093/eurheartj/ehy784.

129. PRODUCT MONOGRAPH PrXARELTO® rivaroxaban tablets 2.5 mg, 10 mg, 15 mg and 20 mg Anticoagulant (ATC Classification: B01AF01) Bayer Inc. 2920 Matheson Boulevard East Mississauga, Ontario L4W 5R6 Canada http://www.bayer.ca. Date of Revision: September 18, 2018.

130. Young AM, Marshall A, Thirlwall J, Chapman O, Lokare A, Hill C, Hale D, Dunn JA, Lyman GH, Hutchinson C, MacCallum P, Kakkar A, Hobbs FDR, Petrou S, Dale J, Poole CJ, Maraveyas A, Levine M. Comparison of an oral factor Xa inhibitor with low molecular weight heparin in patients with cancer with venous thromboembolism: results of a randomized trial (SELECT-D). J Clin Oncol. 2018;36(20):2017–23.

Chapter 2
Routine Anticoagulation for the Provoked and Unprovoked VTE

Mark Bosch

Abbreviations

APS	Antiphospholipid syndrome
BMI	Body mass index
CVC	Central venous catheter
CVST	Cerebral venous sinus thrombosis
DOACs	Direct oral anticoagulants
DVT	Deep vein thrombosis
HIT	Heparin-induced thrombocytopenia
HITT	Heparin-induced thrombocytopenia and thrombosis
INR	International normalized ratio
IVC	Inferior vena cava
LMWH	Low-molecular-weight heparin
NSAIDs	Nonsteroidal anti-inflammatory drugs
OVT	Ovarian vein thrombosis
PE	Pulmonary embolism
PTS	Post-thrombotic syndrome
UFH	Unfractionated heparin
SVT	Superficial venous thrombosis
VKA	Vitamin K antagonist
VTE	Venous thromboembolism

M. Bosch (✉)
Saskatoon Cancer Centre, College of Medicine, University of Saskatchewan,
Saskatoon, SK, Canada
e-mail: Mark.Bosch@saskcancer.ca

© Springer Nature Switzerland AG 2020
H. Goubran et al. (eds.), *Precision Anticoagulation Medicine*,
https://doi.org/10.1007/978-3-030-25782-8_2

55

Introduction

A major component of a general hematologist practice is the management of venous thromboembolism (VTE). Venous thromboembolism is typically a disease of older people, with the incidence of thrombotic events increasing substantially beyond the age of 60 years [2]. Despite considerable time and effort in addressing this significant medical problem, VTE remains a major cause of morbidity and mortality worldwide.

The incidence of VTE exceeds 1 per 1000, and the 30-day mortality of patients suffering a thrombotic event exceeds 25% [3]. VTE can also lead to considerable morbidity, despite appropriate therapy. This is evident by the development of post-thrombotic syndrome in approximately 30% at 10 years, with 10% of the patients suffering venous stasis ulceration [4]. In addition, up to 30% of survivors will develop recurrent VTE within 5 years [5].

Provoked Versus Unprovoked VTE

When evaluating for venous thromboembolism, the preferred term is provoked or unprovoked. This nomenclature focuses the attention on the environment that precipitated the VTE. Approximately half of all VTE cases are unprovoked [6, 7].

- *Provoked VTE* occurs in a patient with a transient (within 3 months) major clinical risk factor.

  - For example, surgery, trauma, recent leg injuries or immobilization (e.g., within 6 weeks flight of >8 hours), pregnancy or puerperium, or in a patient on hormonal therapy (oral contraceptive or hormone replacement therapy) [5].

In patients with a provoked VTE, it is important to differentiate whether or not the factors are transient or persistent, for example, those factors that may resolve, i.e., surgery or estrogen therapy versus a stroke or episodic flares of inflammatory autoimmune disease.

- *Unprovoked* (also termed "idiopathic") *VTE* occurs in a patient with:
  - No major clinical risk factor for VTE, active cancer, thrombophilia, or a family history of VTE.

Treatment of Provoked or Unprovoked VTE

Provoked or unprovoked VTE can be treated with many different anticoagulants and is summarized in Fig. 2.1.

	Dosing	Dosing	Monitoring	Renal/Liver	Considerations
Unfractionated heparin	Unfractionated heparin $$$	Intravenous: 80 U/kg bolus and then 18 U/kg per hour infusion. Subcutaneous: 333 U/kg and then 250 U/kg twice daily	Nomogram aPTT ratio of 1.5–2.5 ULN	May be less effective in liver disease due to decrease production of ATIII	HIT monitoring required (may be seen in up to 5%). If a bolus is given, it is the quickest acting anticoagulant. Short half-life allows quick on and off action and has a reversible agent protamine
LMWH	Enoxaparin $$$	Subcutaneous: 1 mg/kg twice daily or 1.5 mg/kg once daily	Anti-fXa level (0.3–0.7 IU/mL)	Caution if CrCl <30 mL/min (risk of LMWH accumulation)	Twice daily administration. Infrequent HIT monitoring not recommend due to the low incidence of HIT
	Dalteparin $$$$	Subcutaneous: 200 U/kg once daily	Anti-fXa level (0.3–0.7 IU/mL)	Caution if CrCl <30 mL/min (risk of LMWH accumulation)	
	Tinzaparin $$$	Subcutaneous: 200 U/kg once daily	Anti-fXa level (0.3–0.7 IU/mL)	Caution if CrCl <20 mL/min (risk of LMWH accumulation)	
	Nadroparin $$	Subcutaneous: 171 U/kg once daily or Subcutaneous: 86 U/kg twice daily	Anti-fXa level (0.2–0.4 IU/mL)	Caution if CrCl <50 mL/min (risk of LMWH accumulation)	
pentasaccharide factor Xa inhibitor	Fondaparinux $$$	Subcutaneous: Based on weight: <50 kg ¼ 5 mg once daily; 50–100 kg ¼ 7.5 mg once daily; >100 kg ¼ 10 mg once daily	Anti-fXa level (0.3–0.7 IU/mL)	Caution if CrCl <30 mL/min (risk of LMWH accumulation)	No data in pregnancy

Fig. 2.1 *Treatment of VTE* (for full dosing, please refer to Chap. 1)

	Dosing	Dosing	Monitoring	Renal/Liver	Considerations
Vitamin K Antagonist	Warfarin $	Mandatory Concurrent: LMWH or UFH With Oral: Initial dosing typically 5 mg once daily titrated for a goal of INR 2–3	Frequent INR measurements		Lower starting dose in elderly patients, poor nutritional status, concurrent medications affecting metabolism, or underlying renal and liver disease. Requires frequent monitoring Cheapest alternative Frequent drug interactions that may necessity more frequent testing NSAID and other anti-platelet agents should also be avoided
DOAC (anti-Xa)	Rivaroxaban $$	Oral: 15 mg twice daily for 21 days and then 20 mg once daily	None	Dose reduce if CrCl 30–15 mL/min	Avoid for pregnant or nursing patients Reduce dose in
	Apixaban $$	Oral: 10 mg twice daily for 7 days followed by 5 mg twice daily	None	Avoid if CrCl <15 mL/min Avoid if moderate-to-severe liver disease	12-hour half-life and is eliminated through renal, hepatic, and enteral route
	Edoxaban $$	Oral: 60 mg Once Daily if CrCl >50 mL/min 30 mg Once Daily if one or more of the following: CrCl 30–50 mL/min Body weight ≤ 60 kg Concomitant P-glycoprotein inhibition (excluding amiodarone or verapamil)		Contraindicated if CrCl <30 mL/min	In acute treatment of VTE: Must be preceded by 5–10 days of parenteral anticoagulant Not recommended in hemodynamically unstable acute PE or those requiring thrombectomy or thrombolysis
DOAC (direct thrombin inhibitor)	Dabigatran $$	150 mg twice daily after minimum 5 days of LMWH (RECOVER)	None	Avoid if CrCl <30 mL/min	Should not be used in pregnant, breastfeeding women or in those with severe renal dysfunction

aPTT activated partial thromboplastin time, HIT heparin-induced thrombocytopenia, INR international normalized ratio, DOAC direct oral anticoagulant, LMWH low-molecular-weight heparin, VTE venous thromboembolism, CrCl creatinine clearance, PE pulmonary emboliom, $ denotes the relative cost of the treatment compared to each other, the more $ the greater the cost in Canada, more details can be found in the Appendix A

Fig. 2.1 (continued)

Warfarin Management

Warfarin is approved for multiple indications and has been used for over 60 years. When appropriately managed in compliant, stable patients, warfarin is safe and effective. For more details, refer to Chap. 1.

- When warfarin is used in VTE treatment, it requires bridge therapy:
  - Start the LMWH, fondaparinux, or UFH as soon as possible, and continue it for at least 5 days or until the international normalized ratio (INR) is 2 or above for at least 24 hours (Fig. 2.2).
  - When the INR is stable, check weekly for 2 weeks, then every 2 weeks until stable for 1 month, and then monthly. If stable for 3 months, consider every 12 weeks checks.
- Should the INR fall below 2.0 during the first 3 months of therapy after a DVT, therapeutic LMWH should be instituted and warfarin adjusted until the INR is >2.0 for two consecutive days.
- Initiating warfarin by nomogram is best practice [8] (Figs. 2.2 and 2.3).

Fig. 2.2 5-mg warfarin initiation nomogram [8]

Day	INR	Dosage
1		5 mg
2	<1.5 1.5–2.0 2.0–2.5 >2.5	5 mg 2.5–5 mg 0–2.5 mg 0 mg
3	<1.5 1.5–1.9 2.0–3.0 >3.0	5–10 mg 2.5–5 mg 0–2.5 mg 0 mg
4	<1.5 1.5–1.9 2.0–3.0 >3.0	10 mg 5–7.5 mg 0–5 mg 0 mg
5	<1.5 1.5–1.9 2.0–3.0 >3.0	10 mg 5–7.5 mg 0–5 mg 0 mg
6	<1.5 1.5–1.9 2.0–3.0 >3.0	7.5–12.5 mg 5–10 mg 0–7.5 mg 0 mg
Data from Crowther et al. [8]		

Fig. 2.3 Maintenance
of warfarin nomogram

Target INR 2–3	Action
<1.5	Extra dose, ↑ weekly dose by 10–20%
1.5–1.9	↑ weekly dose by 5–10%
2–3	No change
3.1–3.5	↓ weekly dose by 5–10%
3.6–4.9	Hold 1 dose,↓ weekly dose by 10–20%
5–9	Hold 2 doses,↓ weekly dose by 10–20%
>9	Urgent evaluation

Fig. 2.3 Maintenance of warfarin nomogram

Duration of Anticoagulation

There is a consensus that a DVT or PE that is provoked by either surgery or a transient risk factor should be treated with a minimum duration of treatment in 3 months (Fig. 2.4). In the setting of an unprovoked proximal DVT or PE, the duration of anticoagulation is more complex. Most hematologists will determine the duration based on the risk of bleeding for the individual patient.

Discontinue Versus Extend Anticoagulation

The risk of VTE recurrence after stopping anticoagulation is not significantly influenced by the duration of initial treatment (i.e., 3 months vs 6 months) [12]. The risk of recurrent VTE after cessation of anticoagulation is estimated to be 5–10% after 1 year and 30% after 5 years [5] with a case-fatality rate of 3.6% [13]. In recent studies, extending treatment with vitamin K antagonists (VKAs) or direct oral anticoagulants (DOACs: rivaroxaban, apixaban, dabigatran), beyond the initial 3 months, reduces the risk of recurrence by 80–90% [14].

Based on the projected long-term mortality rates associated with recurrent VTE and major bleeding, some guidelines suggest discontinuation of anticoagulation when the annual risk of recurrence is lower than 5% in the first year and 15% in the first 5 years after stopping treatment [15] (Fig. 2.5).

Most guidelines recommend that for patients at low-to-moderate risk for bleeding, extended therapy is recommended. Moreover, for those with a high risk of bleeding, anticoagulation may be discontinued after 3 months. Some guidelines also suggest consideration of low-dose aspirin therapy in this high-risk group (Fig. 2.4).

Unfortunately assessing the bleeding risk is complex and challenging in the clinical setting. Current evaluation relies on the summation of a number of variables (Table 2.1), and a number of risk calculation tools have been developed but are not validated. Also, it is clear that the severity of a single factor may be a better predictor of bleeding than many less severe factors (e.g., the degree of thrombocytopenia) or the temporal relationship to specific events (e.g., major trauma or surgery).

Duration of anticoagulation	ACCP 2016 [5]	NICE [9]	ESC [10]	Thrombosis Canada [11]
Provoked				
First Provoked VTE Event	3 months	3 months	3 months	3 months
Unprovoked				
First Unprovoked VTE Event	Minimum 3 months with indefinite anticoagulation provided low/moderate bleeding risk	Minimum 3 months with extended anticoagulation after assessment of recurrent VTE and bleeding risk	Minimum 3 months with extended anticoagulation to be considered if low bleeding risk	Minimum 3 months and then reassess. Patient not on extended anticoagulation should be considered for low dose as prophylaxis
Second unprovoked VTE event	Indefinite[†] for low/moderate bleeding risk; 3 months for high bleeding risk	No specific recommendation. See first VTE event	Indefinite anticoagulation	Same as first unprovoked VTE, strong indication for indefinite AC unless very high bleeding risk
Special considerations				
Cancer Associate VTE	Indefinite anticoagulation[a]	6 months, then reassess, and consider extending	3-6 months, consider indefinite anticoagulation[†]	Minimum 3 months, then reassess and continue if active cancer or continuing anticancer therapy
Isolated distal DVT	3 months	Not discussed	Not discussed	3 months
CVC-associate VTE	Not discussed	Not discussed	Not discussed	3 months; longer if CVC remains in place
Treatment consideration				
DOAC for management of VTE	DOAC recommended over VKA	VKAs are recommended over NOAC. Rivaroxaban may be considered	DOACs should be considered as alternatives to VKA	DOACs are more convenient and have a lower bleeding risk than VKA
Thrombolysis for intermediate- risk PE	Thrombolysis for intermediate- risk PE is not recommended unless there are signs of deterioration	Do not offer thrombolysis to patients with intermediate-risk PE	Thrombolysis for intermediate-risk PE is not recommended unless there are signs of hemodynamic decompensation	Should not be used routinely in patients with submassive PE

Fig. 2.4 Duration of anticoagulation

Duration of anticoagulation	ACCP 2016 [5]	NICE [9]	ESC [10]	Thrombosis Canada [11]
Thrombolysis for high-risk PE	Thrombolysis is recommended in patients without high bleeding risk	Thrombolysis should be considered	Thrombolysis is recommended	Thrombolysis could be considered
Anticoagulation of asymptomatic SSPE	Not recommended unless there is concomitant DVT or a high risk of VTE recurrence	Not discussed	No specifi recommendation	Not Recommended in isolated subsegmental pulmonary embolism
Aspirin after cessation of anticoagulation for unprovoked PE	Aspirin is recommended	Not discussed	Aspirin should be considered	Aspirin is recommended

°Clinical risk of recurrent VTE no longer outweighs the risk of bleeding, *DVT* deep venous throm-bosis, *PE* pulmonary embolism, *SSPE* subsegmental pulmonary embolism, *VTE* venous thromboembolism, *VKA* vitamin K antagonist, *DOAC* direct oral anticoagulant
[†]Please see Table 2.1 for Risk Stratification

Fig. 2.4 (continued)

Classification	Risk	Extended therapy recommended
Provoked VTE by surgery (a major transient risk factor)	3% recurrence at 5 years [16]	No
Provoked by a nonsurgical transient risk factor (e.g., estrogen therapy, pregnancy, leg injury, flight of >8 hours), recent Ig injuries or immobilization (e.g., within 6 weeks)	15% recurrence at 5 years [16]	No
Unprovoked VTE; not meeting criteria for provoked by a transient risk factor or by cancer	30% recurrence at 5 years [12, 17]	Yes
VTE associated with cancer (also termed "cancer-associated thrombosis")	15% annualized risk of recurrence; recurrence at 5 years not estimated because of high mortality from cancer [18, 19]	Yes

Fig. 2.5 Risk of recurrence based on VTE provocation

From Table 2.1, it is clear that the risk of bleeding during anticoagulant therapy differs among patients and their comorbidities and with the duration of therapy. In general, bleeding rates of VTE patient on anticoagulation vary from low (0.8%/year) to moderate (1.6%/year) to high (>6.5%/year) risk. It has been noted that the highest risk is seen in older patients and during the first month of anticoagulation.

Table 2.1 Risk factors for bleeding [5]

Age >65 years	Liver failure	Poor anticoagulant control
Age >75 years	Thrombocytopenia	Comorbidity and reduced functional capacity
Previous bleeding	Previous stroke	Recent surgery
Cancer	Diabetes	Frequent falls
Metastatic cancer	Anemia	Alcohol abuse
Renal failure	Antiplatelet therapy	Nonsteroidal anti-inflammatory drug

Estimated absolute risk of major bleeding after first 3 months

	Low risk (0 risk factor)	*Moderate risk (1 risk factor)*	*High risk (≥2 risk factors)*
Total risk (%/ year)	0.8	1.6	≥6.5

Drug class	Drug	Comment	Trial
Vitamin K antagonist	Warfarin	Often considered the standard treatment on all extension trials	
NOAC (anti-Xa)	Rivaroxaban	Continuation of rivaroxaban resulted in reduced recurrent thrombotic events compared with placebo (1.3% vs 7.1%) yet similar bleeding rates (0.7% vs 0%)	EINSTEIN-EXTEND [20]
	Apixaban	Received 1 of 2 doses of apixaban (2.5 mg or 5 mg twice daily) or placebo for an additional 12 months. Both apixaban doses reduced recurrent VTE without increasing major bleeding	AMPLIFY-EXTEND [21]
DOAC (direct thrombin inhibitor)	Dabigatran	150 mg twice daily resulted in a lower risk of major or clinically relevant bleeding than warfarin but a higher risk than placebo	RE-MEDY, RE-SONATE [22]
Antiplatelet	ASA	Aspirin 100 mg once daily reduced the risk of recurrence (6.6% vs 11.2% per year) in patients with unprovoked VTE after an initial treatment period of 6–18 months with a vitamin K antagonist In the similarly designed ASPIRE trial, low-dose aspirin resulted in a trend toward reduced VTE recurrence rates	WARFASA [23] ASPIRE [24]

Fig. 2.6 Anticoagulants used in extended duration

Anticoagulants Used in Extended Duration

Although there is variability between guidelines, anticoagulant therapy should be stopped when the benefits no longer outweigh the risks or when educated patients want to stop even if continuing treatment is expected to be of net benefit. For patients on active therapy, the patient's preferences should be regularly reviewed on an ongoing basis (Fig. 2.6).

VTE by Location

Deep Vein Thrombosis (DVT)/Pulmonary Embolism (PE)

Important Facts
- Only 25% of patients presenting with DVT symptoms have a DVT. If present, 80% are proximal and 20% distal.
- 50% with proximal DVT will also have a PE.
- 20–30% of distal DVTs will extend within 1–2 weeks of presentation.

In the absence of any contraindications, warfarin historically has been the treatment of choice for DVT/PE with a target INR of 2.0–3.0. Therapeutic heparin therapy (either UFH or LMWH) must be initiated concomitantly with warfarin. LMWH is preferable to intravenous UFH due to its favorable pharmacokinetic profile and ease of use in the outpatient setting.

From the latest clinical evidence, it is also clear that direct oral anticoagulants (DOACs) are non-inferior to warfarin therapy, and recent guidelines prefer DOAC therapy due to their convenience and lower bleeding risk (see Fig. 2.4).

Alternative treatment to warfarin may be found in Fig. 2.1.

Acute Isolated Distal DVT and Superficial Thrombophlebitis

An isolated distal DVT is defined as DVT confined to the deep veins of the calf (posterior or anterior tibial, peroneal, solely, or gastrocnemius veins).

- Anticoagulation for acute isolated distal leg DVT is controversial.
- The decision to initiate anticoagulation is often made based on the risk of bleeding, if anticoagulation is initiated; 3 months is recommended.
- Since the majority of thrombi progresses within the first 2 weeks, serial imaging can be performed at 1 and 2 weeks without anticoagulation [5].
- In the event of progression on imaging, or risk factors of extension (Table 2.2), anticoagulation initiation is recommended.

Table 2.2 Risk factors for extension	
	Thrombus length greater than 5 cm
	Multiple veins involved
	Unprovoked event
	Close to the popliteal vein
	Cancer
	Previous VTE
	Hospitalization
	Recent surgery
	Positive d-dimer

Superficial Venous Thrombosis (SVT)

Superficial "phlebitis" or thrombosis is a common form of thrombosis. Superficial venous thrombosis (SVT) is defined by the location of the thrombosis (Fig. 2.7).

- Approximately 25% of the patients will also have underlying venous thrombo-embolism, mandating appropriate imaging to exclude a more sinister thrombosis. Figure 2.7 illustrates superficial venous system of the lower extremity.
- In clinical practice, anticoagulation is reserved only for those with severe pain, extensive venous involvement, or evidence of thrombus propagation (Table 2.3).
- The majority of these events may be treated without anticoagulation as these types of thrombosis are thought to have a low risk of development of pulmonary embolism (1.3%). When treatment is required, treatment is similar to other VTE (Fig. 2.8).

Catheter-Related Thrombosis

- The deep veins of the upper extremity include the brachial, axillary, subclavian, and innominate veins.
- Catheter-related thrombosis is a relatively common complication of central venous catheter insertion and is seen in up to 14–18% [26].

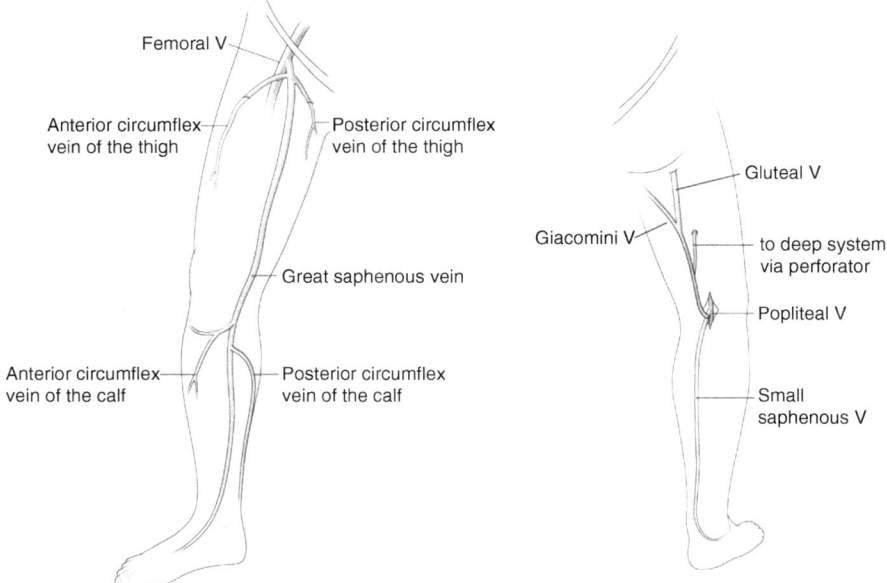

Fig. 2.7 Superficial venous system of the lower extremity [1]

Table 2.3 When to treat superficial venous thrombosis

Isolated SVT >5 cm	*Therapeutic doses of anticoagulation* for 3 months
Isolated SVT which extends to *within 3 cm of the* saphenofemoral junction	*Therapeutic doses of anticoagulation* for 3 months
Isolated SVT≥5 cm in length located >3 cm from the saphenofemoral junction	*Prophylactic doses of fondaparinux (2.5 mg subcutaneously per day), rivaroxaban 10 mg PO daily or prophylactic/ intermediate doses of LMWH (see* Fig. 2.1) for 45 days
Isolated SVT <5 cm in length located >3 cm from the saphenofemoral junction	Patients may receive topical nonsteroidal anti-inflammatory drugs (NSAIDS) and compression therapy for symptomatic relief in conjunction with anticoagulation Consider therapy for those with severe pain, extensive venous involvement, or evidence of thrombus propagation
SVT associated with IV cannulation	Anticoagulation not recommended. Supportive measures should include warm compresses and topical NSAIDs for symptom relief

Data from Thrombosis Canada [25]

Drug class	Suggested dosing	Duration of treatment
LMWH	Dalteparin 5000–10,000 units SC daily Enoxaparin 40–80 mg SC daily Tinzaparin 4500–10,000 units SC daily	45 days
Fondaparinux	2.5 mg SC daily	45 days
Rivaroxaban	10 mg PO daily	45 days
Oral NSAIDs	Ibuprofen 400 mg PO TID Naproxen 500 mg PO BID	7 days
Topical NSAIDs	Topical diclofenac apply 2–4 g to affected area 3 or 4 times daily	7–14 days

Fig. 2.8 Treatment options of superficial venous thrombosis

- The consequences of catheter-related thrombosis are not insubstantial; complications may include pulmonary embolism, loss of venous access, infection, post-thrombotic syndrome (PTS), and delays in treatment [26].
- Catheter removal is not necessary as long as it remains functional and required for clinical care [5]. Close surveillance for resolution of symptoms is recommended; if symptoms persist despite appropriate treatment, the catheter may require removal.
- Despite appropriate treatment, the CVC may require removal.
- Therapeutic anticoagulation is indicated typically for 3 months and should be continued as long as the catheter is in place [5].
- To date, there is insufficient evidence to support prophylactic anticoagulation in the prevention of catheter-related thrombosis.
- Superficial thrombosis of the cephalic and basilic veins does not require anticoagulant therapy.
- In patients with malignancy, LMWH is the preferred anticoagulant, with warfarin being an alternative in patients without malignancy once their critical illness has resolved.

Inferior Vena Cava (IVC) Filters

IVC filters should only be placed only in three situations:

1. Absolute contraindication to therapeutic anticoagulation.

   Bleeding diathesis (e.g., coagulation defects, severe thrombocytopenia [platelet count < 50,000/μL]), uncontrollable active bleeding (e.g., gastrointestinal bleeding from any cause), and acute hemorrhagic stroke, cerebral lesions at high risk of bleeding, severe uncontrolled hypertension, and severe renal and hepatic dysfunction.

2. life-threatening hemorrhage on anticoagulation
3. Failure of anticoagulation when there is acute proximal venous thrombosis:

   Inability to maintain therapeutic levels of anticoagulation and documented progression of VTE while on therapeutic anticoagulation
   - Anticoagulation must be resumed as soon as possible after filter insertion because the filter alone is not an effective treatment of venous thromboembolism [27]. Unfortunately, many patients in whom filters are inserted have contraindications to anticoagulation; therefore, achieving this goal is challenging.
   - Non-retrieved devices pose a major health concern because longer indwelling times are associated with higher risk of potential complications, including vein perforation or thrombosis, filter fracture and fragment embolization, cardiac perforation, and death [28, 29].
   - The risk versus benefit profile favors device removal between 29 and 54 days post insertion [30].

Splanchnic Venous Thrombosis

- The splanchnic venous system includes the portal, hepatic, splenic, superior, and inferior mesenteric veins.
- When a clot affects the hepatic veins, it is also known as Budd-Chiari syndrome.
- Complications may include bowel or splenic infarction or portal hypertension.
- Anticoagulation initiation depends on symptoms, extent, and acuity of thrombus formation. If the patient develops symptoms or has extensive disease, that is considered acute; anticoagulation therapy should be considered [5].
- For incidentally found asymptomatic splanchnic vein thrombosis, no anticoagulation may be required.
- In the absence of randomized trial data, most hematologists treat splanchnic vein thrombosis for 3–6 months.

Ovarian Vein Thrombosis (OVT)

- OVT is a rare condition associated with the postpartum period, malignancy, abdominal and pelvic surgery, pelvic inflammatory disease, and inflammatory bowel disease [31–33].
- Ovarian vein thrombosis treatment is controversial.
- Incidentally detected OVT does not necessarily warrant anticoagulation therapy. However, concurrent DVT/PE must be ruled out.
- In symptomatic OVT, that is, pelvic pain, fever, and a right-sided abdominal mass, the combination of anticoagulant and intravenous (IV) antibiotic therapy is the treatment of choice.

Cerebral Venous Sinus Thrombosis (CVST)

- Cerebral venous and sinus thrombosis (CVST) is a rare disease that accounts for <1% of all strokes.
- Symptoms of CVST include headache, abnormal vision, symptoms of stroke such as weakness of the face and limbs, and seizures.
- Anticoagulation for CVT is controversial [34–37].
- When anticoagulation is used, LMWH is preferable to UFH.

Special Populations

Heparin-Induced Thrombocytopenia and Thrombosis (HITT)

- Heparin-induced thrombocytopenia (HIT) is the development of thrombocytopenia, due to the administration of heparin. When thrombosis occurs, it is called heparin-induced thrombocytopenia and thrombosis (HITT).
- The incidence of HITT has been determined to be between 1% and 5% [38–41]. It is lower in patient and higher in surgical patients receiving prolonged postoperative thromboprophylaxis, i.e., following orthopedic surgery [42] or after coronary artery bypass and/or valve replacement surgery [41].
- Thrombosis occurs in greater than 50% of patients with HIT [43].
- The mortality rate is approximately 20%, and 10% of patients require amputations or suffer other major morbidity [44–46].
- Only argatroban or bivalirudin should be used for the critically ill, high bleeding risk patients, or patients who may need surgery.
- All other anticoagulation agents may be considered but are not approved for the treatment of HIT (Fig. 2.9). For dosing, refer to Chap. 1.
- Argatroban and DOAC should not be used in patient with hepatic.

Fig. 2.9 Non-heparin anticoagulants for the treatment of acute HIT [47]

Approved in HIT	Drug
Yes	Argatroban
	Bivalirudin
No[a]	Fondaparinux
	Apixaban
	Dabigatran
	Rivaroxaban
[a]Limited data on the use and dosage in HIT	

- After correction of thrombocytopenia, patients are transited to an oral agent. For detail about this transition, refer to Chap. 12.

Treatment of VTE in Pregnancy

- Pregnant women diagnosed with a VTE should be treated with full dose LMWH for the remainder of their pregnancy. Please refer to Chap. 6 on VTE and pregnancy.
- Patients should complete at least 6 months of anticoagulation including treatment throughout pregnancy and 6 weeks postpartum.
- Warfarin is contraindicated during the first trimester of pregnancy because of the risk of teratogenicity.
- Anticoagulation postpartum can be either warfarin or LMWH, as neither is excreted in breast milk, and both are safe for the newborn.

Thrombosis in Antiphospholipid Syndrome (APS)

All venous and arterial thrombotic events in the setting of a lupus anticoagulant or an anticardiolipin antibody should be treated with lifelong warfarin therapy. For more details, please refer to Chap. 8 on APS.

- INR should be maintained between 2.0 and 3.0.

Extremes of Body Weight

- Limited data are available on dosing of the LMWHs in morbidly obese patients, especially those who weigh >150 kg or < 45 kg (Fig. 2.10).
- Consider periodic monitoring of anti-factor Xa activity during treatment with LMWHs.
- In patients with BMI <40 or weight < 120 kg , use DOAC as standard doses, and consider VKA above these ranges [48].

Body weight	Preparation/dose	Monitoring	Target level
Actual body weight >150 kg	UH as per VTE protocol	PTT	×2–2.5 baseline PTT
	Enoxaparin 1 mg/kg SC q12h Use adjusted body weight[a] Minimum initial dose is 150 mg SC q12h. Do not use single-daily dosing regimen	An anti-Xa level should be obtained 4 hours after the 1st or 2nd dose	Titrate dose to maintain an anti -Xa level of 0.5–1 units/mL
	Tinzaparin 175 IU/kg SC if BMI > 40 kg/m2		Titrate dose to maintain an anti -Xa level of 0.5–1 units/mL
	Dalteparin 200 IU/kg SC q24h		Titrate dose to maintain an anti -Xa level of 1–2 units/mL
Actual body weight <45 kg	UH	PTT	x 2–2.5 baseline PTT
	Enoxaparin 1.5 mg/kg SC q24h actual body weight	anti-Xa level should be obtained 4 hours after the 3rd AM dose	Titrate dosage to maintain an anti-Xa level of 1–1.5 units/mL
	Tinzaparin 175 IU/kg SC q24h actual weight		Titrate dose to maintain an anti -Xa level of 0.5–1 units/mL
	Dalteparin 200 IU/kg SC q24h actual body weight		Titrate dose to maintain an anti -Xa level of 1–2 units/mL
Ideal BW for men, 50 kg + 2.3 kg (height in cm − 152.4)/2.54; women, 45.5 kg + 2.3 kg (height in cm − 152.4)/2.54 [a]Adjusted body weight = Ideal BW + 0.4 (Actual BW − Ideal BW)			

Fig. 2.10 Dosing and monitoring guidelines for treatment of VTE in patients with extremes of body weight [49]

Patients with Renal Insufficiency

- Anticoagulant therapy in the renal patient is complicated by an increased hemorrhagic risk due to the qualitative platelet defect associated with uremia. For more details, please refer to Chap. 9 – Anticoagulation in renal patients.
- Many anticoagulants are cleared by the kidneys, including the LMWHs and DOAC, danaparoid, hirudin, and bivalirudin, and all these agents need to be dose-adjusted and monitored very closely in these patients (if used at all).
- Despite high-bleeding risks and lack of high-quality evidence in this population, warfarin is still recommended for VTE treatment as it can be quickly and effectively reversed in this high-bleeding risk group.
- Bridging with UFH in patients with severe kidney disease is commonly used not because of lower bleeding risk, but rather due to short therapeutic half-life and reversibility with protamine.
- Due to the accumulation of LMWH in severe renal dysfunction, caution is required when dosing in renal impairment. If required a dose reduction and monitoring of anti-factor Xa levels may be useful (Fig. 2.11).
- NOACs are not typically recommended below <30–15 mL/min (see Fig. 2.12).

The Thrombocytopenic Patient

When deciding to anticoagulate in the setting of thrombocytopenia, clinicians must considered the clinical context, the presence of additional risk factors, and the consequences of thrombosis and bleeding.

Consider the following when anticoagulation is used in the setting of thrombocytopenia:

1. A low platelet count is not protective from thrombosis.
2. In general, thrombotic complications are more dangerous than bleeding complications.
3. Not all etiologies of thrombocytopenia have the same bleeding risk, i.e., ITP versus chemotherapy-related thrombocytosis.

   - The greatest risk of recurrent thrombosis is seen in the first 3 months following thrombosis. During this time frame, every attempt should be made to provide safe anticoagulation.
   - Current practice is to modify treatment based on the severity of thrombocytopaenia which must be monitored closely.
   - LMWH is most often used, and a number of guidelines support reduced dosing based on the platelet count (see Fig. 2.13) [54, 55].
   - Intravenous unfractionated heparin can also be considered in patients with PE or extensive thrombosis.

Initial anti-Xa test	
Pre-dose level (trough) 2–4 hours post-dose (peak)	Before and after the third dose
Subsequent monitoring once in therapeutic range	Twice a week (peak and trough)
Target anti-Xa level	Pre-dose level (trough) < 0.1–0.3 IU/mL[a] 2–4 hours post-dose (peak)0.5–1 IU/mL[a]
[a]Anti-Xa levels out of range should be discussed with a hematologist	

Fig. 2.11 Monitoring of anti-Xa levels with LMWH in renal impairment[50]

	Rivaroxaban [51]	Apixaban [52]	Dabigatran [53]
Half-life (h)	5–13	12	12–14 (27 in CKD4/5)
Renal clearance (%)	33	27	85
Approved for CrCl[a] <30 mL/min	Yes	Yes	No
CrCl[a] 15–29 mL/min	Reduce dose 15 mg daily	Reduce dose 2.5 mg twice daily	
CrCl[a]<15 mL/min	No	No	
[a]As determined by the Cockcroft and Gault' formula for dosing and monitoring			

Fig. 2.12 NOAC in renal failure

Fig. 2.13 Dose reduction of anticoagulation by platelet count

Platelet count	Treatment options
>50 × 10^9	Full-dose therapeutic anticoagulation [57, 58]
25–50 × 10^9	50% dose of LMWH [54, 59]
<25 × 10^9	No anticoagulation [54, 56]

- The use of supportive platelet transfusion to allow for full-dose anticoagulation once the platelet count is greater than 50×10^9/L may also be utilized in the proper clinical context [56].

Patients with Hepatic Insufficiency

- Data on the safety, efficacy, and monitoring of full-dose anticoagulation therapy in VTE in patients with cirrhosis is limited.
- Warfarin is difficult to manage, and the risk of a significant hemorrhagic complication is high as the INR may already be elevated before warfarin use.
- The INR is not well studied in liver disease, with small studies suggesting that the standard range of 2.0–3.0 is achievable [60].
- Use of DOAC is too limited to provide specific advice.

Appendix A

	Dosing	Dosing	Daily cost (80 kg) CDN ($)	First 30-days CDN ($)
LMWH	Enoxaparin	Subcutaneous: 1 mg/kg twice daily or 1.5 mg/kg once daily	26.47	825.50
	Dalteparin	Subcutaneous: 200 U/kg once daily	38.97	1200.50
	Tinzaparin	Subcutaneous: 175 U/kg once daily	28.68	891.80
Vitamin K antagonist	Warfarin	Mandatory concurrent: LMWH or UFH With Oral: Initial dosing typically 5 mg once daily titrated for a goal of INR 2–3	29.81 (days 1–7) then $0.07	214.11
DOAC (anti-Xa)	Rivaroxaban	Oral: 15 mg twice daily for 21 days and then 20 mg once daily	5.74 (days 1–21) then $2.87	173.58
	Apixaban	Oral: 10 mg twice daily for 7 days followed by 5 mg twice daily	6.53 (days 1–7) then $3.27	148.13
DOAC (direct thrombin inhibitor)	Dabigatran	150 mg twice daily after minimum 5 days of LMWH	29.81 (days 1–7) then $3.34	316.89

Taken from the Saskatchewan Drug Plan, http://formulary.drugplan.ehealthsask.ca/Search Formulary, 2018
Note: 30-day pricing include pharmacy mark up (max $20) and a dispensing fee $11.40

References

1. Khilnani NM, et al. Multi-society consensus quality improvement guidelines for the treatment of lower-extremity superficial venous insufficiency with endovenous thermal ablation from the Society of Interventional Radiology, Cardiovascular Interventional Radiological Society of Europe, American College of Phlebology and Canadian Interventional Radiology Association. J Vasc Interv Radiol. 2010;21(1):14–31.
2. Silverstein MD, et al. Trends in the incidence of deep vein thrombosis and pulmonary embolism: a 25-year population-based study. Arch Intern Med. 1998;158(6):585–93.
3. Heit JA, et al. Predictors of survival after deep vein thrombosis and pulmonary embolism: a population-based, cohort study. Arch Intern Med. 1999;159(5):445–53.
4. Mohr DN, et al. The venous stasis syndrome after deep venous thrombosis or pulmonary embolism: a population-based study. Mayo Clin Proc. 2000;75(12):1249–56.
5. Kearon C, et al. Antithrombotic therapy for VTE disease: CHEST guideline and expert panel report. Chest. 2016;149(2):315–52.
6. Di Nisio M, van Es N, Buller HR. Deep vein thrombosis and pulmonary embolism. Lancet. 2016;388(10063):3060–73.
7. Heit JA. Epidemiology of venous thromboembolism. Nat Rev Cardiol. 2015;12(8):464–74.
8. Crowther M. Warfarin: less may be better. Ann Intern Med. 1997;127(4):332; author reply 333.
9. National Clinical Guideline, C. National Institute for Health and Clinical excellence: guidance. In: Venous thromboembolic diseases: the management of venous thromboembolic diseases and the role of thrombophilia testing. London: Royal College of Physicians (UK) National Clinical Guideline Centre; 2012.
10. Konstantinides SV, et al. 2014 ESC guidelines on the diagnosis and management of acute pulmonary embolism. Eur Heart J. 2014;35(43):3033–69, 3069a-3069k.
11. Canada T. Clinical guidelines. Available from: http://thrombosiscanada.ca/clinicalguides/.
12. Boutitie F, et al. Influence of preceding length of anticoagulant treatment and initial presentation of venous thromboembolism on risk of recurrence after stopping treatment: analysis of individual participants' data from seven trials. BMJ. 2011;342:d3036.
13. Carrier M, et al. Systematic review: case-fatality rates of recurrent venous thromboembolism and major bleeding events among patients treated for venous thromboembolism. Ann Intern Med. 2010;152(9):578–89.
14. Castellucci LA, et al. Efficacy and safety outcomes of oral anticoagulants and antiplatelet drugs in the secondary prevention of venous thromboembolism: systematic review and network meta-analysis. BMJ. 2013;347:f5133.
15. Kearon C, Iorio A, Palareti G. Risk of recurrent venous thromboembolism after stopping treatment in cohort studies: recommendation for acceptable rates and standardized reporting. J Thromb Haemost. 2010;8(10):2313–5.
16. Iorio A, et al. Risk of recurrence after a first episode of symptomatic venous thromboembolism provoked by a transient risk factor: a systematic review. Arch Intern Med. 2010;170(19):1710–6.
17. Prandoni P, et al. The risk of recurrent venous thromboembolism after discontinuing anticoagulation in patients with acute proximal deep vein thrombosis or pulmonary embolism. A prospective cohort study in 1,626 patients. Haematologica. 2007;92(2):199–205.
18. Prandoni P, et al. The long-term clinical course of acute deep venous thrombosis. Ann Intern Med. 1996;125(1):1–7.
19. Palareti G, et al. A comparison of the safety and efficacy of oral anticoagulation for the treatment of venous thromboembolic disease in patients with or without malignancy. Thromb Haemost. 2000;84(5):805–10.
20. Investigators E, et al. Oral rivaroxaban for symptomatic venous thromboembolism. N Engl J Med. 2010;363(26):2499–510.
21. Agnelli G, et al. Apixaban for extended treatment of venous thromboembolism. N Engl J Med. 2013;368(8):699–708.
22. Schulman S, et al. Extended use of dabigatran, warfarin, or placebo in venous thromboembolism. N Engl J Med. 2013;368(8):709–18.

23. Becattini C, et al. Aspirin for preventing the recurrence of venous thromboembolism. N Engl J Med. 2012;366(21):1959–67.
24. Brighton TA, et al. Low-dose aspirin for preventing recurrent venous thromboembolism. N Engl J Med. 2012;367(21):1979–87.
25. Canada T. Clinical guidelines superficial thrombophlebitis, superficial vein thrombosis. Available from: http://thrombosiscanada.ca/clinicalguides/.
26. Verso M, Agnelli G. Venous thromboembolism associated with long-term use of central venous catheters in cancer patients. J Clin Oncol. 2003;21(19):3665–75.
27. Buller HR, et al. Antithrombotic therapy for venous thromboembolic disease: the seventh ACCP conference on antithrombotic and thrombolytic therapy. Chest. 2004;126(3 Suppl):401S–28S.
28. Joels CS, Sing RF, Heniford BT. Complications of inferior vena cava filters. Am Surg. 2003;69(8):654–9.
29. Kaufman JA, et al. Development of a research agenda for inferior vena cava filters: proceedings from a multidisciplinary research consensus panel. J Vasc Interv Radiol. 2009;20(6):697–707.
30. Morales JP, et al. Decision analysis of retrievable inferior vena cava filters in patients without pulmonary embolism. J Vasc Surg Venous Lymphat Disord. 2013;1(4):376–84.
31. Jacoby WT, et al. Ovarian vein thrombosis in oncology patients: CT detection and clinical significance. AJR Am J Roentgenol. 1990;155(2):291–4.
32. Harris K, et al. Ovarian vein thrombosis in the nonpregnant woman: an overlooked diagnosis. Ther Adv Hematol. 2012;3(5):325–8.
33. Wysokinska EM, Hodge D, McBane RD 2nd. Ovarian vein thrombosis: incidence of recurrent venous thromboembolism and survival. Thromb Haemost. 2006;96(2):126–31.
34. Piazza G. Cerebral venous thrombosis. Circulation. 2012;125(13):1704–9.
35. Saposnik G, et al. Diagnosis and management of cerebral venous thrombosis: a statement for healthcare professionals from the American Heart Association/American Stroke Association. Stroke. 2011;42(4):1158–92.
36. Einhaupl K, et al. EFNS guideline on the treatment of cerebral venous and sinus thrombosis in adult patients. Eur J Neurol. 2010;17(10):1229–35.
37. Cundiff DK. Anticoagulants for cerebral venous thrombosis: harmful to patients? Stroke. 2014;45(1):298–304.
38. Schmitt BP, Adelman B. Heparin-associated thrombocytopenia: a critical review and pooled analysis. Am J Med Sci. 1993;305(4):208–15.
39. Arepally G, Cines DB. Heparin-induced thrombocytopenia and thrombosis. Clin Rev Allergy Immunol. 1998;16(3):237–47.
40. Warkentin TE. Heparin-induced thrombocytopenia: a ten-year retrospective. Annu Rev Med. 1999;50:129–47.
41. Smythe MA, Koerber JM, Mattson JC. The incidence of recognized heparin-induced thrombocytopenia in a large, tertiary care teaching hospital. Chest. 2007;131(6):1644–9.
42. Warkentin TE, Eikelboom JW. Who is (still) getting HIT? Chest. 2007;131(6):1620–2.
43. Warkentin TE, Kelton JG. A 14-year study of heparin-induced thrombocytopenia. Am J Med. 1996;101(5):502–7.
44. Boshkov LK, et al. Heparin-induced thrombocytopenia and thrombosis: clinical and laboratory studies. Br J Haematol. 1993;84(2):322–8.
45. Nand S, et al. Heparin-induced thrombocytopenia with thrombosis: incidence, analysis of risk factors, and clinical outcomes in 108 consecutive patients treated at a single institution. Am J Hematol. 1997;56(1):12–6.
46. Warkentin TE, et al. Heparin-induced thrombocytopenia in medical surgical critical illness. Chest. 2013;144(3):848–58.
47. Pishko AM. Diagnosis and management of Heparin-Induced Thrombocytopenia (HIT) A POCKET GUIDE FOR THE CLINICIAN DECEMBER 2018. 2018: p. 3.
48. Martin K, et al. Use of the direct oral anticoagulants in obese patients: guidance from the SSC of the ISTH. J Thromb Haemost. 2016;14(6):1308–13.
49. Mackay R. Practice guidelines for the management and prophylaxis of thrombosis in cancer patients 2013[cited 2018].

50. Hughes S, et al. Anticoagulation in chronic kidney disease patients-the practical aspects. Clin Kidney J. 2014;7(5):442–9.
51. Bayer. Summary of product characteristics—Xarelto (Rivaroxaban) 2019 29 Aug 2018 [cited 2019; Available from: https://www.medicines.org.uk/emc/medicine/21265/SPC.
52. Squibb-Pfizer B-M. Summary of product characteristics—Eliquis (Apixiban) 19 Mar 2019]; Available from: https://www.medicines.org.uk/emc/medicine/27220/SPC.
53. Limited BI. Summary of product characteristics—Pradaxa (Dagibatran) 09 Jul 2018 2019]; Available from: https://www.medicines.org.uk/emc/medicine/20760/SPC.
54. Mantha S, et al. Enoxaparin dose reduction for thrombocytopenia in patients with cancer: a quality assessment study. J Thromb Thrombolysis. 2017;43(4):514–8.
55. Wall C, Moore J, Thachil J. Catheter-related thrombosis: a practical approach. J Intensive Care Soc. 2016;17(2):160–7.
56. Watson HG, et al. Guideline on aspects of cancer-related venous thrombosis. Br J Haematol. 2015;170(5):640–8.
57. Bishop L, et al. Guidelines on the insertion and management of central venous access devices in adults. Int J Lab Hematol. 2007;29(4):261–78.
58. Baglin T, et al. Guidelines on the use and monitoring of heparin. Br J Haematol. 2006;133(1):19–34.
59. Murray J, Precious E, Alikhan R. Catheter-related thrombosis in cancer patients. Br J Haematol. 2013;162(6):748–57.
60. Tripodi A, et al. Coagulation parameters in patients with cirrhosis and portal vein thrombosis treated sequentially with low molecular weight heparin and vitamin K antagonists. Dig Liver Dis. 2016;48(10):1208–13.

Chapter 3
Anticoagulation in Cardiac Patients

**Haissam Haddad, Udoka Okpalauwaekwe, Nishant Sharma,
Jay S. Shavadia, Alex Zhai, and Tony Haddad**

Abbreviations

ACC	American College of Cardiologists
ACCP	American College of Chest Physicians
AHA	American Heart Association
AF	Atrial fibrillation
ASA	Acetylsalicylic acid
AVR	Aortic valve replacement
BHV	Bioprosthetic heart valve
BMS	Bare metal stent
CAD	Coronary artery disease
CCS	Canadian Cardiovascular Society
CHADS	Scoring system for atrial fibrillation

H. Haddad (✉)
Department of Medicine, Division of Cardiology, University of Saskatchewan,
Saskatoon, SK, Canada
e-mail: haissam.haddad@usask.ca

U. Okpalauwaekwe · N. Sharma · J. S. Shavadia
Division of Cardiology, College of Medicine, University of Saskatchewan,
Saskatoon, SK, Canada
e-mail: Udok.Okpalauwaekwe@usask.ca; Nishant.Sharma@usask.ca;
Jay.Shavadia@mail.usask.ca

A. Zhai
Division of Cardiology, Department of Medicine, University of Saskatchewan,
Saskatoon, SK, Canada
e-mail: Alex.zhai@mail.usask.ca

T. Haddad
Department of Medicine, College of Medicine, University of Saskatchewan,
Saskatoon, SK, Canada
e-mail: Tony.haddad@usask.ca

© Springer Nature Switzerland AG 2020
H. Goubran et al. (eds.), *Precision Anticoagulation Medicine*,
https://doi.org/10.1007/978-3-030-25782-8_3

CHF	Congestive heart failure
DES	Drug-eluting stent
EF	Ejection fraction
ESC	European Society of Cardiology
HFpEF	Heart failure with preserved ejection fraction
HFrEF	Heart failure with reduced ejection fraction
LVEF	Left ventricular ejection fraction
MHVs	Mechanical heart valves
MVR	Mitral valve replacement
MVRep	Mitral valve repair
NOACs	Non-vitamin K antagonist (VKA) oral anticoagulants
NVAF	Nonvalvular atrial fibrillation
OACs	Oral anticoagulants
PCI	Percutaneous coronary intervention
ST	Stent thrombosis
STEMI	ST-segment elevation myocardial infarction
STS	Society of Thoracic Surgeons
TAVR	Transcatheter aortic valve replacement
TE	Thromboembolism
TIA	Transient ischemic attack
VAF	Valvular atrial fibrillation
VHD	Valvular heart disease
VKA	Vitamin K antagonist

Introduction
Haissam Haddad

It is very important to take into consideration the individualized approach to maximize the benefit and minimize the risk.

In this chapter, we tried to cover anticoagulation use in three major cardiac conditions: atrial fibrillation in heart failure, atrial fibrillation in patients with valvular disease and in patients who are on antithrombotic therapy undergoing percutaneous coronary interventions.

Anticoagulation in Patients with Atrial Fibrillation and Artificial Valves: Translating International Guidelines for Clinical Practice
Haissam Haddad and Udoka Okpalauwaekwe

Introduction

Valvular heart disease (VHD) has a significant impact on the global population, affecting more than 100 million people globally [1, 2]. The use of artificial valves in managing VHD is on the rise globally, with figures estimated to fall between

300,000 and 370,000 surgical repairs annually [1, 3]. In North America alone, it is estimated that about 100,000 patients have valve replacement surgeries annually [2]. There are commercially three types of artificial valves or prostheses used in managing VHD, which are mechanical valves, bioprosthetic valves, and the transcatheter valves for endovascular transplantation [1, 2, 4].

A major life-threatening complicative risk in patients with artificial heart valves is thromboembolism that necessitates the need for anticoagulation [1–4]. Thromboembolic phenomena in patients with artificial heart valves vary in the degree of risks depending on the type of prostheses used in managing the valvular heart disease and the position of the prosthetic implant [2, 3]. Mechanical heart valves (MHVs) have been shown to be more thrombogenic than bioprosthetic heart valves (BHVs); and within each prostheses type lies variability in terms of risk for thromboembolism [2, 3]. Basically, there are three types of mechanical valves: caged-ball, tilting disk, and bileaflet valves. These various types of MHVs exhibit individual thrombogenicities which are related to the nature of materials used and their respective engineering design. As such, the caged ball is the most thrombogenic, followed by the tilting disk and then the bileaflet MHV type [2, 3]. Furthermore, the risk of thrombosis in patients with MHV is directly related to the valve position. For example, valves placed in the mitral position have been shown to have more risk for thromboembolism compared with artificial valves positioned in the aortic side [2]. On the other hand, BHVs are heterografts, with more natural hemodynamic properties, and made from porcine or bovine tissues, each with its own relative risks for thromboembolic phenomena [2, 3]. Globally, MHVs are more commonly used (55%) than BHVs (45%) [7].

A common occurrence in patients with VHD is atrial fibrillation (AF). AF in the patients with VHD is typically categorized into valvular AF (VAF), contrasted from nonvalvular AF (NVAF) [5–7]. NVAF is defined as AF in the absence of mechanical heart valves, rheumatic mitral stenosis or moderate to severe non-rheumatic mitral stenosis, while VAF is the reverse [6]. VAF is considered a life-threatening complicative factor for arterial embolization especially in patients with artificial heart valves.

Anticoagulation therapy for patients with artificial heart valves should take into consideration several factors in balancing the risk over the benefits for the patients' presenting conditions. Traditionally, vitamin K antagonists (VKAs) are the principal category of anticoagulants used and proven to be effective in preventing complications in patients with prosthetic heart valves (especially in the case of MHVs) [1, 2, 8, 9]. According to cardiovascular society guidelines by the AHA/ACC/ACCP, ESC, and CCS, postoperative anticoagulation with VKAs for a short period (3–6 months) is reasonably safe to prevent thromboembolism in patients with artificial heart valves [7, 10–14]. However, there are a few areas of obscurity and uncertainty in defining the guidelines for antithrombotic therapy in preventing artificial heart valve thrombotic phenomena in a setting of comorbid AF. The increasing use of non-vitamin K antagonist oral anticoagulants (NOACs) has also been implicated in this dilemma, raising questions on safety, clinical relevance, and optimality [1, 2].

Guidelines for anticoagulation therapy have been recommended by major cardiovascular societies such as the Canadian Cardiovascular Society (CCS), the American College of Cardiology (ACC), the American Heart Association (AHA), the Heart Rhythm Society (HRS), the American College of Chest Physicians (ACCP), and the European Society of Cardiology (ESC). These guidelines provide recommendations based on the optimal balance of thrombotic and hemorrhagic risk. We intend to compare, contrast, and provide recommendations based on these guidelines for optimal balance of associated risks in patients with AF and artificial heart valves.

Guiding Principles for Anticoagulation Management in Patients with Artificial Heart Valves

Risk Assessment and Stratification

One of the most crucial guiding principles recommended by most if not all the major cardiovascular societies in the anticoagulation management of patients with artificial heart valves is an estimation of the individual risk of bleeding and thromboembolic phenomena. A noteworthy rule of thumb is to recall that MHVs are highly thrombogenic and hence require lifelong commitment to anticoagulant therapy compared to BHVs. Each artificial heart valve has its own unique thrombogenic profile.

Several risk scores developed by major cardiovascular societies have been used to predict the possibility for risk of bleeding. They include some of the following: the $CHADS_2 65$ developed and used by the CCS; the CHA_2DS_2-VASc used by the ACC/AHA/HRS; and the modified CHA_2DS_2-VASc used by the ESC (see Figs. 3.1 and 3.2) [6, 14]. These risk estimation algorithms were developed to help predict bleeding events, most of which were also developed to assess risk in

	AHA/ACC/HRS	CCS	ESC
	CHA_2DS_2-VASc	$CHADS_2 65$	Modified CHA_2DS_2-VASc
Congestive heart failure	1	1	1
Hypertension	1	1	1
Age ≥75 years	2	1[a]	2
Diabetes mellitus	1	1	1
Stroke, TIA, or systemic embolism	2	1	2
Vascular disease (peripheral or coronary)	1	N/A	1
Age 65–74 years	1	1	1
Sex category (female)	1	N/A	1[b]

ACC American College of Cardiology, AHA American Heart Association, CCS Canadian Cardiovascular Society, CHADS$_2$65 indicates congestive heart failure, hypertension, age ≥65 years, diabetes mellitus, prior stroke, or transient ischaemic attack (TIA); CHA$_2$DS$_2$-VASc indicates congestive heart failure, hypertension, age ≥75 years (assigned score of 2), diabetes mellitus, prior stroke or transient ischemic attack (TIA) or thromboembolism (assigned score of 2), vascular disease, age 65–74 years, sex category; ESC European Society of Cardiology, HRS Heart Rhythm Society, N/A not applicable
[a]Included as part of age >65 years
[b]Not counted in the absence of other risk factors

Fig. 3.1 Risk prediction algorithm by society guidelines

Stroke risk score	CCS	ACC/AHA/HRS	ESC
0	No anticoagulants (conditional recommendation)	No anticoagulants (class IIa)	No anticoagulants (class III)
1	OAC (strong recommendation)	OAC or ASA or no anticoagulants (class IIb)	OAC for men (IIa)
≥ 2	OAC (strong recommendation)	OAC (class I)	OAC for men and women (class I)

ASA Aspirin, CCS Canadian Cardiovascular Society, ACC American College of Cardiology, AHA American Heart Association, HRS Heart Rhythm Society, ESC European Society of Cardiology, OAC oral anticoagulant

Fig. 3.2 Summary of anticoagulation recommendations based on risk scores [6]

patients with AF. The AHA/ACC/HRS guidelines for anticoagulation management in AF patients used the CHA_2DS_2-VASc [6, 11], which was first adopted by the ESC but later modified to emphasize the female sex category as a stronger independent risk factor for assessing the risk of bleeding or stroke [6, 12]. The CCS, on the other hand, did not consider the female sex or vascular disease as indications for anticoagulation therapy; rather, it retained the original $CHADS_2$ algorithmic framework, lowering the age criterion to 65 years (hence the new acronym, $CHADS_2$65) [7, 15]. The justification given for this change was based on a Danish national cohort study [16], where patients followed up for 10 years at ages ≥65 years were shown to be the third strongest predictor of stroke, although other empirical evidence still showed that the risk of bleeding or stroke steadily increased in patients >75 years [2, 6].

With regards to risk stratification, several major society guidelines categorize patients with artificial heart valves according to their risk of developing thromboembolic phenomena. According to the ACCP guidelines [17], high-risk patients for thromboembolism include those with mitral valve prostheses, patients with caged-ball or single-disk aortic valve prostheses, or patients with a history of stroke/TIA within the previous 6 months. Moderate-risk patients for thromboembolism include patients with a bileaflet aortic valve with any of the following: AF, previous stroke/TIA, and other risk factors for stroke (i.e., hypertension, diabetes, CHF, or age >75 years). Low-risk patients for thromboembolism are those with bileaflet aortic valves and no other risk factor for stroke [17]. According to the ACC/AHA guidelines, risk stratification is based on risk factors for a thromboembolic event that include AF, previous thromboembolism, left ventricular systolic dysfunction <35%, and any hypercoagulable condition [10, 11]. The ESC guidelines risk stratification for patients with artificial heart valves considers patients with mechanical valves in the mitral position as having higher risk for thromboembolism regardless of valve type [12]. Another high-risk factor considered under the ESC guidelines includes the presence of one of the following: previous thromboembolism, AF, left atrial diameter > 50 mm, left atrial dense spontaneous echo contrast, mitral stenosis of any degree, left ventricular ejection fraction (LVEF) < 35%, and any hypercoagulable state [12].

Valve type	Target INR			
	Aortic position		Mitral position	
	Uncomplicated/ without risk factors	With risk factors[a]	Uncomplicated/ without risk factors	With risk factors[a]
Mechanical HVs[b]				
Bileaflet	2.0–3.0	2.5–3.5	2.5–3.5	2.5–3.5
Tilting discs	2.0–3.0	2.5–3.5	2.5–3.5	2.5–3.5
Caged ball	2.5–3.5	2.5–3.5	2.5–3.5	2.5–3.5
Caged-disc valve	2.5–3.5	2.5–3.5	2.5–3.5	2.5–3.5
Bioprosthetic HVs[c]				
Xenografts	2.0–3.0	2.0–3.0	2.0–3.0	2.0–3.0

[a]Risk factors include AF, previous thromboembolism, LV dysfunction, or hypercoagulable conditions
[b]ACC recommends VKA plus aspirin (75–100 mg) (class I), ACCP recommends aspirin (50–100 mg) only in high-risk patients
[c]ACC recommends VKA for 3 months except in uncomplicated aortic valve replacement. ACCP recommends aspirin over VKA which should be continued if there is no other indication of anticoagulation. Postoperatively, ACC recommends aspirin (80–100 mg), while ACCP recommends aspirin 3 months after replacement

Fig. 3.3 Target INR values for patients with artificial valves on VKAs according to international guidelines [1]

Anticoagulation Intensity Goal

Anticoagulation intensity is measured using the international normalized ratio (INR). The INR recommended by major cardiovascular societies to achieve an optimal risk-benefit ratio between bleeding and thrombosis is targeted at an INR between 2.0 and 3.5. This range also varies with artificial heart valve type, associated risks, and presence or absence of complications (see Fig. 3.3).

Anticoagulation Timing

Although there are dissimilar views addressing this issue on anticoagulation timing, all major guidelines recommend commencing anticoagulation therapy in the first 24–48 hours after artificial valvular surgery for MHVs and for the first 3 months following implantation for BHVs. However, some major society guidelines tend to differ in certain conditions where aspirin may be used as an alternative to VKA or used in combination with clopidogrel or other forms of VKAs besides warfarin (see Fig. 3.4).

Society	Recommendations
Anticoagulation therapy in mechanical heart valves	
ACC/ AHA	Anticoagulation with VKA (INR of 2.5 for AVR with no risk factors for TE; INR of 3.0 for AVR with risk factors for TE or MVR) plus aspirin 75–100 mg daily (class I)
ACCP	(i) VKA (INR of 2.5 for AVR and 3.0 for MVR) indicated; no VKA for long-term management (Grade 1B) (ii) Aspirin 50–100 mg indicated in patients at low risk of bleeding (Grade 1B)
ESC	(i) Anticoagulation with VKA (target INR according to prosthesis thrombogenicity and patient-related risk factors (class I)) (ii) Aspirin ≤100 mg daily if concomitant atherosclerotic disease and/or TE despite adequate INR (class IIa)
Anticoagulation therapy in bioprosthetic heart valves	
ACC/ AHA	Anticoagulation with VKA (INR of 2.5) plus aspirin 75–100 mg for the first 3 months followed by aspirin 75–100 mg daily alone (class IIa/IIb)
ACCP	(i) Aspirin 50–100 mg indicated in the first 3 months (Grade 2C) (ii) Aspirin 50–100 mg indicated over VKA and over no APT for the first 3 months after AVR in patients in sinus rhythm (Grade 2C) (iii) VKA (INR of 2.5) indicated over no VKA for the first 3 months after MVR (Grade 2C)
ESC	(i) Anticoagulation with VKA for the first 3 months after MVR, MVRep, or TVR (class IIa) (ii) Anticoagulation with VKA for the first 3 months after AVR (class IIb) (iii) Aspirin ≤100 mg daily for the first 3 months after AVR (class IIa)
Anticoagulation therapy in TAVR	
CCS	Indefinite low-dose aspirin plus thienopyridine for 1–3 months. No clopidogrel if warfarin is indicated
ACC/ AHA	Clopidogrel 75 mg plus aspirin 75–100 mg for 6 months followed by aspirin 75–100 mg daily alone (class IIb)
ACCP	Aspirin 50–100 mg plus clopidogrel 75 mg/dl indicated over VKA and over no APT for the first 3 months (Grade 2C)
ACC/ STS	Aspirin 81 mg/day for indefinite period plus clopidogrel 75 mg/day for 3–6 months. Avoid triple therapy unless definite indication exists.

ACC American College of Cardiology, *ACCP* American College of Chest Physicians, *AHA* American Heart Association, *APT* antiplatelet therapy, *AVR* aortic valve replacement, *CCS* Canadian Cardiovascular Society, *ESC* European Society of Cardiology, *INR* international normalized ratio, *MVR* mitral valve replacement, *MVRep* mitral valve repair, *STS* Society of Thoracic Surgeons, *TAVR* transcatheter aortic valve replacement, *TE* thromboembolism, *TVR* target vessel revascularization, *VKA* vitamin K antagonist

Fig. 3.4 Anticoagulation therapy in artificial valves

Bridging Therapy

This refers to a short-term interruption of anticoagulation therapy in at-risk patients for clinical or surgical reasons. The use of bridging therapy is commonly considered in patients with high risk for thromboembolic phenomena. Based on guideline recommendations, there seems to be no common consensus on the estimated risk of thromboembolism, which could guide informed decision making in clinical practice. However, a consensual recommendation by major cardiovascular societies is to consider the need to use unfractionated heparin (UFH) or low-molecular-weight heparin (LMWH) in patients with artificial heart valves if VKA is interrupted [7, 11, 12, 14].

Anticoagulation Therapy in Artificial Valves

VKA remains the standard of anticoagulation care for patients carrying artificial heart valves [3, 7, 8, 11, 12, 14]. Warfarin is a common VKA used internationally with others like phenprocoumon, fluindione, and acenocoumarol commonly used in Europe and South America, with differences among these drugs based on their half-life (acenocoumarol having the shortest and phenprocoumon having the longest half-life). Few studies have shown warfarin to be better than acenocoumarol in preventing extreme anticoagulation, while phenprocoumon has been shown to produce preferably better international normalized ratio (INR) stabilities and fewer bleeding episodes compared to warfarin and acenocoumarol [4]. However, largely, VKAs work by inhibiting vitamin-K-dependent gamma-carboxylation of coagulation factors II, VII, IX, and X. A thumbnail summary based on society guidelines is described in the following sub-paragraphs.

Mechanical, Bioprosthetic, and Endovascular Heart Valves Anticoagulation Therapy

Because patients with MHVs are at higher risk for thromboembolism, VKAs are recommended by major guidelines for use in anticoagulation care. For patients with MHVs and presence of an additional risk factor, including aspirin has been proven to confer greater clinical benefits [7, 14]. The inclusion of aspirin has also been shown to produce clinical benefits in patients with BHVs in the mitral position who later develop AF. Patients with BHVs, however, are seldom treated with systemic anticoagulants for a short period following valve transplantation. For transcatheter valves placed endovascularly, current guideline recommendations from major cardiovascular societies suggest the use of anticoagulant pretreatment and during treatment in combination of lifelong aspirin (75–100 mg) daily and clopidogrel 75 mg daily for 3–6 months [1, 3]. AHA/ACC and ESC guidelines for BHVs recommend anticoagulation with VKA during the first 3 months post-artificial heart surgery [11]. ACCP guidelines recommend anticoagulation with VKAs for BHVs when the implant is done in the mitral position [17]. This recommendation is considered weak as it is based on dated reports.

Besides recent studies reveal that physicians can achieve beneficial results post BHV implantation with APT instead of VKAs [18]. Thus, the bone of contention among clinicians, and a point of disagreement with guidelines with regard to anticoagulation therapy with BHVs, lies on whether or not anticoagulation is necessary in early postoperative period. See Fig. 3.4 for summary on international guidelines. Dosage recommendations for VKAs by international guidelines have also been debatable due to response variability in patients from several studies. Hence, there are considered no universal dosage recommendations, but rather tailoring antithrombotic therapy to each patient's INR monitoring [7, 14] (see Fig. 3.3).

Concomitant Atrial Fibrillation Anticoagulation Therapy

VAF in the setting of artificial heart valves is considered a life-threatening risk factor for arterial embolism. For patient with MHVs and the prensence of other risk factors, Apirin 75–100mg is recommended. This management strategy is supported by almost all major society guidelines (CCS, ACC/AHA/HRS, ACCP, and ESC). Addition of aspirin to VKA therapy is also shown to be beneficial for patients with BHVs in the mitral position who develop AF, reducing risk of stroke, and mortality. It is vital to note that the concurrence of AF in patients with artificial valves (especially with BHVs) is an indication for chronic VKA use [7, 11, 12]. See Fig. 3.4.

Antithrombotic Therapy in Patients with Artificial Valve Thrombosis

Artificial valve thrombosis is a common and fatal complication directly associated with artificial valve implantation. Its degree of severity varies with the type of valve and its position in the heart. Managing artificial valve thrombosis is considered an emergency as there are limited clinical trials addressing this condition. Management recommendations remain controversial bordering around thrombolytic therapy or surgical interventions. ACC/AHA guidelines recommend early surgical intervention for patients with thrombosed left-sided artificial valves and New York heart association (NYHA) functional class III/IV symptoms [10, 11]. According to ACC/AHA, thrombolytic therapy should be considered for patients in whom surgery carries a high risk or for whom surgery is absolutely contraindicated [10, 11]. For patients with small artificial heart valve clot burden who are NYHA functional class I or II, treatment with short-term intravenous UFH or continuous infusion of fibrinolytic therapy may be beneficial. Patients who have right-sided artificial heart valves with large clot burden and who are NYHA class III/IV will benefit from fibrinolytic therapy [10, 11].

Conversely, the ESC guidelines recommend emergent valve replacement as choice of treatment for obstructive thrombosis in critically ill patients without serious comorbidities. The ESC further recommends a valve replacement of thrombosed artificial heart valve to a less thrombogenic type in cases of obstructive prosthetic valve thrombosis [12, 13]. According to the ESC, fibrinolysis is considered only in the following situations: critically ill patients developing valve thrombosis; situations where surgery is not readily available or patient cannot be transferred; and thrombosis of tricuspid or pulmonary artificial heart valve [12, 13].

Management of Over-anticoagulation and Bleeding

Another major complicative risk of anticoagulation therapy is over-anticoagulation causing major bleeding. This is particularly common with many systemic anticoagulants including VKA. The risk for major bleeding with anticoagulants begins to rise when the INR value increases ≥ 5, although bleeding can still occur at therapeutic or subtherapeutic INR values. The recommendations for managing this complication are consistent across major society guidelines which recommend an individualized approach based largely on the patient's condition and expert opinion, as rapid reversal of anticoagulation could increase the risks of prosthetic valve thrombosis or other thromboembolic phenomena [7, 11, 12].

Recommendations and Conclusions

In the management of thromboembolism in patients with artificial heart valves, it is important to take into consideration the individualized approach to treatment for the patient. This will be based on a number of variables like the type of artificial valve implanted, the risk stratification of the patient, the target anticoagulation intensity, and duration of closed management. VKA remains the standard of anticoagulation care for patients carrying artificial heart valves. Although the role of non-VKA oral anticoagulants (NOACs) is used in some settings, the role of these novel drugs is yet to be established in the setting of artificial heart valves. Therefore, knowledge of these guidelines for anticoagulation therapy in patients with artificial valves is essential to balance between thrombosis and bleeding in complex patient populations.

Appendix

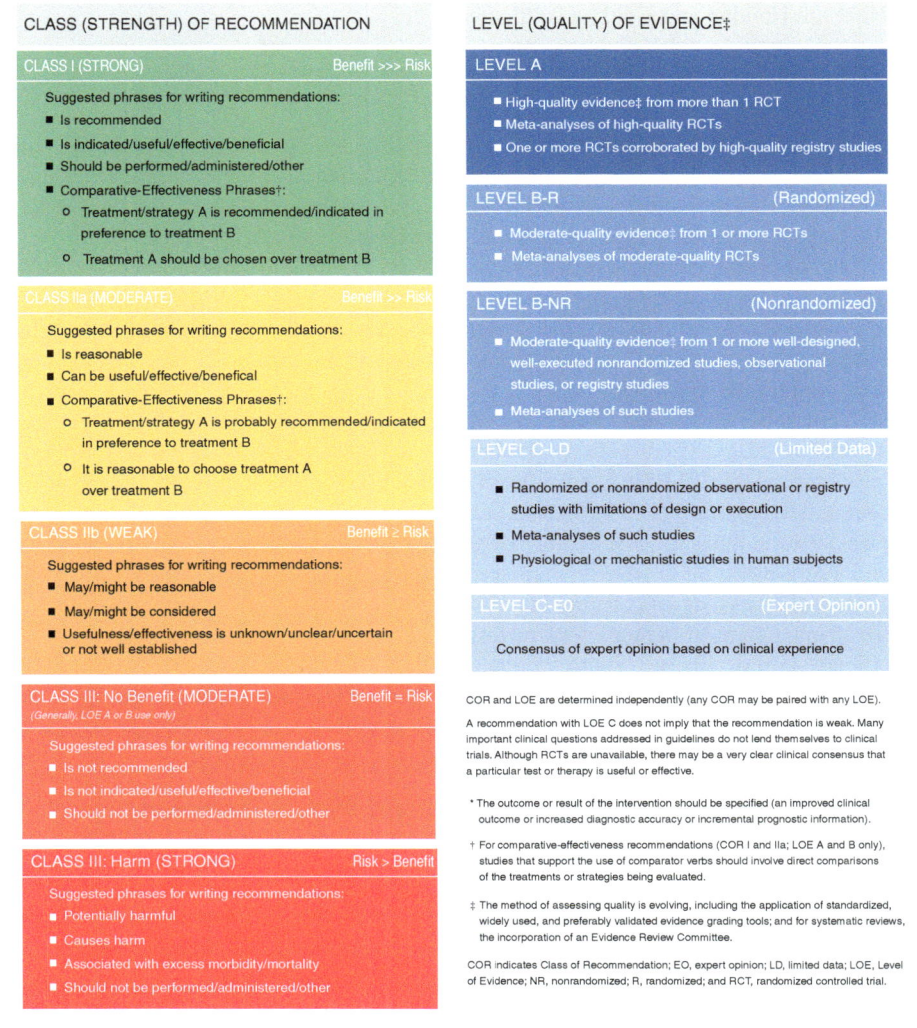

Classes of Recommendation and Levels of Evidence to Clinical Strategies, Interventions, Treatments, or Diagnostic Testing in Patient Care
Adapted from the ESC/EACTS Guidelines for the management of valvular heart disease

Atrial Fibrillation and Combination Antithrombotic Therapies in Patients Undergoing PCI (C, D, & A)

Haissam Haddad and Udoka Okpalauwaekwe

Introduction

Atrial fibrillation (AF) is the most common adult cardiac arrhythmia globally, with its prevalence in the United States projected to double over the next half decade. In large part, this projected increase relates to an increase in the aging population, and the burden of comorbidities traditionally associated with AF [19].

Not surprisingly, the drivers of AF such as hypertension, diabetes mellitus, sleep apnea, obesity, and smoking overlap significantly with the predisposition for coronary artery disease (CAD) [20]. Therefore, with parallel increases in the global burden of AF and CAD, a significant increase is anticipated in the patient with concomitant AF and CAD.

Contemporary AF and CAD trials and large nationwide registries have estimated an approximate 18% of patients undergoing percutaneous coronary intervention to have clinical AF [21]. As approximately 80% of patients will have an indication for oral anticoagulation (OAC), optimal choice and duration of antithrombotic strategies aimed at mitigating ischemic events (both embolic stroke and stent thrombosis) and major bleeding have been at the crux of recent clinical trials [22].

The objective of this chapter is to review the contemporary evidence focused on the management of patients with atrial fibrillation with concomitant CAD and specifically in those treated with percutaneous coronary intervention (PCI) in whom a risk-benefit assessment of ischemia and bleeding needs strong consideration.

Ischemic and Bleeding Risks in Patients with AF Treated with PCI

In the general population, the overall risk for an AF-related thromboembolic event has a 5-fold higher risk with gradation in this risk based on several patient-level factors [23]. Different variations of common denominator variables exist within the available risk-stratifying schema; in general, increasing age (RR per decade: 1.5; 95% CI: 1.3–1.7) and prior TIA/stroke portend the greatest stroke risk (RR: 2.5; 95% CI: 1.8–3.5); other predisposing factors include congestive heart failure (RR: 4.22; CI: 2.1, 8.03), hypertension (RR: 2.0; 95% CI: 1.6–2.5), and diabetes mellitus (RR: 1.7; 95% CI: 1.4–2.0) [24].

PCI invariably predisposes patients to the risk of stent thrombosis (ST). While ST incident rates ranging from 0.6% to 3.2% for bare metal stents (BMS) and 0.6–3.4% for drug-eluted stent (DES) have previously been reported [25], the risk of ST has substantially been reduced to <1% with thinner stent strut DES iterations.

Nevertheless, even with improved DES iterations, some combination of antithrombotic therapy is therefore required in patients with AF treated with PCI. As such, while increasingly potent antithrombotic agents are now available to mitigate the potentially catastrophic events of ST and embolic stroke, the consequent risk of major bleeding is substantially increased.

Similarly, in patients with AF on OAC, while DOACs have reduced the risk of major (HR: 0.86; 95% CI: 0.73–1.0; $p = 0.06$) and intracranial bleeding (HR: 0.49; 95% CI: 0.39–0.59; $p < 0.0001$), and increased risk for gastrointestinal bleeding (HR: 1.25; 95% CI: 1.01–1.55; $p = 0.043$) is evident [26].

Therefore, the combination of dual antiplatelet therapy with OAC ("triple therapy"), while attractive to mitigate ischemic events, significantly increases the predisposition to major bleeding.

Combining Antithrombotic Agents: The Evidence

Triple therapy with the vitamin K antagonist (VKA) warfarin has thus far been the standard of care in patients with AF treated with PCI. The *WOEST trial* (What is the Optimal Antiplatelet and Anticoagulant Therapy in Patients with Oral Anticoagulation and Coronary Stenting) examined the concept of long-term aspirin (ASA) discontinuation in 573 AF patients requiring PCI. At 1 year, patients randomized to triple therapy (warfarin + ASA + clopidogrel) were noted to have higher bleeding event rates compared to the dual pathway strategy of warfarin and clopidogrel (44.4% vs 19.4%; HR: 0.36; 95% CI: 0.26–0.5). This trial was, however, not powered for efficacy [27].

The *PIONEER AF-PCI* trial (Prevention of Bleeding in Patients with Atrial Fibrillation Undergoing PCI) tested the use of DOACs in exchange for warfarin and additionally eliminating ASA in favor of the "dual pathway" (OAC + clopidogrel). This trial randomized patients with AF treated with PCI into three schema: Rivaroxaban 10–15 mg PO OD + P2Y12-inhibitor for 12 months (group 1); Rivaroxaban 2.5 mg PO BID + DAPT for 1, 6, and 12 months (group 2); and warfarin + DAPT for 1, 6, and 12 months (group 3). At 12 months, clinically significant bleeding was lower in both the rivaroxaban groups compared to warfarin (group 1 vs 3: HR: 0.59; 95% CI: 0.47–0.76 and group 2 vs 3: HR: 0.63; 95% CI: 0.50–0.80) [28]. In addition, there was no significant difference in the rate of major adverse cardiovascular events (although the trial was not powered to detect differences in efficacy).

Similarly, the *RE-DUAL PCI* trial (Randomized Evaluation of Dual Antithrombotic Therapy with Dabigatran versus Triple Therapy with Warfarin in Patients with Non-valvular Atrial Fibrillation Undergoing PCI) randomized patients with AF undergoing PCI to the "dual" pathway at two different dabigatran doses of

(110 mg PO BID and 150 mg PO BID, plus P2Y12 inhibitor) and traditional triple therapy (warfarin + P2Y12 inhibitor + ASA). At 14 months, the triple therapy group had a 11.5% absolute increase in bleeding events in the dabigatran 110 BID dual pathway (HR: 0.52; 95% CI: 0.42–0.63) and 5.5% absolute increase in the dabigatran 150 BID dual pathway (HR: 0.72; 95% CI: 0.58–0.88). Furthermore, thrombotic events (MI, stroke, systemic embolism, death, or unplanned revascularization) were similar across all groups [29].

Further high-quality evidence on the role and risks associated with a dual pathway strategy will emerge with completion of the *AUGUSTUS* trial (Apixaban versus Warfarin in Patients with Atrial Fibrillation and Acute Coronary Syndromes or PCI, NCT02415400) in which patients on a P2Y12 inhibitor have been randomized in a 2 × 2 factorial design to apixaban or VKA, and ASA with placebo [30]. Specifically, the unique 2 × 2 trial design would separate the bleeding effects of the combination of antiplatelet and anticoagulation agents. In a similar group of patients, the *ENTRUST-AF-PCI* trial (Edoxaban Treatment versus Vitamin K Antagonist in Patients with Atrial Fibrillation Undergoing PCI, NCT02866175) will also provide an examination of the safety and efficacy of an edoxaban-based antithrombotic strategy.

For patients who have valvular atrial fibrillation or having mechanical heart valves and requiring concomitant antiplatelet therapy, high-quality data exists to support the use of VKA as the OAC of choice. In fact, from the learning of the *RE-ALIGN* trial (Randomized Evaluation of Long-Term Anticoagulant Therapy), DOACs are harmful in this patient population [31, 32].

Minimizing Risks

In AF patients anticipated to be on combination antithrombotic therapies, various potentially modifiable measures could be implemented to minimize bleeding risks.

Periprocedural Factors

Vascular Access Radial compared with femoral arterial access should be considered as default in all patients on an OAC undergoing cardiac catheterization, and particularly so, in those with an emergent/urgent indication in whom the bleeding risks are the greatest and the time to interrupt and allow OAC washout prior to the procedure is often insufficient. Several randomized trials and robust registry data exist to support the use of a default radial strategy in STEMI patients treated with a primary PCI or pharmacoinvasive strategy [33–36]; intuitively, this data should extrapolate even more to STEMI patients on OAC presenting for PCI.

Stent Selection The higher risk of stent thrombosis related to first generation DES has previously led to recommendations favoring the use of bare metal stents in patients requiring combination antithrombotic therapies. However, with improved efficacy and safety associated with newer generation DES, their use is now almost universally accepted across all patient subsets.

More recently, the development of ultrathin bare metal stents in the *NORSTENT* trial (Norwegian Coronary Stent) demonstrated much lower adverse event rates than observed in prior bare metal stent trials and provides an important alternative to patients in whom antiplatelet therapy interruption is anticipated within a very short duration from stent implantation [37].

Post-Procedural Factors

Triple Therapy In patients being considered for triple therapy, lower doses of aspirin (<100 mg) should be used, as the incremental benefit in use of higher aspirin dosing is limited, yet associated with a significantly higher risk for bleeding [38]. Additionally, the P2Y12 antagonist of choice is clopidogrel as the newer P2Y12 inhibitors, prasugrel or ticagrelor, have not been evaluated as part of triple therapy. The use of newer P2Y12 receptor antagonists as part of triple therapy could be considered in patients with documented clopidogrel resistance.

Proton Pump Inhibitors (PPI) In patients on triple therapy or in those considered to be high at-risk for bleeding, concomitant proton pump inhibitor use is recommended. As the clinical implications of the pharmacodynamics interactions between clopidogrel and PPI use are unclear, the use of PPIs with weaker CYP2C19 inhibition (such as pantoprazole) is preferred.

Duration The duration of dual antiplatelet therapy (DAPT) in general and as part of triple therapy has been the focus of several recent clinical trials. Emerging evidence appears to support the use of a dual strategy over triple therapy [39]. However, individualizing treatment durations on balance of ischemic-bleeding risk need careful consideration. In general, 1 year of single antiplatelet therapy (SAPT) + OAC is applicable to most patients, following which continued OAC for stroke prevention is recommended. In patients with high-risk clinical presentations for recurrent ischemic events such as ACS presentation, diabetes mellitus, prior stent thrombosis, or high-risk angiographic/procedural characteristics such as lesion characteristics or stent burden, up to 6 months of triple therapy may be acceptable. More importantly, decisions regarding the duration of combination antithrombotic therapy are dynamic and need to be regularly reviewed on the patient's clinical background.

Summary

The number of patients with concomitant AF and CAD requiring combination antithrombotic therapy is increasing. Contemporary evidence supports the use of a dual pathway compared to triple therapy, as the latter strategy significantly predisposes patients to major bleeding. The use of a DOAC is preferred over warfarin as part of a dual strategy. Invariably, there will be patients at high risk of recurrent ischemia and in whom triple therapy may be prudent. However, the choice and duration of combination antithrombotic therapy should be individualized and most importantly regularly reevaluated as individual patients' ischemic and bleeding risks are dynamic. Figure 3.5 illustrates the treatment algorithm whereas Fig. 3.6 illustrates the landmark trials in atrial fibrillation and combination antithrombotic therapies in patients undergoing PCI.

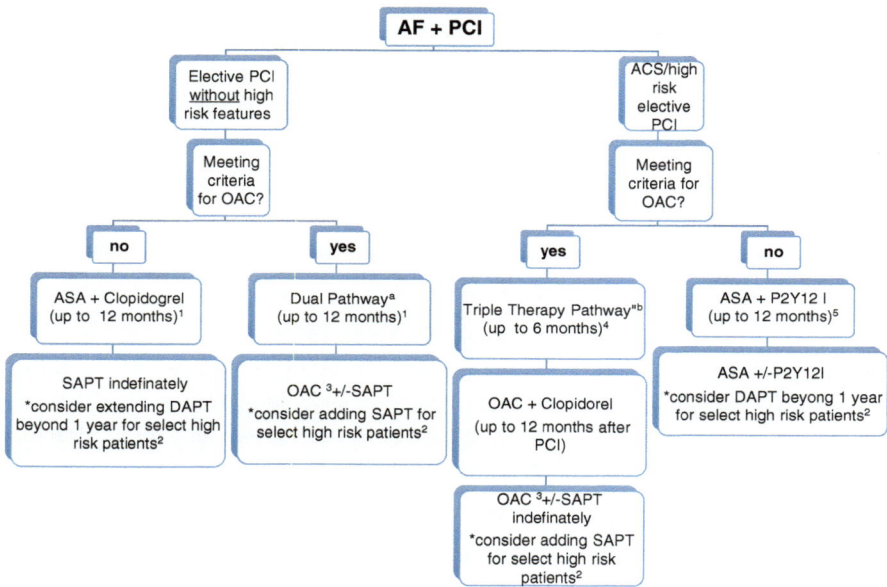

Fig. 3.5 Treatment algorithm. (Adapted from CCS 2018 Antiplatelet guidelines) [40]
[a]Dual pathway:
   Rivaroxaban 15 mg OD + clopidogrel 75 mg OD
   Dabigatran 110 mg or 150 mg BID + clopidogrel 75 mg OD
   Warfarin + clopidogrel 75 mg OD
[b]Triple therapy:
   Rivaroxaban 2.5 mg BID + ASA 81 mg + clopidogrel 75 mg OD
   Warfarin (INR of 2.0–2.5) + ASA 81 mg + clopidogrel 75 mg OD
[1]BMS: at least 1 month; DES: at least 3 months
[2]Reference Fig. 3.1
[3]Dose of OAC beyond 12 months should be adjusted to standard stroke prevention doses
[4]Consider 1 month if high-risk bleeding (ESC 2017; reference Fig. 3.2); can discontinue at any time
[5]Ticagrelor and Prasugrel preferred over Clopidogrel

Trial	N	Follow-up, months	Treatment arm	Primary outcome	Secondary outcome
WOEST (2013) [27]	563	12 months	Warfarin + Clopidogrel 75 mg (double therapy) Warfarin + Clopidogrel 75 mg + ASA 80–100 mg (triple therapy)	Any bleeding at 1 year: 19.4% vs 44.4% (p < 0.001)	Death, MI, stroke, stent thrombosis, TVR: 11.1% vs 17.6% (p = 0.025)
PIONEER AF-PCI (2016) [28]	2124	12 months	*Group1:* Rivaroxaban 10–15 mg OD + P2Y12 inhibitor (12 months), n = 709 *Group 2:* Rivaroxaban 2.5 mg BID + DAPT (1, 6, or 12 months), n = 709 *Group 3:* Warfarin + DAPT (1, 6, or 12 months), n = 706	Clinically significant bleeding: 16.8% (group 1) vs 18.0% (group 2) vs 26.7% (group 3) *(HR: 0.59, p < 0.001 for group 1 vs 3; HR: 0.63, p < 0.001 for group 2 vs 3)*	Major bleeding: 2.1% (group 1) vs 1.9% (group 2) vs 3.3% (group 3) *(HR 0.66, p = 0.23 for group 1 vs 3; HR 0.57, p = 0.11 for group 2 vs 3)* Adverse cardiac event: 6.5% (group 1) vs 5.6% (group 2) vs 6.0% (group 3) *(HR 1.08, p = 0.75 for group 1 vs 3; HR 0.93, p = 0.76 for group 2 vs 3)* Stent thrombosis: 0.8% (group 1) vs 0.9% (group 2) vs 0.7% (group 3) *(HR 1.20, p = 0.79 for group 1 vs 3; HR 1.44, p = 0.57 for group 2 vs 3)* All-cause death or recurrent hospitalizations: 35% (group 1) vs 32% (group 2) vs 42% (group 3) *(HR: 0.79, p = 0.008 for group 1 vs 3; HR: 0.75, p = 0.002 for group 2 vs 3)*
RE-DUAL PCI (2017) [29]	2725	14 months	Dabigatran 110 mg BID + clopidogrel/ticagrelor Dabigatran 150 mg BID + clopidogrel/ticagrelor Warfarin + Clopidogrel + low-dose ASA (1 or 3 months)	ISTH major/CRNM bleeding: 15.4% (110-mg dual therapy group) vs 26.9% (triple therapy group) *(HR: 0.52, p < 0.001 for noninferiority, p < 0.001 for superiority)* 20.2% (150–mg dual therapy group) vs 25.7% (triple therapy group) *(HR: 0.72; p < 0.001 for noninferiority)*	Composite of all-cause death, thrombotic events, and unplanned revascularization: 13.7% (both dual therapy groups combined) vs 13.4% (triple therapy group) *(HR: 1.04, p = 0.005 for noninferiority)*

Fig. 3.6 Landmark trials in atrial fibrillation and combination antithrombotic therapies in patients undergoing PCI

Anticoagulation in Heart Failure and Atrial Fibrillation (E & F)

Atrial Fibrillation and Heart Failure

Heart failure and atrial fibrillation frequently co-exist. Atrial fibrillation can precipitate acute exacerbation of heart failure symptoms; chronically, atrial fibrillation may perpetuate progression of heart failure through rate-related LV dysfunction or through maladaptive neurohormonal activation. On the other hand, heart failure with reduced ejection fraction (HFrEF, LVEF <40%) or preserved ejection (HFpEF, LVEF >50%) can independently increase the risk for the development of atrial fibrillation (HR: 1.43; CI: 0.85–2.40) [41, 42]. Prevalence of atrial fibrillation progressively increases with more symptomatic heart failure: atrial fibrillation is present in up to 40% of patients who are in NYHA class IV heart failure, compared to 4% in patients who are NYHA I [43]. The presence of atrial fibrillation is associated with worse prognosis for HF patients with both HFrEF and HFpEF [44].

Risk Stratification and Decision for Anticoagulation

While there is no established role for anticoagulation in the management of HF patients in sinus rhythm, most HF patients with atrial fibrillation should be considered for systemic anticoagulation. Both HFrEF and HFpEF have been shown to have strong association with increased risk of stroke and thromboembolism in patients with nonvalvular atrial fibrillation [45–48]. Indeed, the presence of heart failure is a key feature in ischemic stroke risk stratification tools such as the ATRIA Stroke Risk Score [49] (diabetes, hypertension, female, Congestive HF, proteinuria, eGFR <45 or ESRD and variable points for age depending on previous stroke), $CHADS_2$ [50] (Congestive HF, hypertension, age >75 years, diabetes mellitus, double risk for prior stroke or TIA or thromboembolism), or CHA_2DS_2-VASc [51] (Congestive HF, hypertension, double risk for age >75 years, diabetes mellitus, double risk for prior stroke or TIA or thromboembolism, vascular disease, age 65–74 years, sex category). These risk stratification schemes have been well validated in numerous nonvalvular AF cohorts [52–54], in spite of slight differences in the definition of heart failure in these scoring systems (CHF in ATRIA and $CHADS_2$ scores is defined as recent HF exacerbation, whereas CHF in CHA_2DS_2-VASc refers to recently decompensated HF irrespective of EF, or moderate to severe systolic dysfunction on imaging even if asymptomatic).

As a result, a number of professional societies base their recommendations for anticoagulation in AF patients on these risk stratification tools. Both the 2014 AHA/ACC/HRS Guidelines [10] and the 2016 ESC Guidelines recommended the use of CHA_2DS_2-VASc risk score. There is consensus with both sets of guidelines recommending oral anticoagulation for patients at higher thromboembolic risk, with

CHA$_2$DS$_2$-VASc score of 2 or above. However, for AF patients with HF but no other risk factors (CHA$_2$DS$_2$-VASc score of 1), the AHA/ACC/HRS Guidelines provides a class IIb recommendation for a choice between oral anticoagulation, aspirin, or no antithrombotic therapy; on the other hand, the ESC Guidelines [13] recommends consideration of oral anticoagulation, accounting for individual characteristics and patient preferences, for male patients with CHA$_2$DS$_2$-VASc score of 1 and female patients of 2. In contrast, the 2014 CCS Guidelines [15] recommended an alternative algorithm incorporating different elements of CHADS$_2$ and CHA$_2$DS$_2$-VASc scores. According to the CHADS-65 (congestive heart failure, hypertension, age, diabetes, stroke or TIA or thromboembolism) risk stratification system, all AF patients with HF should receive antithrombotic therapy.

Choice of Anticoagulation in AF with HF

The choice of oral anticoagulation therapy for atrial fibrillation patients with heart failure is not different from that of the general population. Since the 1950s, warfarin and other vitamin-K antagonist agents were the standard of care in terms of antithrombotic therapy for AF patients with increased thrombotic risk factors until recently [55]. Vitamin K antagonists have multiple sites of action in the coagulation cascades. Meta-analyses including studies with up to 31% of subjects with coexisting HF [56] show that therapy with adjusted-dose warfarin reduced stroke by up to 64%, compared to controls [57, 58]. This is an absolute risk reduction of 2.6–2.7% per year, corresponding to a number needed to treat of 37–38, in order to prevent one stroke [57, 59]. When compared to antiplatelet agents, warfarin use was associated with significant reduction in stroke risk, increased risk of intracranial hemorrhage, but not major extracranial hemorrhages [60, 61].

However, AF patients with HF taking warfarin had lower overall time in therapeutic window [62], which may impact the effectiveness of warfarin in the prevention of thromboembolic events. Over the past decade, the availability of novel, direct, NOAC, including direct thrombin antagonists (dabigatran [63]) or factor Xa inhibitors (rivaroxaban [64], apixaban [65], and edoxaban [66]), has dramatically changed the management of thromboembolic risks for patients with atrial fibrillation. While dedicated large, randomized trials of these medications in the subpopulation of AF patients with HF are not available, the analysis of these large trials which include HF subpopulation does provide support for their use in the prevention of thromboembolic events.

In the multicenter RE-LY trial [63] comparing dabigatran with warfarin, 4904 of the total 18,113 patients recruited (27.1%) had a history of heart failure, defined as NYHA class II or higher HF symptoms before screening. In the HF subgroup analysis of the RE-LY study [67], dabigatran at either the 110 mg or 150 mg dose was shown to be comparable, or better than warfarin at reducing the annual rate of stroke or systemic embolism (1.90% or 1.44%, compared with 1.92%, respectively). Moreover, dabigatran at either dose was superior to warfarin in the annual rate of major bleeding (3.9% for warfarin, compared with 3.26% at 110 mg and 3.1% at 150 mg).

The ARISTOTLE trial compared apixaban with dose-adjusted warfarin [68]. In this study, approximately 35% of the trial population, or 6451 of 18,201 patients recruited, had HF (defined as symptomatic heart failure within 3 months prior to study initiation, or LVEF less than 40%). Analysis of this subpopulation demonstrated that apixaban was better than warfarin for stroke and systemic embolism prevention (1.4%, compared with 1.6% per year), as well as incidence of major bleeding (1.9% compared with 3.1% per year, respectively).

The therapeutic effect and safety of rivaroxaban was compared with dose-adjusted warfarin in the ROCKET-AF study [64]. In this multicenter, randomized, double-blind trial, 9033 patients (63.7% of total) had HF, defined as clinic HF or LVEF ≤35%. In the HF subgroup analysis of the ROCKET-AF trial, rivaroxaban was found to be non-inferior when compared with warfarin in terms of prevention of stroke and systemic embolic events (1.90 per 100 patient years, compared with 2.09, respectively), with a similar bleeding risk (14.22 vs 14.02 per 100 patient years, respectively) and a lower hemorrhagic stroke.

Edoxaban at either high (60 mg daily) or low (30 mg daily) was compared with warfarin in the ENGAGE-AF-TIMI 48 trial [29]. Among the 14,071 patients randomized to well-controlled warfarin or the high-dose edoxaban regime, 8145 patients had class I–IV HF (presence or history of stage C or D HF, according to ACC/AHA definitions [69]), accounting for 57.9% of total [70]. In this patient population, edoxaban was consistently associated with lower risk of major bleeding (NYHA class I–II – HR: 0.79, 95% CI: 0.65–0.96; NYHA class III–IV – HR: 0.79, 95% CI: 0.54–1.17) and comparable efficacy compared with warfarin in terms of prevention of stroke and systemic thromboembolism (NYHA class I–II – HR: 0.88, 95% CI: 0.69–1.12; NYHA class III–IV – HR: 0.83, 95% CI: 0.55–1.25) [70].

In the absence of dedicated clinical trials, a number of meta-analyses helped provide reassurance regarding the use of NOAC in HF patients with AF, based on aggregate trial-level data from these phase III studies. Among the 32,512 AF patients with HF included in the first three trials (RE-LY, ARISTOTLE, and ROCKET-AF) [71], 19,122 patients received NOAC, while 13,390 received dose-adjusted warfarin therapy. Compared to warfarin, patients receiving single-dose/high-dose NOAC therapy had 14% lower risk of stroke or thromboembolic events and had a 24% lower risk of major bleeding. On the other hand, low-dose NOAC regimens were comparable to warfarin in the prevention of stroke and thromboembolic events, but had a non-significant trend toward lower risk of major bleeding [33]. Similarly, a more recent analysis that included the results from all four trials (RE-LY, ARISTOTLE, ROCKET-AF, and ENGAGE-AF-TIMI [48]) showed that NOAC therapies significantly reduced thromboembolic events, major bleeding, as well as intracranial hemorrhage in HF patients with AF [72]. Consistent with these analyses, both AHA/ACC/HRS [10] and ESC [13] guidelines consider NOAC therapy to be an adequate option for anticoagulation of AF patients in general, whereas the CCS Guidelines [15] suggest the use of NOAC in preference to warfarin for nonvalvular AF.

Summary

Heart failure significantly impacts the mortality and morbidity of patients with atrial fibrillation. In order to minimize the elevated risk of stroke and thromboembolic events in AF patients with HF, anticoagulation should be considered. Risk stratification scores such as the CHA_2DS_2-VASc score can be utilized to facilitate this decision. The oral vitamin K antagonist, warfarin, has been used successfully as the anticoagulant of choice for many decades; however, more recently a number of phase III clinical trials have highlighted the potential of NOACs to replace warfarin in nonvalvular AF. While there are no dedicated trials of NOAC in HF patients with AF, subgroup analyses of the current phase III NOAC clinical trials, as well as pooled meta-analysis based on these studies, suggest that NOAC therapy is at least as safe and effective, if not better, than warfarin. However, in clinical practice, the choice of anticoagulation therapy for AF patient with HF is frequently influenced by other factors including cost [73, 74], comorbidities such as renal insufficiency [74], as well as the availability of reversal agents [75].

References

1. Saksena D, Muralidharan S, Mishra YK, Kanhere V, Mohanty BB, Srivastava CP, Mange J, Puranik M, Nair MP, Goel P, Srivastava P. Anticoagulation management in patients with valve replacement. J Assoc Physicians India. 2018;66(1):59–74.
2. O'Callaghan M, Chester R, Scheckel C, Lee JZ, Fernandes R, Shamoun F. Bioprosthetic valve thrombosis while on anovel oral anticoagulant for atrial fibrillation. CASE. 2018;2(2):54.
3. Dangas GD, Weitz JI, Giustino G, Makkar R, Mehran R. Prosthetic heart valve thrombosis. J Am Coll Cardiol. 2016;68(24):2670–89.
4. Leiria TL, Lopes RD, Williams JB, Katz JN, Kalil RA, Alexander JH. Antithrombotic therapies in patients with prosthetic heart valves: guidelines translated for the clinician. J Thromb Thrombolysis. 2011;31(4):514–22.
5. Molteni M, Polo Friz H, Primitz L, Marano G, Boracchi P, Cimminiello C. The definition of valvular and non-valvular atrial fibrillation: results of a physicians'survey. Europace. 2014;16(12):1720–5.
6. Andrade JG, Macle L, Nattel S, Verma A, Cairns J. Contemporary atrial fibrillation management: a comparison of the current AHA/ACC/HRS, CCS, and ESC guidelines. Can J Cardiol. 2017;33(8):965–76.
7. Andrade JG, Verma A, Mitchell LB, Parkash R, Leblanc K, Atzema C, Healey JS, Bell A, Cairns J, Connolly S, Cox J. 2018 Focused Update of the Canadian Cardiovascular Society Guidelines for the management of atrial fibrillation. Can J Cardiol. 2018;34(11):1371–92.
8. Verheugt FW. Anticoagulation in patients with mechanical heart valves: follow the guidelines. Neth Hear J. 2015;23(2):109–10.
9. Whitlock RP, Sun JC, Fremes SE, Rubens FD, Teoh KH. Antithrombotic and thrombolytic therapy for valvular disease: antithrombotic therapy and prevention of thrombosis: American College of Chest Physicians Evidence-Based Clinical Practice Guidelines. Chest. 2012;141(2):e576S–600S.
10. January CT, Wann LS, Alpert JS, Calkins H, Cigarroa JE, Conti JB, Ellinor PT, Ezekowitz MD, Field ME, Murray KT, Sacco RL. 2014 AHA/ACC/HRS guideline for the management of patients with atrial fibrillation: a report of the American College of Cardiology/American

Heart Association Task Force on Practice Guidelines and the Heart Rhythm Society. J Am Coll Cardiol. 2014;64(21):e1–76.

11. Nishimura RA, Otto CM, Bonow RO, Carabello BA, Erwin JP, Fleisher LA, Jneid H, Mack MJ, McLeod CJ, O'gara PT, Rigolin VH. 2017 AHA/ACC focused update of the 2014 AHA/ ACC guideline for the management of patients with valvular heart disease: a report of the American College of Cardiology/American Heart Association Task Force on Clinical Practice Guidelines. J Am Coll Cardiol. 2017;70(2):252–89.

12. Authors/Task Force Members, Falk V, Baumgartner H, Bax JJ, De Bonis M, Hamm C, Holm PJ, Iung B, Lancellotti P, Lansac E, Muñoz DR. 2017 ESC/EACTS Guidelines for the management of valvular heart disease. Eur J Cardiothorac Surg. 2017;52(4):616–64.

13. Kirchhof P, Benussi S, Kotecha D, Ahlsson A, Atar D, Casadei B, Castella M, Diener HC, Heidbuchel H, Hendriks J, Hindricks G. 2016 ESC Guidelines for the management of atrial fibrillation developed in collaboration with EACTS. Eur Heart J. 2016;37(38):2893–962.

14. Macle L, Cairns JA, Andrade JG, Mitchell LB, Nattel S, Verma A, Andrade J, Atzema C, Bell A, Connolly S, Cox JL. The 2014 atrial fibrillation guidelines companion: a practical approach to the use of the Canadian Cardiovascular Society guidelines. Can J Cardiol. 2015;31(10):1207–18.

15. Verma A, Cairns JA, Mitchell LB, Macle L, Stiell IG, Gladstone D, McMurtry MS, Connolly S, Cox JL, Dorian P, Ivers N. 2014 focused update of the Canadian Cardiovascular Society Guidelines for the management of atrial fibrillation. Can J Cardiol. 2014;30(10):1114–30.

16. Olesen JB, Lip GY, Hansen ML, Hansen PR, Tolstrup JS, Lindhardsen J, Selmer C, Ahlehoff O, Olsen AM, Gislason GH, Torp-Pedersen C. Validation of risk stratification schemes for predicting stroke and thromboembolism in patients with atrial fibrillation: nationwide cohort study. BMJ. 2011;342:d124.

17. Douketis JD. The 2016 American College of Chest Physicians treatment guidelines for venous thromboembolism: a review and critical appraisal. Intern Emerg Med. 2016;11(8):1031–5.

18. Fiedler KA, Maeng M, Mehilli J, Schulz-Schüpke S, Byrne RA, Sibbing D, Hoppmann P, Schneider S, Fusaro M, Ott I, Kristensen SD. Duration of triple therapy in patients requiring oral anticoagulation after drug-eluting stent implantation: the ISAR-TRIPLE trial. J Am Coll Cardiol. 2015;65(16):1619–29.

19. Chugh SS, Havmoeller R, Narayanan K, Singh D, Rienstra M, Benjamin EJ, Gillum RF, Kim YH, McAnulty JH Jr, Zheng ZJ, Forouzanfar MH, Naghavi M, Mensah GA, Ezzati M, Murray CJ. Worldwide epidemiology of atrial fibrillation: a Global Burden of Disease 2010 Study. Circulation. 2014;129(8):837–47.

20. Benjamin EJ, Levy D, Vaziri SM, D'Agostino RB, Belanger AJ, Wolf PA. Independent risk factors for atrial fibrillation in a population-based cohort.The Framingham Heart Study. JAMA. 1994;271(11):840–4.

21. Rubenstein JC, Cinquegrani MP, Wright J. Atrial fibrillation in acute coronary syndrome. J Atr Fibrill. 2012;5(1):551. Published 2012 Jun 15. https://doi.org/10.4022/jafib.551.

22. Nieuwlaat R, Capucci A, Camm AJ, Olsson SB, Andresen D, Davies DW, Cobbe S, Breithardt G, Le Heuzey JY, Prins MH, Lévy S, Crijns HJ, European Heart Survey Investigators. Atrial fibrillation management: a prospective survey in ESC member countries: the Euro Heart Survey on Atrial Fibrillation. Eur Heart J. 2005;26:2422–34.

23. Wolf PA, Abbott RD, Kannel WB. Atrial fibrillation as an independent risk factor for stroke: the Framingham Study. Stroke. 1991;22:983–8.

24. Risk factors for stroke and efficacy of antithrombotic therapy in atrial fibrillation. Analysis of pooled data from five randomized controlled trials. Arch Intern Med. 1994;154:1449–57.

25. Claessen BE, Henriques JPS, Jaffer FA, Mehran R, Piek JJ, Dangas GD. Stent thrombosis. J Am Coll Cardiol Intv. 2014;7(10):1081–92. https://doi.org/10.1016/j.jcin.2014.05.016.

26. Ruff CT, Giugliano RP, Braunwald E, Hoffman EB, Deenadayalu N, Ezekowitz MD, Camm AJ, Weitz JI, Lewis BS, Parkhomenko A, Yamashita T, Antman EM. Comparison of the efficacy and safety of new oral anticoagulants with warfarin in patients with atrial fibrillation: a meta-analysis of randomised trials. Lancet. 2014;383(9921):955–62.

27. Dewilde WJ, Oirbans T, Verheugt FW, et al. on behalf of the WOEST Investigators. Use of clopidogrel with or without aspirin in patients taking oral anticoagulant therapy and undergoing percutaneous coronary intervention: an open-label, randomised, controlled trial. Lancet. 2013;381:1107–15.
28. Gibson CM, Mehran R, Bode C, et al. Prevention of bleeding in patients with atrial fibrillation undergoing PCI. N Engl J Med. 2016;375:2423–34.
29. Cannon CP, Bhatt DL, Oldgren J, et al. on behalf of the RE-DUAL PCI Steering Committee and Investigators. Dual antithrombotic therapy with dabigatran after PCI in atrial fibrillation. N Engl J Med. 2017;377:1513–24.
30. Lopes RD, Vora AN, Liaw D, Granger CB, Darius H, Goodman SG, et al. An open-Label, 2 × 2 factorial, randomized controlled trial to evaluate the safety of apixaban vs. vitamin K antagonist and aspirin vs. placebo in patients with atrial fibrillation and acute coronary syndrome and/or percutaneous coronary intervention: Rationale and design of the AUGUSTUS trial. Am Heart J. 2018;200:17–23.
31. Van de Werf F, Brueckmann M, Connolly SJ, Friedman J, Granger CB, Härtter S, Harper R, Kappetein AP, Lehr T, Mack MJ, Noack H, Eikelboom JW. A comparison of dabigatranetexilate with warfarin in patients with mechanical heart valves: THE Randomized, phase II study to evaluate the safety and pharmacokinetics of oral dabigatranetexilate in patients after heart valve replacement (RE-ALIGN). Am Heart J. 2012;163(6):931–7.
32. Eikelboom JW, Connolly SJ, Brueckmann M, Granger CB, Kappetein AP, Mack MJ, et al. Dabigatran versus warfarin in patients with mechanical heart valves. N Engl J Med. 2013;369(13):1206–14.
33. Shavadia J, Welsh R, Gershlick A, Zheng Y, Huber K, Halvorsen S, et al. Relationship between arterial access and outcomes in ST-elevation myocardial infarction with a pharmacoinvasive versus primary percutaneous coronary intervention strategy: insights from the Strategic Reperfusion Early After Myocardial Infarction (STREAM) Study. J Am Heart Assoc. 2016;5
34. Mamas A, Ratib K, Routledge H, Fath-Ordoubadi F, Neyses L, Louvard Y, et al. Influence of arterial access site selection on outcomes in primary percutaneous coronary intervention: are the results of randomized trials achievable in clinical practice? J Am Coll Cardiol Intv. 2013;6(7):707–8.
35. Romagnoli E, Biondi-Zoccai G, Sciahbasi A, et al. Radialversus femoral randomized investigation in ST-segment elevation acute coronary syndrome: the RIFLE-STEACS (Radial Versus Femoral Randomized Investigation in ST-Elevation Acute Coronary Syndrome) study. J Am Coll Cardiol. 2012;60:2481–9.
36. Valgimigli M, Gagnor A, Calabró P, et al. on behalf of the MATRIX Trial Investigators. Radial versus femoral access in patients with acute coronary syndromes undergoing invasive management: a randomisedmulticentre trial. Lancet. 2015;385:2465–76.
37. Jolly SS, Yusuf S, Cairns J, et al. Radial versus femoral access for coronary angiography and intervention in patients with acute coronary syndromes (RIVAL): a randomised, parallel group, multicentre trial. Lancet. 2011;377:1409–20. Bonaa KH, et al. Drug-eluting or bare-metal stents for coronary artery disease. N Engl J Med. 2016;375:1242–52.
38. Levine GN, O'Gara PT, Bates ER, et al. 2015 ACC/AHA/SCAI focused update on primary percutaneous coronary intervention for patients with ST-elevation myocardial infarction: an update of the 2011 ACCF/AHA/SCAI Guideline for Percutaneous Coronary Intervention and the 2013 ACCF/AHA guideline for the management of ST-elevation myocardial infarction. J Am Coll Cardiol. 2016; https://doi.org/10.1016/j.jacc.2016.03.513.
39. Golwala HB, Cannon CP, Steg PG, Doros G, Qamar A, Ellis SG, Oldgren J, Ten Berg JM, Kimura T, Hohnloser SH, Lip GYH, Bhatt DL. Safety and efficacy of dual vs. triple antithrombotic therapy in patients with atrial fibrillation following percutaneous coronary intervention: a systematic review and meta-analysis of randomized clinical trials. Eur Heart J. 2018;39(19):1726.

40. Mehta SR, Bainey KR, Cantor WJ, Lordkipanidzé M, Marquis-Gravel G, Robinson SD, et al. 2018 Canadian cardiovascular society/Canadian association of interventional cardiology focused update of the guidelines for the use of antiplatelet therapy. Can J Cardiol. 2018;34(3):214–33.
41. Kishore A, Vail A, Majid A, Dawson J, Lees KR, Tyrrell PJ, Smith CJ. Detection of atrial fibrillation after ischemic stroke or transient ischemic attack: a systematic review and meta-analysis. Stroke. 2014;45:520–5261.
42. Tsang TS, Gersh BJ, Appleton CP, Tajik AJ, Barnes ME, Bailey KR, Oh JK, Leibson C, Montgomery SC, Seward JB. Left ventricular diastolic dysfunction as a predictor of the first diagnosed nonvalvular atrial fibrillation in 840 elderly men and women. J Am Coll Cardiol. 2002;40:1636–44.
43. Maisel WH, Stevenson LW. Atrial fibrillation in heart failure: epidemiology, pathophysiology, and rationale for therapy. Am J Cardiol. 2003;91:2D–8D.
44. Olsson LG, Swedberg K, Ducharme A, Granger CB, Michelson EL, McMurray JJ, Puu M, Yusuf S, Pfeffer MA, Investigators C. Atrial fibrillation and risk of clinical events in chronic heart failure with and without left ventricular systolic dysfunction: results from the candesartan in heart failure-assessment of reduction in mortality and morbidity (charm) program. J Am Coll Cardiol. 2006;47:1997–2004.
45. Divani AA, Vazquez G, Asadollahi M, Qureshi AI, Pullicino P. Nationwide frequency and association of heart failure on stroke outcomes in the united states. J Card Fail. 2009;15:11–6.
46. Friberg L, Rosenqvist M, Lip GY. Evaluation of risk stratification schemes for ischaemic stroke and bleeding in 182 678 patients with atrial fibrillation: the swedish atrial fibrillation cohort study. Eur Heart J. 2012;33:1500–10.
47. Agarwal M, Apostolakis S, Lane DA, Lip GY. The impact of heart failure and left ventricular dysfunction in predicting stroke, thromboembolism, and mortality in atrial fibrillation patients: a systematic review. Clin Ther. 2014;36:1135–44.
48. Hays AG, Sacco RL, Rundek T, Sciacca RR, Jin Z, Liu R, Homma S, Di Tullio MR. Left ventricular systolic dysfunction and the risk of ischemic stroke in a multiethnic population. Stroke. 2006;37:1715–9.
49. Singer DE, Chang Y, Borowsky LH, Fang MC, Pomernacki NK, Udaltsova N, Reynolds K, Go AS. A new risk scheme to predict ischemic stroke and other thromboembolism in atrial fibrillation: the atria study stroke risk score. J Am Heart Assoc. 2013;2:e000250.
50. Gage BF, Waterman AD, Shannon W, Boechler M, Rich MW, Radford MJ. Validation of clinical classification schemes for predicting stroke: results from the national registry of atrial fibrillation. JAMA. 2001;285:2864–70.
51. Lip GY, Nieuwlaat R, Pisters R, Lane DA, Crijns HJ. Refining clinical risk stratification for predicting stroke and thromboembolism in atrial fibrillation using a novel risk factor-based approach: the euro heart survey on atrial fibrillation. Chest. 2010;137:263–72.
52. Aspberg S, Chang Y, Atterman A, Bottai M, Go AS, Singer DE. Comparison of the atria, chads2, and cha2ds2-vasc stroke risk scores in predicting ischaemic stroke in a large swedish cohort of patients with atrial fibrillation. Eur Heart J. 2016;37:3203–10.
53. van den Ham HA, Klungel OH, Singer DE, Leufkens HG, van Staa TP. Comparative performance of atria, chads2, and cha2ds2-vasc risk scores predicting stroke in patients with atrial fibrillation: results from a national primary care database. J Am Coll Cardiol. 2015;66:1851–9.
54. Guo Y, Apostolakis S, Blann AD, Wang H, Zhao X, Zhang Y, Zhang D, Ma J, Wang Y, Lip GY. Validation of contemporary stroke and bleeding risk stratification scores in non-anticoagulatedchinese patients with atrial fibrillation. Int J Cardiol. 2013;168:904–9.
55. Cleland JG, Mumtaz S, Cecchini L. Role of antithrombotic agents in heart failure. Curr Cardiol Rep. 2012;14:314–25.
56. IConnolly S, Pogue J, Hart R, Pfeffer M, Hohnloser S, Chrolavicius S, Pfeffer M, Hohnloser S, Yusuf S. Clopidogrel plus aspirin versus oral anticoagulation for atrial fibrillation in the atrial fibrillation clopidogrel trial with irbesartan for prevention of vascular events (active w): arandomised controlled trial. Lancet. 2006;367:1903–12.

57. Hart RG, Pearce LA, Aguilar MI. Meta-analysis: antithrombotic therapy to prevent stroke in patients who have nonvalvular atrial fibrillation. Ann Intern Med. 2007;146:857–67.
58. Saxena R, Koudstaal PJ. Anticoagulants for preventing stroke in patients with nonrheumatic atrial fibrillation and a history of stroke or transient ischaemic attack. Cochrane Database Syst Rev. 2004:CD000185.
59. Aguilar MI, Hart R. Oral anticoagulants for preventing stroke in patients with non-valvular atrial fibrillation and no previous history of stroke or transient ischemic attacks. Cochrane Database Syst Rev. 2005:CD001927.
60. Aguilar MI, Hart R, Pearce LA. Oral anticoagulants versus antiplatelet therapy for preventing stroke in patients with non-valvular atrial fibrillation and no history of stroke or transient ischemic attacks. Cochrane Database Syst Rev. 2007:CD006186.
61. Saxena R, Koudstaal P. Anticoagulants versus antiplatelet therapy for preventing stroke in patients with nonrheumatic atrial fibrillation and a history of stroke or transient ischemic attack. Cochrane Database Syst Rev. 2004:CD000187.
62. Apostolakis S, Sullivan RM, Olshansky B, Lip GYH. Factors affecting quality of anticoagulation control among patients with atrial fibrillation on warfarin: the same-tt(2)r(2) score. Chest. 2013;144:1555–63.
63. Connolly SJ, Ezekowitz MD, Yusuf S, Eikelboom J, Oldgren J, Parekh A, Pogue J, Reilly PA, Themeles E, Varrone J, Wang S, Alings M, Xavier D, Zhu J, Diaz R, Lewis BS, Darius H, Diener HC, Joyner CD, Wallentin L, Committee R-LS, Investigators. Dabigatran versus warfarin in patients with atrial fibrillation. N Engl J Med. 2009;361:1139–51.
64. Patel MR, Mahaffey KW, Garg J, Pan G, Singer DE, Hacke W, Breithardt G, Halperin JL, Hankey GJ, Piccini JP, Becker RC, Nessel CC, Paolini JF, Berkowitz SD, Fox KA, Califf RM, Investigators RA. Rivaroxaban versus warfarin in nonvalvular atrial fibrillation. N Engl J Med. 2011;365:883–91.
65. Granger CB, Alexander JH, McMurray JJ, Lopes RD, Hylek EM, Hanna M, Al-Khalidi HR, Ansell J, Atar D, Avezum A, Bahit MC, Diaz R, Easton JD, Ezekowitz JA, Flaker G, Garcia D, Geraldes M, Gersh BJ, Golitsyn S, Goto S, Hermosillo AG, Hohnloser SH, Horowitz J, Mohan P, Jansky P, Lewis BS, Lopez-Sendon JL, Pais P, Parkhomenko A, Verheugt FW, Zhu J, Wallentin L, Committees A, Investigators. Apixaban versus warfarin in patients with atrial fibrillation. N Engl J Med. 2011;365:981–92.
66. Giugliano RP, Ruff CT, Braunwald E, Murphy SA, Wiviott SD, Halperin JL, Waldo AL, Ezekowitz MD, Weitz JI, Spinar J, Ruzyllo W, Ruda M, Koretsune Y, Betcher J, Shi M, Grip LT, Patel SP, Patel I, Hanyok JJ, Mercuri M, Antman EM, Investigators EA-T. Edoxaban versus warfarin in patients with atrial fibrillation. N Engl J Med. 2013;369:2093–104.
67. Ferreira J, Ezekowitz MD, Connolly SJ, Brueckmann M, Fraessdorf M, Reilly PA, Yusuf S, Wallentin L, Investigators R-L. Dabigatran compared with warfarin in patients with atrial fibrillation and symptomatic heart failure: a subgroup analysis of the re-ly trial. Eur J Heart Fail. 2013;15:1053–61.
68. Goto S, Zhu J, Liu L, Oh BH, Wojdyla DM, Aylward P, Bahit MC, Gersh BJ, Hanna M, Horowitz J, Lopes RD, Wallentin L, Xavier D, Alexander JH, ARISTOTLE Investigators. Efficacy and safety of apixaban compared with warfarin for stroke prevention in patients with atrial fibrillation from East Asia: a subanalysis of the Apixaban for Reduction in Stroke and Other Thromboembolic Events in Atrial Fibrillation (ARISTOTLE) Trial. Am Heart J. 2014;168(3):303–9.
69. Yancy CW, Jessup M, Bozkurt B, Butler J, Casey DE Jr, Drazner MH, Fonarow GC, Geraci SA, Horwich T, Januzzi JL, Johnson MR, Kasper EK, Levy WC, Masoudi FA, McBride PE, McMurray JJ, Mitchell JE, Peterson PN, Riegel B, Sam F, Stevenson LW, Tang WH, Tsai EJ, Wilkoff BL. 2013 accf/aha guideline for the management of heart failure: a report of the american college of cardiology foundation/american heart association task force on practice guidelines. J Am Coll Cardiol. 2013;62:e147–239.

70. Magnani G, Giugliano RP, Ruff CT, Murphy SA, Nordio F, Metra M, Moccetti T, Mitrovic V, Shi M, Mercuri M, Antman EM, Braunwald E. Efficacy and safety of edoxaban compared with warfarin in patients with atrial fibrillation and heart failure: insights from engage af-timi 48. Eur J Heart Fail. 2016;18:1153–61.
71. Xiong Q, Lau YC, Senoo K, Lane DA, Hong K, Lip GY. Non-vitamin k antagonist oral anti-coagulants (noacs) in patients with concomitant atrial fibrillation and heart failure: a systemic review and meta-analysis of randomized trials. Eur J Heart Fail. 2015;17:1192–200.
72. Savarese G, Giugliano RP, Rosano GM, McMurray J, Magnani G, Filippatos G, Dellegrottaglie S, Lund LH, Trimarco B, Perrone-Filardi P. Efficacy and safety of novel oral anticoagulants in patients with atrial fibrillation and heart failure: a meta-analysis. JACC Heart Fail. 2016;4:870–80.
73. Deitelzweig S, Amin A, Jing Y, Makenbaeva D, Wiederkehr D, Lin J, Graham J. Medical cost reductions associated with the usage of novel oral anticoagulants vs warfarin among atrial fibrillation patients, based on the re-ly, rocket-af, and aristotle trials. J Med Econ. 2012;15:776–85.
74. Heywood JT, Fonarow GC, Costanzo MR, Mathur VS, Wigneswaran JR, Wynne J, Committee ASA, Investigators. High prevalence of renal dysfunction and its impact on outcome in 118,465 patients hospitalized with acute decompensated heart failure: a report from the adhere database. J Card Fail. 2007;13:422–30.
75. Pollack CV Jr, Reilly PA, Eikelboom J, Glund S, Verhamme P, Bernstein RA, Dubiel R, Huisman MV, Hylek EM, Kamphuisen PW, Kreuzer J, Levy JH, Sellke FW, Stangier J, Steiner T, Wang B, Kam CW, Weitz JI. Idarucizumab for dabigatran reversal. N Engl J Med. 2015;373:511–20.

Chapter 4
Thrombosis and Anticoagulation in Children

Ahmed Maher Kaddah and Iman Fathy Iskander

Abbreviations

aPL	Antiphospholipid antibodies
aPTT	Activated partial thromboplastin time
AT	Antithrombin
CSVT	Cerebral sinus venous thrombosis
CT	Computerized tomography
CTPA	Computed tomographic pulmonary angiography
CVADs	Central venous access devices
CVCs	Central venous catheters
DVT	Deep vein thrombosis
FFP	Fresh frozen plasma
HIT	Heparin-induced thrombocytopenia
INR	International normalized ratio
IT	Inherited thrombophilia
LMWH	Low-molecular-weight heparin
MRV	Magnetic resonance venography
OCP	Oral contraceptive pill
PCC	Prothrombin complex concentrate
PE	Pulmonary embolism
PICCs	Peripherally inserted central catheters
PT	Prothrombin time
PTS	Postthrombotic syndrome
PVT	Portal vein thrombosis
RVT	Renal vein thrombosis
SLE	Systemic lupus erythematosus
TPA	Recombinant tissue plasminogen activator
TPN	Total parenteral nutrition

A. M. Kaddah (✉)
Pediatrics and Pediatric Hematology, College of Medicine, Cairo University, Giza, Egypt

I. F. Iskander
Pediatrics & Neonatology, College of Medicine, Cairo University, Giza, Egypt

© Springer Nature Switzerland AG 2020
H. Goubran et al. (eds.), *Precision Anticoagulation Medicine*,
https://doi.org/10.1007/978-3-030-25782-8_4

103

UFH   Unfractionated heparin
VKA   Vitamin K antagonist
VTE   Venous thromboembolism

Epidemiology

The incidence of venous thromboembolism (VTE) in children is lower than adults. However, it is being increasingly recognized in the pediatric population as a complication of health care.

Estimates of the annual incidence of VTE in the general pediatric population range from 0.14 to 0.21 per 10,000 children [1, 2]. Among hospitalized pediatric patients, the incidence of VTE is approximately 20–60 per 10,000 admissions [3–5]. Rates are highest among children with underlying medical conditions, such as malignancy and cardiac disease [3, 5].

Risk of VTE in children versus adults The risk of VTE is substantially lower in children. Several factors may contribute to the relatively low incidence of VTE throughout childhood:

- Children less commonly develop diseases causing damage to the vascular endothelium, e.g., diabetes, dyslipidemias, and hypertension.
- Children are less frequently exposed to acquired prothrombotic risk factors (e.g., oral contraceptives, hormone replacement therapy, pregnancy and puerperium, smoking, malignancy, orthopedic surgery).
- As compared to adults, plasma concentrations of all vitamin K-dependent factors, almost all contact factors, and the capacity to generate thrombin are decreased throughout childhood [6, 7].
- The capacity to inhibit thrombin is enhanced throughout childhood due to increased plasma concentrations of the thrombin inhibitor alpha-2-macroglobulin [6–8].

Among children, the commonest age groups are neonates and teenagers, due to the associated underlying diseases and interventions.

The risk factor for thrombosis in this vulnerable population can be stratified into inherited, including factor V Leiden mutation, prothrombin G20210A mutation, and protein C, S, and antithrombin (AT) deficiencies [10] and acquired.

The commonest acquired precipitating factor is the presence of a central venous access device (CVAD), which is related to almost 90% of VTE in neonates and >60% in older children [9].

Other factors include infection, trauma, immobilization, surgery, malignancy, chronic inflammatory conditions, antiphospholipid syndrome, myeloproliferative neoplasms, proteinuria, and paroxysmal nocturnal hemoglobinuria. Heart failure and congenital heart diseases can also lead to venous thromboembolism [10].

Central Venous Access Devices (CVADs)

CVADs are the most important risk factor for VTE. Approximately one- to two-thirds of VTEs in children are associated with CVADs [1, 5, 11]. CVADs are extremely important for the long- and short-term management of pediatric patients with a variety of severe diseases (e.g., total parenteral nutrition, intensive fluid management, administration of blood products, antibiotics, and chemotherapy). CVAD-associated VTEs can occur in the upper venous system (in association with central venous catheters (CVCs) inserted percutaneously through a jugular or subclavian vein) or in the lower extremity (in association with CVCs placed in the femoral vein) [12, 13]. Peripherally inserted central catheters (PICCs) also may be associated with VTE. Central venous catheters (CVCs) are a risk factor because they present an extrinsic intravascular surface, injure vessel walls, and interfere with blood flow.

Inherited Thrombophilia (IT)

The most common IT disorders include factor V Leiden; prothrombin G20210A mutation, deficiencies of antithrombin, protein C, and protein S; and increased lipoprotein (a).

In children with VTE, the prevalence of IT ranges from 10% to 59% [2, 14–21].

Other Conditions

Acquired conditions that are frequently associated with VTEs in children include:

- Infection.
- Malignancy VTE can occur as a complication of any pediatric malignancy. VTE is a particularly common in children with acute lymphoblastic leukemia who are treated with asparaginase.
- Congenital heart disease.
- Trauma: The risk of VTE increases following major traumatic injury; however, risk in children is substantially lower compared to adult trauma patients. The risk is highest among patients with a major vascular injury and those requiring orthopedic surgery.
- Nephrotic syndrome.
- Inflammatory bowel disease [22].
- SLE [1, 23, 24].

These risk factors are characterized by either a protein-losing state, inflammatory state, or vascular disruption, which are consistent with Virchow's triad describing VTE risk.

Clinical manifestations Clinical manifestations of VTE in children vary, depending on both the location and extension of the thrombus.

Central venous line Central venous catheter (CVC)-related VTE is usually asymptomatic or manifests with chronic symptoms, including repeated loss of CVC patency, CVC-related sepsis, and prominent collateral circulation in the skin over the chest, back, neck, and face [23, 25, 26]. VTE presents acutely with swelling and discoloration of the limb, facial swelling, pulmonary embolism, chylous pleural effusion, and/or superior vena cava syndrome (presents by dyspnea, a sensation of head fullness, congested neck veins, and mediastinal broadening on chest x-ray) [27–30].

Deep vein thrombosis (DVT) Non-CVC-related VTEs can occur in any venous system but most commonly present in the lower extremities, especially in the iliac, femoral, and/or popliteal veins. DVT manifests with unilateral leg, buttock, inguinal, and/or abdominal pain associated with swelling and/or reddish or purple discoloration of the legs. Larger calf diameter in the affected leg compared with the contralateral leg may also be noted. Homans' sign (calf pain on passive dorsiflexion of the foot) is unreliable for the presence of DVT in children [31].

Outside of the setting of CVC-related VTE, upper extremity DVT is rare in children. Upper extremity DVT manifests with unilateral swelling and discoloration of the arm and hand [31]. Swelling of the face may be noted if the thrombus extends into the superior vena cava. Patients may complain of pain in the affected arm.

Pulmonary embolism Pulmonary embolism (PE) is rare in children [32–34]. PE can manifest with pleuritic chest pain, tachypnea, cough, tachycardia, acute dyspnea, hypoxia, and sudden collapse. Clinical signs of DVT may also be present.

Most commonly, however, the clinical manifestations of PE in children, especially young children, are nonspecific and often mimic the clinical symptoms of the underlying disease. For this reason, and because younger children cannot verbalize their symptoms, PE should be considered in the differential diagnosis of cardiorespiratory deterioration in all critically ill children [35]. Commonly reported risk factors for PE in children include trauma, immobility, recent surgery, CVCs, oral contraceptive use, and inflammatory conditions [36–38]. Other predisposing causes include malignancy, heart disease, dehydration, hypercoagulable states, and obesity [39, 40].

Renal vein thrombosis In children, renal vein thrombosis (RVT) most commonly occurs secondary to nephrotic syndrome and renal transplantation [41–43]. RVT may manifest with hematuria, anuria, vomiting, hypovolemia, proteinuria, and thrombocytopenia. However, RVT most often has an insidious onset and produces no symptoms referable to the kidney. In this case, the RVT may first be diagnosed when the patient presents with a thromboembolic event (e.g., PE). If the thrombus extends from the renal vein into the inferior vena cava, both lower extremities may become cyanotic and edematous.

RVT is the most prevalent non-catheter-related VTE during the neonatal period and accounts for up to 20% of all thromboembolic events in newborns [44].

Portal vein thrombosis Portal vein thrombosis (PVT) may be precipitated by liver transplantation, splenectomy, sickle cell disease, chemotherapy, infections, or antiphospholipid syndrome [45–50]. PVT may present acutely with an acute abdomen, particularly in adolescents [51], or may be asymptomatic for long periods until features of chronic portal hypertension occur (e.g., splenomegaly or GIT bleeding secondary to esophageal varices) [35]. In neonates, PVT is mostly related to umbilical catheterization and sepsis [52].

Diagnosis

Ultrasonography is the preferred initial diagnostic study in most children with suspected venous thrombosis. *Noncompressibility* of the vein with or without visible intraluminal thrombus confirms the diagnosis. Alternative imaging modalities are available (e.g., *contrast venography*, contrast magnetic resonance venography [*MRV*], computerized tomography [*CT*] venography); however, they are rarely necessary.

Duplex ultrasonography is the preferred initial test because it is noninvasive, readily available, does not require sedation, and does not expose the child to ionizing radiation. Diagnostic approach varies depending on the location of the suspected thrombus [53]:

- **Lower extremity** – Compression ultrasonography is recommended for initial evaluation of DVT in the lower extremities. If ultrasonography is normal and the clinical suspicion of DVT remains high, the study can be repeated after a week [53]. In children with suspected proximal extension of femoral DVT, MRV is the appropriate diagnostic study. CT is also a reasonable choice if MRV is not available; however, CT has the disadvantage of exposing the child to radiation.
- **Upper extremity** – Evaluation of the peripheral upper extremity, axillary, subclavian, and internal jugular veins should be done with ultrasonography; however, this may be relatively insensitive for detection of central intrathoracic VTE. It can yield false-negative results due to the position of the clavicles (which hinder the view of the distal subclavian veins) and the thoracic cage (which hinders compression of veins in a central location) [54]. Assessment of the central veins for VTE can be performed using MRV, CT, or contrast venography; we prefer MRV because it does not expose the child to radiation.
  In patients with *non-catheter-related upper extremity DVT*, a diagnosis of thoracic outlet syndrome (also referred to as Paget-Schroetter syndrome or "effort" thrombosis) should be considered. *Catheter-associated* – Patients with signs or symptoms of large vessel thrombosis (e.g., swelling and/or discoloration of the related limb) should be evaluated with duplex ultrasound. For mechanical catheter problems, instillation of intravenous contrast into the lumen of the catheter under fluoroscopy may readily demonstrate the presence of thrombus at the tip of the catheter.
- **Pulmonary embolism – Computed tomographic pulmonary angiography (CTPA)** is the imaging modality of choice for diagnosis of PE in children [55].

Differential diagnosis The differential diagnosis of VTE depends of the location of the thrombus.

Deep vein thrombosis (DVT) Mimics of upper or lower extremity DVT include conditions that present with swelling, erythema/discoloration, and tenderness of the extremity:

• Baker's cyst
• Cellulitis
• Musculoskeletal injury
• Lymphangitis or lymph obstruction
• Superficial thrombophlebitis

The history and physical examination findings can often distinguish DVT from these conditions, though ultrasonography is ultimately required to make the diagnosis.

Treatment

The goals of treating VTE are to:

• Prevent local extension and embolization of the thrombus
• Aid in resolving the existing thrombus
• Prevent VTE recurrence
• Minimize long-term complications (e.g., postthrombotic syndrome)

Antithrombotic therapy consists of the administration of anticoagulant agents (unfractionated heparin [UFH], low-molecular-weight heparin [LMWH], or vitamin K antagonists [VKA, e.g., warfarin]). Figure 4.1 illustrates the comparison between the different anticoagulants used in children.

- LMWH is generally preferred over UFH in most circumstances. LMWH also is generally preferred over VKA because the response to VKAs in children tends to be unpredictable and requires frequent monitoring and dose adjustment. Nonetheless, VKA may be preferred by patients requiring long-term therapy because they are administered orally. Other anticoagulants (e.g., factor Xa inhibitors and direct thrombin inhibitors) are rarely used in children.
- The ASH guidelines suggests antithrombin [AT] replacement with standard anticoagulation and not only anticoagulation alone in pediatric patients with DVT/cerebral sinus venous thrombosis (CSVT)/PE failing to improve clinically to standard anticoagulation and if measurement of AT concentrations reveals low AT level in relation to age [56].

	Unfractionated heparin	LMWH	Vitamin K antagonist
Administration	Intravenous	Subcutaneous	Oral: affected by diet
Need for monitoring and dose adjustment	Frequent monitoring and dose adjustment	Periodic monitoring Usually fixed dose	Frequent monitoring and dose adjustment
Renal failure	No dose adjustment	Mild: dose adjustment and close monitoring Severe: not indicated	No dose adjustment
Hepatic failure	No dose adjustment	No dose adjustment	Mild and/or raised baseline prothrombin time: dose adjustment and close monitoring Severe: not indicated

Fig. 4.1 Comparison of different anticoagulants in children

– Thrombolytic agents (e.g., recombinant tissue plasminogen activator [TPA], uro-kinase) are used only in selected patients with major vessel occlusion, e.g., pulmonary embolism with hemodynamic compromise or compromise of organs or limbs.

Provoked VTE
Thrombosis during childhood is almost exclusively "provoked," meaning that it develops due to identifiable underlying conditions and risk factors. Of these risk factors, the most common is an indwelling central venous catheter. Other risk factors include surgery, trauma, infection, immobilization, malignancy, use of estrogen-containing oral contraceptive pills (OCPs), inflammatory conditions (e.g., systemic lupus erythematosus), structural venous abnormalities, and inherited thrombophilia.

For children with provoked VTE, we suggest initial anticoagulation with either low-molecular-weight heparin (LMWH) or unfractionated heparin (UFH) for 5–10 days, followed by 3 months of either LMWH or a VKA [53, 57].

LMWH is generally preferred for the reasons summarized in Fig. 4.1.

However, *UFH* may be preferred for initial therapy in some circumstances, such as in patients with renal failure or those with bleeding risks who require finely tuned titration and the ability to quickly turn on or off the infusion (e.g., patients requiring multiple surgeries or other invasive procedures).

If VKA is used, the treatment should overlap with UFH/LMWH until the international normalized ratio (INR) is in the therapeutic range (*i.e.*, *2.0–3.0*) on two consecutive days. Data on DOACs is also emerging.

Special considerations and/or modifications of this regimen are warranted in the following circumstances:

- **CVC-related VTE** – In addition to standard anticoagulation therapy, CVC should be removed after 3–5 days of treatment if clinically feasible. If CVC is required and still functioning, prophylactic dose of LMWH should be given to prevent recurrent VTE following therapeutic anticoagulation until CVC is removed. In children with ongoing but potentially reversible risk factors (e.g., nephrotic syndrome or Kawasaki), anticoagulant therapy is extended beyond 3 months until the risk factor has resolved [57].
- **Malignancy** – Management of thromboembolism in children with cancer needs special consideration because these patients typically have CVCs, are undergoing treatment with drugs that may affect anticoagulation decisions, and often need surgical procedures.
- **SLE** – Episodes of VTE in children with SLE are treated in similar manner as VTE due to other causes; however, some children may require prolonged or even lifelong anticoagulant therapy. The duration of therapy depends upon the persistent presence of antiphospholipid antibodies (aPL) and, to a lesser extent, the location of the thrombus. The most common approach in children with a first VTE is indefinite anticoagulant therapy as long as aPL are present. In children with recurrent VTE and aPL, lifelong anticoagulant therapy is recommended. Presence of lupus anticoagulants in plasma may interfere with the coagulation tests used to monitor heparin and VKA. If lupus anticoagulants interfere with aPTT, either an insensitive aPTT reagent or a heparin assay should be used to monitor heparin therapy. If lupus anticoagulants interfere with prothrombin time (PT), plasma concentration of prothrombin can be used to monitor VKA therapy [58].

Unprovoked VTE

VTE is considered unprovoked if there is no identifiable disorder or risk factor (including CVC) that predisposes the patient to thrombosis. Unprovoked thrombosis in children is rare. Children with unprovoked VTE should be screened for inherited thrombophilias (Fig. 4.2) [57, 70–72].

Treatment of unprovoked VTE is similar to that of provoked VTE, except the duration of treatment is longer (6–12 months rather than 3 months). Children with recurrent unprovoked VTE are treated indefinitely [57].

Figure 4.3 illustrates the therapeutic approach to children with active or remote VTE and to those with family history of venous thromboembolism.

The commonly used thrombophilia testing includes DNA-based PCR testing for factor V Leiden mutation as well as prothrombin gene mutation G20210A and pro-

Clinical condition	Recommendation	Impact
First CVC thrombosis	Not recommended	No change of treatment
Non-CVC-related	Considered	Impact on treatment duration
Recurrent with or without CVC or other risk factors	Strongly considered	Impact on treatment duration and counseling family members
Family history	Individualized	Adolescent females taking oral contraceptives
Acquired risk factors without VTE	Not recommended	No treatment offered

Fig. 4.2 Testing for inherited thrombophilia

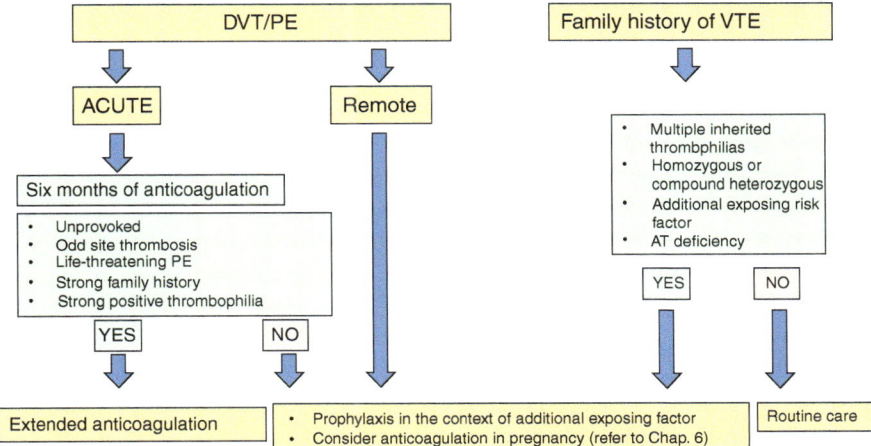

Fig. 4.3 Therapeutic approach to children with active or previous clots and those with family history of clotting

tein C, S, and AT deficiency testing by chromogenic or clotting assay which usually bears a strong association with thromboembolism. Testing for hyperhomocysteinemia or DNA testing for methyl tetrahydrofolate reductase confers a weak risk for thrombosis, whereas antiphospholipid antibody testing based on coagulation assay or ELISA testing for anticardiolipins or beta2 glycoproteins is associated with higher risks [10]. Details of the antiphospholipid syndrome are described in Chap. 8.

Blocked CVC When a CVC is blocked but no definite thrombus is identified, recombinant tissue plasminogen activator (tPA, alteplase) may be used to lyse intraluminal thrombus and restore catheter patency.

For this purpose, acceptable dosing regimens of recombinant tPA include:

- Children ≤10 kg – Alteplase 0.5 mg/mL; instill a volume equal to the internal volume of the lumen catheter (maximum 1 mL/lumen)
- Children >10 kg – Alteplase 1 mg/mL; instill a volume equal to the internal volume of the lumen catheter (maximum 2 mL/lumen)

After a dwell time of 1–2 hours, aspiration from the catheter should be attempted (the lumen should not be used until the tPA is withdrawn). If the first attempt is unsuccessful, the CVC may be treated with a second course of tPA [57, 59]. If the CVC remains blocked after two doses of tPA, an imaging study (ultrasound or contrast venography) should be performed to determine if there is a catheter-related thrombosis.

Prospective and retrospective studies in children have demonstrated that alteplase is safe and effective in the restoration of function to occluded CVC in infants and children [60–63].

Pulmonary Embolism

Treatment of pulmonary embolism (PE) includes initial administration of LMWH or UFH for 7–10 days and then long-term anticoagulation with either LMWH or VKA. For children with PE associated with a transient risk factor (e.g., surgery), anticoagulation therapy is continued for a minimum of 3 months; for unprovoked PE, the duration of treatment is 6 months [36, 64]. If VKA is chosen for long-term therapy, it can be started 1 or 2 days after initiation of therapeutic heparin.

The decision to use thrombolytic agents (e.g., tPA or urokinase) should be individualized and considered only in children with extensive and hemodynamically compromising PE [57]. Consultation with a pediatric hematologist is recommended.

Major vessel occlusion For infants and children with major vessel occlusion causing compromise of organs or limbs, systemic or catheter-directed thrombolytic therapy may be warranted [57]. Recombinant tPA (alteplase) is the thrombolytic agent used most commonly in children; urokinase (not available in the United States) is used infrequently.

Data on the efficacy, dose, and safety of thrombolytic agents in this setting are limited and indications for thrombolytic therapy remain highly individualized [57, 65–69]. Consultation with a vascular specialist and/or pediatric hematologist is suggested.

Thrombolytic therapy is not recommended in patients with right-to-left cardiac shunts because of the risk of arterial emboli to the central nervous system.

- **Systemic thrombolysis** – The optimal dose of recombinant tPA for systemic thrombolysis in children is not established. The available evidence is limited to case reports and single-institution case series. The doses used in these reports ranged from 0.1 to 0.6 mg/kg per hour for a duration of 6 hours [57]. Some patients may require a longer or shorter duration of therapy. Some experts suggest that a low-dose infusion of recombinant tPA (0.01–0.06 mg/kg per hour for up to 96 hours) may have a decreased incidence of major bleeding and can be considered [67, 69]. UFH therapy is typically discontinued or provided at a low dose (e.g., 10 units/kg per hour) during thrombolytic infusion.

- **Catheter-directed thrombolysis** – Catheter-directed thrombolysis refers to a low-dose infusion of recombinant tPA through a catheter with the tip situated within the thrombus. This approach may offer several advantages over systemic thrombolysis, including higher response rate and decreased rate of major bleeding complications [65]. The recommended dose for catheter-directed thrombolysis with recombinant tPA is 0.01 mg/kg per hour for 24 hours. UFH therapy is typically provided at a low dose (e.g., 10 units/kg per hour) during thrombolytic infusion.

- **Monitoring** – Routinely measure fibrinogen level prior to starting thrombolytic therapy. Fresh frozen plasma (FFP) should be administered to patients with low fibrinogen (<100 mg/dL) since the efficacy of thrombolytic agents is reduced in this setting. Endogenous plasminogen also is depleted by thrombolytic agents, an effect known as "plasminogen steal." Therefore, patients who are receiving thrombolytic therapy should have fibrinogen levels monitored every 6 hours and FFP should be provided for fibrinogen levels <100 mg/dL.

- **Prevention and management of bleeding** – The major complication of thrombolytic therapy is bleeding. Before thrombolytic therapy is initiated, any derangements that may increase the risk of bleeding (e.g., thrombocytopenia, vitamin K deficiency) should be corrected. In patients who are at high risk for bleeding, thrombolytic therapy should be avoided [66]. Mild hemorrhagic complications of thrombolytic therapy can be treated with local pressure and topical thrombin preparations. Major bleeding from a local site is managed by stopping thrombolytic therapy and administration of FFP or cryoprecipitate along with other blood products if necessary. If bleeding is life threatening, addition of an antifibrinolytic agent (e.g., aminocaproic acid) may help restore hemostasis.

VTE Prophylaxis

Prophylactic pharmacologic therapy is limited to children who have multiple risk factors for VTE [3, 17]. LMWH is generally the preferred agent for providing thromboprophylaxis in the acute setting (Fig. 4.6). Prophylactic doses for different LMWH agents in children are presented in Fig. 4.4.

For therapeutic treatment, the dose is adjusted as needed to achieve anti-factor Xa levels between 0.5 and 1 units/mL in samples taken 4–6 hours after the last subcutaneous injection. For prophylaxis, there is no need for monitoring or dose adjustment. All doses are given subcutaneously.

There are no established standards of practice regarding when to initiate thromboprophylaxis in hospitalized children; decisions are individualized based chiefly on the number and nature of underlying risk factors. Important predictors of VTE in this setting include critical illness, mechanical ventilation, systemic infection, hospitalization duration of ≥5 days, age (risk is higher among postpubertal adolescents), oral

Age-dependent dosage		<2 months	≥2 months
Enoxaparin	Initial	1.5 mg/kg/12 hours (can also use 1.75 mg/kg/dose for term infants and 2 mg/kg/dose for preterm)	1 mg/kg/12 hours (can also use 1.75 mg/kg/dose for term infants and 2 mg/kg/dose for preterm)
	Prophylactic	0.75 mg/kg/12 hours	0.5 mg/kg/12 hours
Tinzaparin	Initial	275 units/kg/24 hours	−2 to 12 months: 250 units/kg/24 hours −1 to 5 years: 240 units/kg/24 hours
	Prophylactic	Not applicable	Not applicable
Weight-adjusted dosage		<5 kg	≥5 kg
Dalteparin	Initial	129 ± 43 units/kg/24 hours	
	Prophylactic	92 ± 52 units/kg/24 hours	
Reviparin	Initial	150 units/kg/12 hours	100 units/kg/12 hours
	Prophylactic	50 units/kg/12 hours	30 units/kg/12 hours

Fig. 4.4 LMWH dose adjustment table [57, 70–72]

contraceptive use, known thrombophilia, prior history of VTE, severe obesity, surgery (particularly orthopedic surgery), trauma, and prolonged immobility [18–21].

Routine use of antithrombotic therapy is not recommended for the following groups of patients, unless there are additional clinically relevant risk factors (e.g., known inherited thrombophilia or history of prior VTE) [57]:

- Children with CVC
- Children with cancer and CVCs

When prophylactic LMWH is provided, it should be continued only so long as important clinically relevant risk factors persist. For example, an adolescent patient started on LMWH for risk factors including bloodstream infection, mechanical ventilation, CVC, and immobility can have prophylaxis discontinued once she/he is extubated, ambulating, and no longer bacteremic (note that the presence of a CVC alone is not a reason for continuing prophylaxis).

- Children with certain chronic conditions who have long-lasting risk of VTE may require long-term prophylactic antithrombotic therapy (typically with warfarin); this includes the following conditions [57]: children receiving long-term home *total parenteral nutrition* (TPN) [73, 74], children undergoing hemodialysis via an arteriovenous fistula or central venous access device [75], and children with certain types of cardiac disease (aspirin may be a reasonable alternative to anticoagulation in some of these patients except those with mechanical valve replacement). Cases include:

  - Univentricular heart following palliation with cavop
  - Severe cardiomyopathy
  - Pulmonary hypertension
  - Selected cases with congenital and infantile nephrotic syndrome

Secondary Prevention

For patients with a prior episode of provoked VTE, long-term antithrombotic therapy (at prophylactic or therapeutic doses) may be warranted if the patient has VTE risk factor(s) other than CVC that persist or recur. Indications include:

- Children with one of the chronic conditions requiring long-term primary prophylaxis, as listed above (long-term TPN dependency, hemodialysis dependency, certain forms of heart disease, congenital nephrotic syndrome). Inflammatory bowel disease, during a flare of the disease.
- SLE, during a flare of the disease and/or if there are persistent aPL. For children with a prior episode of unprovoked VTE who develop a second episode, treatment is continued indefinitely.

Anticoagulant agents The anticoagulant agents used most commonly in children include low-molecular-weight heparins (LMWH), unfractionated heparin (UFH), and vitamin K antagonists VKA (e.g., warfarin).

Low-Molecular-Weight Heparin

Advantages of LMWH LMWHs offer several advantages over UFH and vitamin K antagonists (VKA) and are particularly suited to the efficient and safe treatment of children with or at risk for VTE 10:

- **More predictable anticoagulant response** – *The superior bioavailability of LMWH*, longer half-life, and dose-independent clearance result in a more predictable anticoagulant response [76]. *Less laboratory monitoring and dose adjustment* – Because of the more predictable pharmacokinetics, LMWH therapy requires less laboratory monitoring and dose adjustment. By contrast, treatment with UFH and particularly VKA requires frequent monitoring and dose adjustment. *Less effect of diet (compared with VKA)* – Children's diets have a wide range of vitamin K intake which can impact the effectiveness of VKA. This is not a concern with LMWH or UFH.
- **Easier administration (compared with UFH)** – LMWHs can be administered subcutaneously, which is critically important for infants and young children with poor venous access. Subcutaneous catheters that can remain in place for 7 days can reduce the number of injections to as few as one per week [77].

Dose, monitoring, and adverse effects (For a full description of the pharmacological properties, refer to Chap. 1.)

Dose Guidelines for therapeutic and prophylactic dosing of LMWH (including enoxaparin, dalteparin, reviparin, and tinzaparin) in children are presented in the Fig. 4.4 [78–81].

The therapeutic dose of LMWH is age-dependent, with newborns having increased dose requirements per body weight compared with older children [82]. Higher doses may also be necessary in critically ill children [83]. Dose adjustment and close monitoring of anti-factor Xa levels are necessary in children with renal insufficiency. If renal insufficiency is severe, LMWH should be avoided.

Monitoring Monitoring of LMWH therapy is only possible using an anti-factor Xa assay and not by activated partial thromboplastin time (aPTT) values. The approach depends on whether the drug is used for treatment or prophylaxis:

- **Treatment** – Because of individual variation in responsiveness, patients receiving treatment doses of LMWH should be monitored periodically by checking anti-factor Xa levels. Samples should be taken 4–6 hours after the last subcutaneous injection; with this timing, the therapeutic range is between 0.5 and 1.0 units/mL.
- **Prophylaxis** – Laboratory monitoring is generally not necessary when LMWH is used at prophylactic dosing.

Adverse effects The risk of clinically significant bleeding in children treated with LMWH is approximately 2–3% [84].

In 1997 the Food and Drug Administration (FDA) Public Health Advisory drew awareness to the formation of spinal epidural hematomas following prophylactic LMWH in patients with epidural catheters. For children undergoing lumbar puncture, at least two scheduled doses of LMWH should be omitted prior to the procedure.

Other complications, including heparin-induced thrombocytopenia (HIT) and osteoporosis, are relatively rare with LMWH compared with UFH [85, 86].

Reversal If clinically significant bleeding occurs with LMWH therapy, *protamine sulfate* should be administered intravenously (IV) and will neutralize approximately 75% of the anti-factor Xa activity and reduce or eliminate bleeding [87]. The dose of protamine sulfate required is based upon the amount of the dose of LMWH received in the previous 3–4 hours; 1 mg protamine sulfate can inactivate 100 units of LMWH [88].

Unfractionated Heparin: Dose, Monitoring, and Adverse Effects

Dose

When UFH is used for treatment of VTE, therapy is typically initiated with a loading dose of 75 units/kg IV over 10 minutes. Boluses should be reduced or withheld for patients with significant bleeding risks (e.g., children recovering from a neurosurgical procedure or with other risks for intracranial bleeding). The loading dose is followed by a maintenance dose of UFH, which depends on the age of the patient [57, 88]:

- Infants – 28 units/kg per hour
- Children (≥1 year old) and adolescents – 20 units/kg per hour

The increased requirement for UFH in the young reflects a faster clearance of UFH, due to a larger volume of distribution [89, 90]. For children who are overweight or obese, one study suggests that actual body weight can be used to calculate the loading dose, up to a maximum of 5000 units/loading dose, and 1000/units/hour for the initial continuous infusion [91]. This maximum dose is consistent with the alternative dosing regimen used in adults [92].

Monitoring

UFH therapy in children is monitored by measuring anti-factor Xa activity; the target range for therapeutic heparinization is 0.35–0.7 units/mL [57]. aPTT testing can help with dose adjustments, but only after determining the aPTT range corresponding to the target anti-factor Xa activity range in the patient (Fig. 4.5).

1. UFH bolus dose: 75 units/kg IV over 10 minutes				
2. Initial maintenance dose Infants <1 year: 28 units/kg per hour Children 21 year: 20 units/kg per hour				
3. Adjust UFH to reach anti-factor Xa activity of 0.35–0.7 units/mL. Repeat test every 4 hours and then daily when two consecutive readings are in range In most children, this corresponds to a goal aPTT of 60–85 seconds aPTT testing can be used to help dose adjustments but only after determining the aPTT range corresponding to target anti-factor Xa range in the patient Initial testing is performed 4–6 hours after starting the infusion				
Anti-Xa (units/mL)	aPTT (seconds)	Bolus (units/kg)	Hold infusion (minutes)	Rate change
0.1	<50	50	0	Increased by 10%
0.11–0.34	50–59	0	0	Increased by 10%
0.35–0.7	60–85	0	0	No change
0.71–0.99	86–95	0	0	Decrease by 10%
1–1.19	96–120	0	30	Decrease by 10%
≥1.2	>120	0	60	Decrease by 15%
4. When anti-Xa/aPTT values are therapeutic, monitor anti-Xa/aPTT and CBC daily.				

Fig. 4.5 Protocol for systemic unfractionated heparin administration and adjustment for children

In infants and children, aPTT monitoring is not a reliable marker for therapeutic UFH levels because there are age variations in the mechanism of action of UFH [57, 88, 93–97].

UFH dosing strategies also should take into account the significance of the clot and the potential risk of bleeding in an individual patient [1, 95, 96].

UFH: unfractionated heparin; IV: intravenous, aPTT: activated partial thromboplastin time

If both anti-Xa activity and aPTT are monitored and there is a disconnect between the two values such that the aPTT is 150, yet the anti-Xa level is subtherapeutic, the UFH should not be increased to achieve the desired therapeutic anti-Xa level because it was reported that this has led to bleeding complications particularly in neonates [57, 97].

Adverse Effects

- **Bleeding**
- **Osteoporosis**
- **HIT**: HIT is caused by heparin-dependent antiplatelet antibodies. In children, HIT seems to be relatively uncommon [98–101] but should always be considered when other causes of thrombocytopenia have been excluded [102, 103]. If HIT is strongly suspected or confirmed, UFH therapy and all other forms of heparin (e.g., heparin flushes) should be stopped and another antithrombotic agent (e.g., argatroban, fondaparinux) employed if ongoing anticoagulation is necessary [79, 104].

Reversal Bleeding complications secondary to the use of UFH are usually controlled by termination of the infusion. If the bleeding is life threatening or immediate reversal is required, heparin can be neutralized rapidly by protamine sulfate given IV. The dose of protamine sulfate is based upon the amount of heparin received in the previous 2 hours; 1 mg of protamine sulfate inactivates 100 units of UFH [57]. For details on reversal, please refer to Chap. 13.

Vitamin K Antagonists: Dose, Monitoring, and Adverse Effects

Dose The initial dose of warfarin is 0.2 mg/kg orally (maximum 5 mg) [57]. In patients with mild liver dysfunction and/or elevated baseline prothrombin time, a lower initial dose should be used (e.g., 0.1 mg/kg). Warfarin should be avoided in patients with severe liver failure. A lower initial dose (0.1 mg/kg) is also appropriate when warfarin is used for VTE prophylaxis (e.g., after the Fontan procedure) [105].

1. Day 1 – If the baseline INR is 1.0–1.3, initial dose of warfarin is 0.2 mg/kg orally in a single dose	
2. Days 2–4 – Adjust warfarin dose according to INR	
INR 1.1–1.3	Keep same dose
INR 1.4–3	Reduce 50% of day 1 dose
INR 3.1–3.5	Reduce 75% of day 1 dose
INR > 3.5	Hold warfarin until INR < 3.5, then restart at 20% reduced dose
3. Maintenance dose according to INR	
INR 1.1–1.4	Increase dose by 20%
INR 1.5–1.9	Increase dose by 10%
INR 2–3	No change
INR 3.1–3.5	Decrease dose by 10%
INR > 3.5	Hold warfarin until INR < 3.5, then restart at 50% reduced dose

INR international normalized ratio
In patients with mild liver dysfunction and/or elevated baseline prothrombin time, a lower initial dose should be used (e.g., 0.1 mg/kg). Warfarin should be avoided in severe liver failure [57, 97].

Fig. 4.6 Suggested warfarin administration dosage and adjustment to keep INR between 2 and 3 for pediatric patients

Monitoring VKA therapy is monitored with the PT, which is reported as an international normalized ratio (INR) in order to assure comparability among various laboratories [106]. The therapeutic range for VKA therapy for treatment of VTE in children is typically an INR of 2.0–3.0; this range is largely based on recommendations for adults. Patients with mechanical heart valves should be treated according to adult recommendations, in which the target INR varies depending on valve position and type.

The INR should be checked daily until levels are in the target range for two or more consecutive days (Fig. 4.6). The interval between testing can be gradually increased if the INR remains stable. In the maintenance phase, the INR is typically checked every 1–2 weeks, depending on the child's clinical stability and age (more frequent testing may be necessary in young children).

Monitoring VKA therapy in children requires more frequent INR measurements and dose adjustments than in adult patients, because children's diets have a wide range of vitamin K intake. Diets with poor sources of vitamin K, such as breast milk, induce sensitivity to VKA. Diets supplemented with vitamin K, such as total parenteral nutrition (TPN) or nutrient formula, induce resistance to VKA [73, 105]. In addition, many children who are treated with VKA are taking other medications that can reduce absorption from the intestine or alter the metabolic clearance of VKA [57, 105].

Adverse effects The major side effect of VKA is bleeding. The risk of bleeding in children treated with VKAs appears to be low (i.e., <2%) [73, 75, 107].

Other side effects of VKA, such as tracheal calcification or hair loss, rarely are seen in children [65]. Teratogenic effects are a potential concern in adolescent females should pregnancy occur.

Reversal When reversal of VKA anticoagulation therapy is required, management consists of *vitamin K* administration with or without transfusion of *prothrombin complex concentrate* (PCC) or FFP.

- **Patients with active bleeding** – In patients with life-threatening bleeding (e.g., intracranial hemorrhage), IV vitamin K can be administered at a dose of 5–10 mg by slow infusion over 10–20 minutes in combination with infusion of PCC (50 units/kg). If PCC is not available, FFP (20 mL/kg) can be used. IV administration of recombinant factor VIIa also may be considered.
  In patients with clinically significant but not life-threatening bleeding, IV vitamin K can be administered at a dose of 0.5–2 mg in combination with transfusion of either PCC or FFP. Details of reversal are covered in Chap. 13.
- **Supratherapeutic INR without active bleeding** – For patients with an excessively elevated INR (e.g., >8) who lack active bleeding, we typically administer small doses of vitamin K (0.5–1 mg orally). The aim is to modestly improve the INR without fully reversing the effect. If the response is not adequate, larger doses (2–5 mg orally) can be given. Lower doses of vitamin K are preferred in patients who will require ongoing VKA therapy since larger doses can make the patient temporarily resistant to the further action of VKA.

Other anticoagulants Other anticoagulants include factor Xa inhibitors (fondaparinux, apixaban, and edoxaban) and direct thrombin inhibitors (argatroban, bivalirudin, and dabigatran). Data on these agents in pediatric patients are extremely limited [68, 69, 73–77]. Use of these agents in children is generally limited to patients with HIT who require cessation of heparin and ongoing anticoagulation with non-heparinoid agents (argatroban and fondaparinux are the agents most commonly used in this setting) [69, 73, 74, 77]. Otherwise, use of these agents in children is limited to clinical trials.

- **Rivaroxaban** Recent data point that treatment with bodyweight-adjusted rivaroxaban appears to be safe in children and will be evaluated in the EINSTEIN-Jr phase 3 trial.

- **Argatroban** Argatroban is a direct thrombin inhibitor approved in the USA and Canada for treatment of thrombosis in adult patients with HIT. Argatroban is eliminated by the liver, and dose reduction should be considered in patients with hepatic dysfunction. There is no available reversal agent for argatroban. *Bivalirudin* – Bivalirudin is another direct thrombin inhibitor that has been subjected to limited clinical trials in pediatric patients. *Fondaparinux* – Fondaparinux is a synthetic antithrombin-dependent inhibitor of factor Xa. *Direct oral anticoagulant (DOAC)* – Novel DOACs that are approved for use in adult patients include the direct thrombin inhibitor dabigatran and the factor Xa inhibitors rivaroxaban, apixaban, edoxaban.

Recurrence

- For pediatric patients with VTE, the risk of recurrence ranges from 7% to 20% [1, 20, 23, 108]. Recurrence risk depends on whether the thrombosis was provoked or unprovoked and the nature of underlying VTE risk factors.

- In children with provoked VTE (e.g., CVC-associated or due to an underlying medical condition), recurrence is uncommon if the underlying cause is removed or resolved.
- By contrast, a prothrombotic state does appear to be a predictor of VTE recurrence among children with unprovoked VTE. However, recurrence risk relating to prothrombotic state is uncertain in children <2 years old.

Postthrombotic syndrome   The postthrombotic syndrome (PTS) is a chronic complication of VTE. It is characterized by chronic venous insufficiency, with symptoms varying from mild edema to chronic pain and ulceration of the affected limb [109]. PTS occurs secondary to a combination of pathophysiologic mechanisms, including an initial inflammatory process within the involved vein, venous outflow obstruction, destruction of venous valves, and venous reflux [110, 111].

Diagnosis of PTS is primarily based upon clinical symptoms including localized edema, pain, alterations in skin temperature, differences in limb circumference, the presence of varicose veins, trophic skin changes (stasis dermatitis), and skin ulceration [112, 113]. Reported rates of PTS after VTE in children range from 10% to 70%; the considerable variation is due mostly to differences in the populations studied and the definition of PTS [19, 25, 114–118].

Mortality   The overall risk of mortality among pediatric patients with any type of VTE ranges from 8% to 17% [1, 3, 4, 23]; the risk for patients with PE is approximately 10–20% [37, 119]. However, these estimates are difficult to interpret since the majority of patients in these studies had associated chronic conditions (e.g., cancer, cardiac disease). In registry studies wherein the cause of death was ascertained, mortality as a direct result of thrombotic complications occurred in 2–4% of patients. The majority of VTE-related deaths in these studies were due to PE.

References

1. van Ommen CH, Heijboer H, Büller HR, et al. Venous thromboembolism in childhood: a prospective two-year registry in The Netherlands. J Pediatr. 2001;139:676.
2. Tuckuviene R, Christensen AL, Helgestad J, et al. Pediatric venous and arterial noncerebral thromboembolism in Denmark: a nationwide population-based study. J Pediatr. 2011;159:663.
3. Raffini L, Huang YS, Witmer C, Feudtner C. Dramatic increase in venous thromboembolism in children's hospitals in the United States from 2001 to 2007. Pediatrics. 2009;124:1001.
4. Setty BA, O'Brien SH, Kerlin BA. Pediatric venous thromboembolism in the United States: a tertiary care complication of chronic diseases. Pediatr Blood Cancer. 2012;59:258.
5. Takemoto CM, Sohi S, Desai K, et al. Hospital-associated venous thromboembolism in children: incidence and clinical characteristics. J Pediatr. 2014;164:332.
6. Andrew M, Vegh P, Johnston M, et al. Maturation of the hemostatic system during childhood. Blood. 1992;80:1998.
7. Massicotte P, Leaker M, Marzinotto V, et al. Enhanced thrombin regulation during warfarin therapy in children compared to adults. Thromb Haemost. 1998;80:570.
8. Mitchell L, Piovella F, Ofosu F, Andrew M. Alpha-2-macroglobulin may provide protection from thromboembolic events in antithrombin III-deficient children. Blood. 1991;78:2299.

9. Virchow R. Phlogose und Thrombose im Gefässsystem. In: Virchow R, editor. Gesammelte Abhandlungen zur Wissenschaftli chen Medizin. Frankfurt: Meidinger Sohn & Comp; 1856. p. 458.
10. Albisetti M, Anthony KC. Venous thrombosis and thromboembolism in children -risk-factors-clinical-manifestations-and-diagnosis: Uptodate; 2018.
11. Kuhle S, Massicotte P, Chan A, et al. Systemic thromboembolism in children. Data from the 1-800-NOCLOTS Consultation Service. Thromb Haemost. 2004;92:722.
12. Massicotte MP, Dix D, Monagle P, et al. Central venous catheter related thrombosis in children: analysis of the Canadian Registry of Venous Thromboembolic Complications. J Pediatr. 1998;133:770.
13. Worly JM, Fortenberry JD, Hansen I, et al. Deep venous thrombosis in children with diabetic ketoacidosis and femoral central venous catheters. Pediatrics. 2004;113:e57.
14. Nowak-Göttl U, Dübbers A, Kececioglu D, et al. Factor V Leiden, protein C, and lipoprotein (a) in catheter related thrombosis in childhood: a prospective study. J Pediatr. 1997;131:608.
15. Bonduel M, Hepner M, Sciuccati G, et al. Prothrombotic abnormalities in children with venous thromboembolism. J Pediatr Hematol Oncol. 2000;22:66.
16. Bonduel M, Hepner M, Sciuccati G, et al. Factor V Leiden and prothrombin gene G20210A mutation in children with venous thromboembolism. Thromb Haemost. 2002;87:972.
17. Lawson SE, Butler D, Enayat MS, Williams MD. Congenital thrombophilia and thrombosis: a study in a single centre. Arch Dis Child. 1999;81:176.
18. van Ommen CH, Peters M. Venous thromboembolic disease in childhood. Semin Thromb Hemost. 2003;29:391.
19. van Ommen CH, Heijboer H, van den Dool EJ, et al. Pediatric venous thromboembolic disease in one single center: congenital prothrombotic disorders and the clinical outcome. J Thromb Haemost. 2003;1:2516.
20. Revel-Vilk S, Chan A, Bauman M, Massicotte P. Prothrombotic conditions in an unselected cohort of children with venous thromboembolic disease. J Thromb Haemost. 2003;1:915.
21. Neshat-Vahid S, Pierce R, Hersey D, et al. Association of thrombophilia and catheter-associated thrombosis in children: a systematic review and meta-analysis. J Thromb Haemost. 2016;14:1749.
22. Nguyen GC, Bernstein CN, Bitton A, et al. Consensus statements on the risk, prevention, and treatment of venous thromboembolism in inflammatory bowel disease: Canadian Association of Gastroenterology. Gastroenterology. 2014;146:835.
23. Andrew M, David M, Adams M, et al. Venous thromboembolic complications (VTE) in children: first analyses of the Canadian Registry of VTE. Blood. 1994;83:1251.
24. Levy DM, Massicotte MP, Harvey E, et al. Thromboembolism in paediatric lupus patients. Lupus. 2003;12:741.
25. Monagle P, Adams M, Mahoney M, et al. Outcome of pediatric thromboembolic disease: a report from the Canadian Childhood Thrombophilia Registry. Pediatr Res. 2000;47:763.
26. Journeycake JM, Buchanan GR. Catheter-related deep venous thrombosis and other catheter complications in children with cancer. J Clin Oncol. 2006;24:4575.
27. Marie I, Lévesque H, Cailleux N, et al. [Deep venous thrombosis of the upper limbs. Apropos of 49 cases]. Rev Med Interne. 1998;19:399.
28. Mulvihill SJ, Fonkalsrud EW. Complications of superior versus inferior vena cava occlusion in infants receiving central total parenteral nutrition. J Pediatr Surg. 1984;19:752.
29. Rockoff MA, Gang DL, Vacanti JP. Fatal pulmonary embolism following removal of a central venous catheter. J Pediatr Surg. 1984;19:307.
30. Derish MT, Smith DW, Frankel LR. Venous catheter thrombus formation and pulmonary embolism in children. Pediatr Pulmonol. 1995;20:349.
31. Pipe S, Goldenberg N. Acquired disorders of hemostasis. In: Orkin SH, Fisher DE, Ginsburg D, Look AT, Lux SE, Nathan DG, editors. Nathan and Oski's hematology and oncology of infancy and childhood, vol. 1. 8th ed. Philadelphia: Saunder; 2015. p. 1103.

32. Byard RW, Cutz E. Sudden and unexpected death in infancy and childhood due to pulmonary thromboembolism. An autopsy study. Arch Pathol Lab Med. 1990;114:142.
33. Matthew DJ, Levin M. Pulmonary thromboembolism in children. Intensive Care Med. 1986;12:404.
34. Agha BS, Sturm JJ, Simon HK, Hirsh DA. Pulmonary embolism in the pediatric emergency department. Pediatrics. 2013;132:663.
35. Andrew M, Monagle P, Brooker LA. Thromboembolic complications during infancy and childhood. Hamilton: BC Decker Inc; 2000.
36. Biss TT, Brandão LR, Kahr WH, et al. Clinical features and outcome of pulmonary embolism in children. Br J Haematol. 2008;142:808.
37. Biss TT, Brandão LR, Kahr WH, et al. Clinical probability score and D-dimer estimation lack utility in the diagnosis of childhood pulmonary embolism. J Thromb Haemost. 2009;7:1633.
38. Hancock HS, Wang M, Gist KM, et al. Cardiac findings and long-term thromboembolic outcomes following pulmonary embolism in children: a combined retrospective-prospective inception cohort study. Cardiol Young. 2013;23:344.
39. Buck JR, Connors RH, Coon WW, et al. Pulmonary embolism in children. J Pediatr Surg. 1981;16:385.
40. Goldsby RE, Saulys AJ, Helton JG. Pediatric pulmonary artery thromboembolism: an illustrative case. Pediatr Emerg Care. 1996;12:105.
41. Tinaztepe K, Buyan N, Tinaztepe B, Akkök N. The association of nephrotic syndrome and renal vein thrombosis: a clinicopathological analysis of eight pediatric patients. Turk J Pediatr. 1989;31:1.
42. Chugh KS, Malik N, Uberoi HS, et al. Renal vein thrombosis in nephrotic syndrome–a prospective study and review. Postgrad Med J. 1981;57:566.
43. Harmon WE, Stablein D, Alexander SR, Tejani A. Graft thrombosis in pediatric renal transplant recipients. A report of the North American Pediatric Renal Transplant Cooperative Study. Transplantation. 1991;51:406.
44. Brandão LR, Simpson EA, Lau KK. Neonatal renal vein thrombosis. Semin Fetal Neonatal Med. 2011;16:323.
45. Brady L, Magilavy D, Black DD. Portal vein thrombosis associated with antiphospholipid antibodies in a child. J Pediatr Gastroenterol Nutr. 1996;23:470.
46. Arav-Boger R, Reif S, Bujanover Y. Portal vein thrombosis caused by protein C and protein S deficiency associated with cytomegalovirus infection. J Pediatr. 1995;126:586.
47. Skarsgard E, Doski J, Jaksic T, et al. Thrombosis of the portal venous system after splenectomy for pediatric hematologic disease. J Pediatr Surg. 1993;28:1109.
48. Arnold KE, Char G, Serjeant GR. Portal vein thrombosis in a child with homozygous sickle-cell disease. West Indian Med J. 1993;42:27.
49. Harper PL, Edgar PF, Luddington RJ, et al. Protein C deficiency and portal thrombosis in liver transplantation in children. Lancet. 1988;2:924.
50. Brisse H, Orbach D, Lassau N, et al. Portal vein thrombosis during antineoplastic chemotherapy in children: report of five cases and review of the literature. Eur J Cancer. 2004;40:2659.
51. Stringer MD, Marshall MM, Muiesan P, et al. Survival and outcome after hepatic artery thrombosis complicating pediatric liver transplantation. J Pediatr Surg. 2001;36:888.
52. Williams S, Chan AK. Neonatal portal vein thrombosis: diagnosis and management. Semin Fetal Neonatal Med. 2011;16:329.
53. Chalmers E, Ganesen V, Liesner R, et al. Guideline on the investigation, management and prevention of venous thrombosis in children. Br J Haematol. 2011;154:196.
54. Male C, Chait P, Ginsberg JS, et al. Comparison of venography and ultrasound for the diagnosis of asymptomatic deep vein thrombosis in the upper body in children: results of the PARKAA study. Prophylactic Antithrombin Replacement in Kids with ALL treated with Asparaginase. Thromb Haemost. 2002;87:593.
55. Tang CX, Schoepf UJ, Chowdhury SM, et al. Multidetector computed tomography pulmonary angiography in childhood acute pulmonary embolism. Pediatr Radiol. 2015;45:1431.

56. Monagle P, Cuello CA, Augustine C, Bonduel M, Brandão LR, Capman T, et al. American Society of Hematology 2018 Guidelines for management of venous thromboembolism: treatment of pediatric venous thromboembolism. Blood Adv. 2018;2:3292–316.
57. Monagle P, Chan AK, Goldenberg NA, et al. Antithrombotic therapy in neonates and children: Antithrombotic Therapy and Prevention of Thrombosis, 9th ed: American College of Chest Physicians Evidence-Based Clinical Practice Guidelines. Chest. 2012;141:e737S.
58. Andrew M, Monagle P, Brooker LA. Thromboembolic complications during infancy and childhood. Hamilton: BC Dekker Inc; 2000.
59. Choi M, Massicotte MP, Marzinotto V, et al. The use of alteplase to restore patency of central venous lines in pediatric patients: a cohort study. J Pediatr. 2001;139:152.
60. Blaney M, Shen V, Kerner JA, et al. Alteplase for the treatment of central venous catheter occlusion in children: results of a prospective, open-label, single-arm study (The Cathflo Activase Pediatric Study). J Vasc Interv Radiol. 2006;17:1745.
61. Shen V, Li X, Murdock M, et al. Recombinant tissue plasminogen activator (alteplase) for restoration of function to occluded central venous catheters in pediatric patients. J Pediatr Hematol Oncol. 2003;25:38.
62. Chesler L, Feusner JH. Use of tissue plasminogen activator (rt-PA) in young children with cancer and dysfunctional central venous catheters. J Pediatr Hematol Oncol. 2002;24:653.
63. Terrill KR, Lemons RS, Goldsby RE. Safety, dose, and timing of reteplase in treating occluded central venous catheters in children with cancer. J Pediatr Hematol Oncol. 2003;25:864.
64. Kearon C, Akl EA, Comerota AJ, et al. Antithrombotic therapy for VTE disease: Antithrombotic Therapy and Prevention of Thrombosis, 9th ed: American College of Chest Physicians Evidence-Based Clinical Practice Guidelines. Chest. 2012;141:e419S.
65. Manco-Johnson MJ, Grabowski EF, Hellgreen M, et al. Recommendations for tPA thrombolysis in children. On behalf of the Scientific Subcommittee on Perinatal and Pediatric Thrombosis of the Scientific and Standardization Committee of the International Society of Thrombosis and Haemostasis. Thromb Haemost. 2002;88:157.
66. Albisetti M. Thrombolytic therapy in children. Thromb Res. 2006;118:95.
67. Wang M, Hays T, Balasa V, et al. Low-dose tissue plasminogen activator thrombolysis in children. J Pediatr Hematol Oncol. 2003;25:379.
68. Gupta AA, Leaker M, Andrew M, et al. Safety and outcomes of thrombolysis with tissue plasminogen activator for treatment of intravascular thrombosis in children. J Pediatr. 2001;139:682.
69. Goldenberg NA, Durham JD, Knapp-Clevenger R, Manco-Johnson MJ. A thrombolytic regimen for high-risk deep venous thrombosis may substantially reduce the risk of postthrombotic syndrome in children. Blood. 2007;110:45.
70. Malowany JL, Monagle P, Knoppert DC, et al. Enoxaparin for neonatal thrombosis: a call for a higher dose for neonates. Thromb Res. 2008;122:826.
71. Sanchez de Toledo J, Gunawardena S, Munoz R, et al. Do neonates, infants and young children need a higher dose of enoxaparin in the cardiac intensive care unit. Cardiol Young. 2010;20:138.
72. Richard AA, Kim S, Moffett BS, et al. Comparison of anti-Xa levels in obese and non-obese pediatric patients receiving treatment doses of enoxaparin. J Pediatr. 2012;162:293.
73. Newall F, Barnes C, Savoia H, et al. Warfarin therapy in children who require long-term total parenteral nutrition. Pediatrics. 2003;112:e386.
74. Vegting IL, Tabbers MM, Benninga MA, et al. Prophylactic anticoagulation decreases catheter-related thrombosis and occlusion in children with home parenteral nutrition. JPEN J Parenter Enteral Nutr. 2012;36:456.
75. Paglialonga F, Artoni A, Braham S, et al. Vitamin K antagonists in children with central venous catheter on chronic haemodialysis: a pilot study. Pediatr Nephrol. 2016;31:827.
76. Albisetti M, Andrew M. Low molecular weight heparin in children. Eur J Pediatr. 2002;161:71.
77. Young E, Wells P, Holloway S, et al. Ex-vivo and in-vitro evidence that low molecular weight heparins exhibit less binding to plasma proteins than unfractionated heparin. Thromb Haemost. 1994;71:300.

78. Massicotte P, Adams M, Marzinotto V, et al. Low-molecular-weight heparin in pediatric patients with thrombotic disease: a dose finding study. J Pediatr. 1996;128:313.
79. Massicotte P, Julian JA, Marzinotto V, et al. Dose-finding and pharmacokinetic profiles of prophylactic doses of a low molecular weight heparin (reviparin sodium) in pediatric patients. Thromb Res. 2003;109:93.
80. Nohe N, Flemmer A, Rümler R, et al. The low molecular weight heparin dalteparin for prophylaxis and therapy of thrombosis in childhood: a report on 48 cases. Eur J Pediatr. 1999;158(Suppl 3):S134.
81. Revel-Vilk S, Chan AK. Anticoagulation therapy in children. Semin Thromb Hemost. 2003;29:425.
82. Kuhle S, Massicotte P, Dinyari M, et al. Dose-finding and pharmacokinetics of therapeutic doses of tinzaparin in pediatric patients with thromboembolic events. Thromb Haemost. 2005;94:1164.
83. Schloemer NJ, Abu-Sultaneh S, Hanson SJ, et al. Higher doses of low-molecular-weight heparin (enoxaparin) are needed to achieve target anti-Xa concentrations in critically ill children. Pediatr Crit Care Med. 2014;15:e294.
84. Bidlingmaier C, Kenet G, Kurnik K, et al. Safety and efficacy of low molecular weight heparins in children: a systematic review of the literature and metaanalysis of single-arm studies. Semin Thromb Hemost. 2011;37:814.
85. Melissari E, Parker CJ, Wilson NV, et al. Use of low molecular weight heparin in pregnancy. Thromb Haemost. 1992;68:652.
86. Warkentin TE, Levine MN, Hirsh J, et al. Heparin-induced thrombocytopenia in patients treated with low-molecular-weight heparin or unfractionated heparin. N Engl J Med. 1995;332:1330.
87. Van Ryn-McKenna J, Cai L, Ofosu FA, et al. Neutralization of enoxaparine-induced bleeding by protamine sulfate. Thromb Haemost. 1990;63:271.
88. Ignjatovic V, Summerhayes R, Than J, et al. Therapeutic range for unfractionated heparin therapy: age-related differences in response in children. J Thromb Haemost. 2006;4:2280.
89. Andrew M, Ofosu F, Schmidt B, et al. Heparin clearance and ex vivo recovery in newborn piglets and adult pigs. Thromb Res. 1988;52:517.
90. McDonald MM, Jacobson LJ, Hay WW Jr, Hathaway WE. Heparin clearance in the newborn. Pediatr Res. 1981;15:1015.
91. Taylor BN, Bork SJ, Kim S, et al. Evaluation of weight-based dosing of unfractionated heparin in obese children. J Pediatr. 2013;163:150.
92. Guyatt GH, Akl EA, Crowther M, et al. Executive summary: Antithrombotic Therapy and Prevention of Thrombosis, 9th ed: American College of Chest Physicians Evidence-Based Clinical Practice Guidelines. Chest. 2012;141:7S.
93. Schechter T, Finkelstein Y, Ali M, et al. Unfractionated heparin dosing in young infants: clinical outcomes in a cohort monitored with anti-factor Xa levels. J Thromb Haemost. 2012;10:368.
94. Hanslik A, Kitzmüller E, Tran US, et al. Monitoring unfractionated heparin in children: a parallel-cohort randomized controlled trial comparing 2 dose protocols. Blood. 2015;126:2091.
95. Andrew M, Marzinotto V, Massicotte P, et al. Heparin therapy in pediatric patients: a prospective cohort study. Pediatr Res. 1994;35:78.
96. Newall F, Johnston L, Ignjatovic V, Monagle P. Unfractionated heparin therapy in infants and children. Pediatrics. 2009;123:e510.
97. Trucco M, Lehmann CU, Mollenkopf N, et al. Retrospective cohort study comparing activated partial thromboplastin time versus anti-factor Xa activity nomograms for therapeutic unfractionated heparin monitoring in pediatrics. J Thromb Haemost. 2015;13:788.
98. Newall F, Barnes C, Ignjatovic V, Monagle P. Heparin-induced thrombocytopenia in children. J Paediatr Child Health. 2003;39:289.
99. Schmugge M, Risch L, Huber AR, et al. Heparin-induced thrombocytopenia-associated thrombosis in pediatric intensive care patients. Pediatrics. 2002;109:E10.

100. Severin T, Sutor AH. Heparin-induced thrombocytopenia in pediatrics. Semin Thromb Hemost. 2001;27:293.
101. Klenner AF, Lubenow N, Raschke R, Greinacher A. Heparin-induced thrombocytopenia in children: 12 new cases and review of the literature. Thromb Haemost. 2004;91:719.
102. Warkentin TE. Heparin-induced thrombocytopenia. Pathogenesis, frequency, avoidance and management. Drug Saf. 1997;17:325.
103. Warkentin TE, Chong BH, Greinacher A. Heparin-induced thrombocytopenia: towards consensus. Thromb Haemost. 1998;79:1.
104. Wilhelm MJ, Schmid C, Kececioglu D, et al. Cardiopulmonary bypass in patients with heparin-induced thrombocytopenia using Org 10172. Ann Thorac Surg. 1996;61:920.
105. Streif W, Andrew M, Marzinotto V, et al. Analysis of warfarin therapy in pediatric patients: a prospective cohort study of 319 patients. Blood. 1999;94:3007.
106. Ansell J, Hirsh J, Hylek E, et al. Pharmacology and management of the vitamin K antagonists: American College of Chest Physicians Evidence-Based Clinical Practice Guidelines (8th Edition). Chest. 2008;133:160S.
107. Moffett BS, Kim S, Bomgaars LR. Readmissions for warfarin-related bleeding in pediatric patients after hospital discharge. Pediatr Blood Cancer. 2013;60:1503.
108. Nowak-Göttl U, Junker R, Kreuz W, et al. Risk of recurrent venous thrombosis in children with combined prothrombotic risk factors. Blood. 2001;97:858.
109. Prandoni P, Lensing AW, Prins MR. The natural history of deep-vein thrombosis. Semin Thromb Hemost. 1997;23:185.
110. Thulesius O. The pathophysiology of post-thrombotic syndrome. Wien Med Wochenschr. 1994;144:196.
111. Immelman EJ, Jeffery PC. The postphlebitic syndrome. Pathophysiology, prevention and management. Clin Chest Med. 1984;5:537.
112. Goldenberg NA, Brandão L, Journeycake J, et al. Definition of post-thrombotic syndrome following lower extremity deep venous thrombosis and standardization of outcome measurement in pediatric clinical investigations. J Thromb Haemost. 2012;10:477.
113. Revel-Vilk S, Brandão LR, Journeycake J, et al. Standardization of post-thrombotic syndrome definition and outcome assessment following upper venous system thrombosis in pediatric practice. J Thromb Haemost. 2012;10:2182.
114. Kuhle S, Koloshuk B, Marzinotto V, et al. A cross-sectional study evaluating post-thrombotic syndrome in children. Thromb Res. 2003;111:227.
115. van Ommen CH, Ottenkamp J, Lam J, et al. The risk of postthrombotic syndrome in children with congenital heart disease. J Pediatr. 2002;141:582.
116. Spentzouris G, Gasparis A, Scriven RJ, et al. Natural history of deep vein thrombosis in children. Phlebology. 2015;30:412.
117. Avila ML, Pullenayegum E, Williams S, et al. Post-thrombotic syndrome and other outcomes of lower extremity deep vein thrombosis in children. Blood. 2016;128(14):1862–9.
118. Goldenberg NA, Donadini MP, Kahn SR, et al. Post-thrombotic syndrome in children: a systematic review of frequency of occurrence, validity of outcome measures, and prognostic factors. Haematologica. 2010;95:1952.
119. Dijk FN, Curtin J, Lord D, Fitzgerald DA. Pulmonary embolism in children. Paediatr Respir Rev. 2012;13:112.

Chapter 5
Cancer-Associated Thrombosis (CAT)

Mohamed Elemary, Otto Moodley, Derek Pearson, and Hadi Goubran

Abbreviation

ASCO	American Society of Clinical Oncology
CAT	Cancer-associated thrombosis
CVC	Central venous catheter
DOACs	Direct oral anticoagulants
DVT	Deep vein thrombosis
LMWH	Low-molecular-weight heparin
NCCN	National Comprehensive Cancer Network
PE	Pulmonary embolism
SSPE	Sub-segmental PE
UFH	Unfractionated heparin
VTE	Venous thromboembolism

Historic Background

The year 2017 marked the 150th anniversary of the publication of the renowned French professor Armand Trousseau (*Phlegmasia Alba Dolens*) [1] in which he described superficial thrombophlebitis (Fig. 5.1) as a forewarning sign of occult visceral malignancy [2]. Coincidentally, he developed a similar finding in himself and died. The term *Trousseau syndrome* was extended to include any thrombosis occurring in the context of malignancy. Interestingly, a similar observation was reported by Bouillard earlier in the nineteenth century [3].

M. Elemary (✉) · O. Moodley · D. Pearson · H. Goubran
Saskatoon Cancer Centre, College of Medicine, University of Saskatchewan, Saskatoon, SK, Canada
e-mail: Mohamed.elemary@saskcancer.ca; Otto.moodley@saskacancer.ca; Derek.pearson@saskcancer.ca; Hadi.goubran@saskcancer.ca

© Springer Nature Switzerland AG 2020
H. Goubran et al. (eds.), *Precision Anticoagulation Medicine*,
https://doi.org/10.1007/978-3-030-25782-8_5

Fig. 5.1 Superficial
thrombophlebitis affecting
the lower extremities

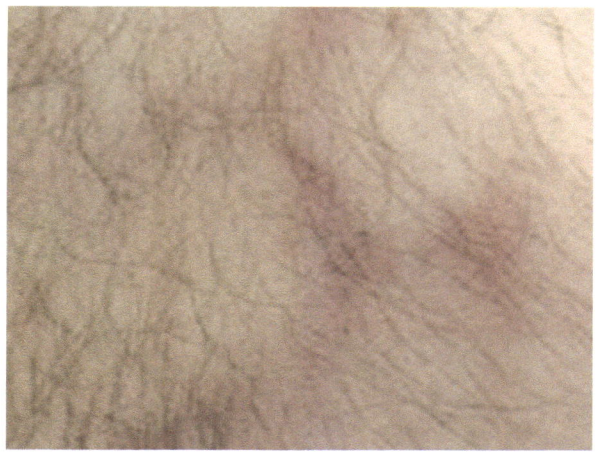

The Amplitude of the Problem

It is widely accepted that cancer is associated with a fourfold increased risk of clot formation. This risk is increased to 6.5-fold when chemotherapy is administered and to 19.8-fold in the presence of metastasis. Combining these estimates with the estimates of venous thromboembolism in the general population (roughly 1/1000), one can assume that the incidence of VTE in cancer patients is in the range of 1/200 [4–6]. Although Horsted et al. estimated that VTE occurs in even greater than 1% of cancer patients each year, this varies widely by cancer type and time since diagnosis [7] with around 20% of VTEs occurring in patients suffering from cancer [5].

Horsted et al. (2012) dissected this association based on the cancer type (Fig. 5.2), pancreatic and brain cancers being on top of the list with breast and prostate being less influential in causing VTE [7].

Patients with cancer who develop VTE have reduced life expectancy. On the basis of long-term, follow-up data of *thrombosis-related mortality*, those with cancer have a four- to eightfold higher risk of dying after an acute thrombotic event than patients without cancer [8, 9]. Furthermore, on the basis of follow-up data of *direct cancer-related mortality*, Sørensen and colleagues demonstrated that the survival of patients with cancer and VTE was 12% compared to 36% (threefold) in those without VTE ($P < 0.001$) when matched for type of cancer, sex, age, and the year of diagnosis [10]. Therefore, it seems evident that VTE represents the second leading cause of death in cancer patients [5].

Furthermore, unprovoked venous thromboembolism [VTE] may be the earliest sign of cancer [11–13]; based on retrospective data, up to 10% of patients with unprovoked venous thromboembolism will receive a diagnosis of cancer in the first year after their VTE [13]. In a very recent meta-analysis, occult cancer was detected in 1:20 patients within 1 year of receiving the diagnosis of unprovoked VTE, older age being associated with higher prevalence (>10% at 80) [14]. Newer prospective

Cancer site   IRR (95% CI)

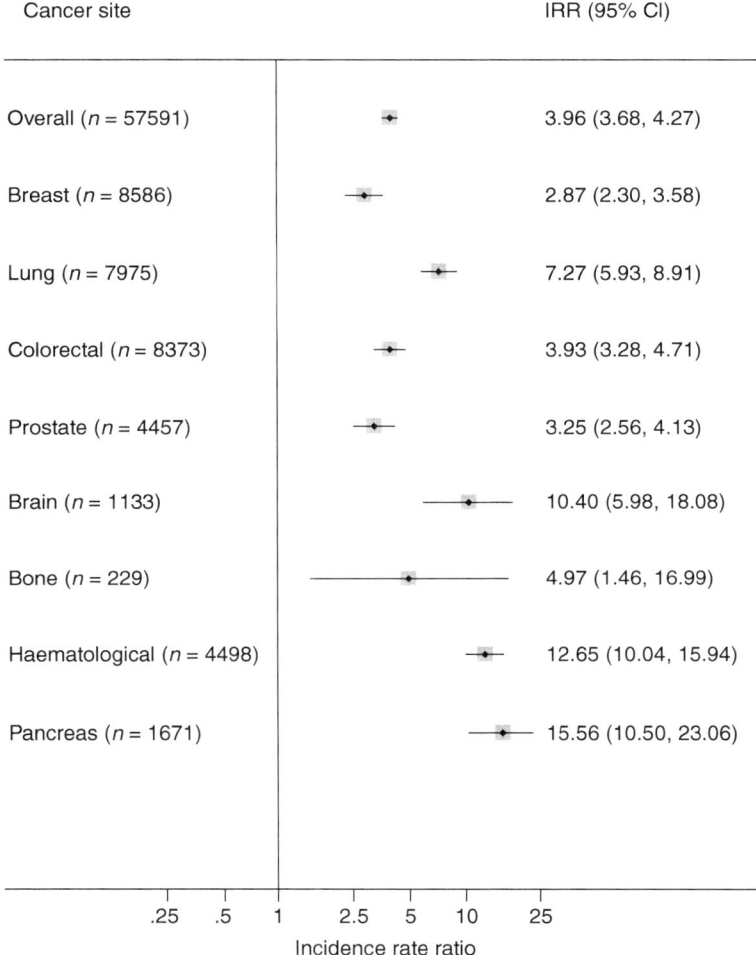

Overall (n = 57591)	3.96 (3.68, 4.27)
Breast (n = 8586)	2.87 (2.30, 3.58)
Lung (n = 7975)	7.27 (5.93, 8.91)
Colorectal (n = 8373)	3.93 (3.28, 4.71)
Prostate (n = 4457)	3.25 (2.56, 4.13)
Brain (n = 1133)	10.40 (5.98, 18.08)
Bone (n = 229)	4.97 (1.46, 16.99)
Haematological (n = 4498)	12.65 (10.04, 15.94)
Pancreas (n = 1671)	15.56 (10.50, 23.06)

.25   .5   1   2.5   5   10   25

Incidence rate ratio

Fig. 5.2 Association between different types of cancer and thrombosis (Horsted et al. [7])

data, however, are putting these numbers into question. Given this relationship between unprovoked VTE and cancer, it is appealing for clinicians to screen their patients with a first episode of acute unprovoked VTE for potential occult malignancy. Five different studies have compared limited (thorough history and physical exam, basic bloodwork) to more extensive occult cancer screening strategies. Extensive screening strategies do not seem to diagnose more occult cancers or improve cancer-related mortality [15] suggesting that an age-appropriate routine screening is the wisest and cost-economic approach.

In a post hoc analysis of a systematic review and individual patient data meta-analysis of adults with unprovoked VTE with at least 12 months of follow-up, cancer types were grouped according to thoracic, abdominopelvic, or other locations. The pooled 12-month period prevalence of cancer in DVT only, PE only, and DVT + PE was 5.6% (95% CI, 4.4–7.2), 4.3% (95% CI, 2.7–6.9), and 5.6% (95% CI, 1.7–15.5), respectively. Most occult cancers were located in the abdomen (68.4%). There was no relationship between VTE type and cancer location [16].

Challenges in Treating CAT

Cancer patients with clots present with specific therapeutic challenges as they have a five- to sixfold risk of bleeding from the burden of cancer and end-organ damage as well as due to the presence of concomitant thrombocytopenia resulting from chemotherapy or bone marrow infiltration. The cumulative incidence of recurrent thromboembolism in these patients is also higher, reported at 20.7% versus 6.8% in patients without cancer [17, 18]. Higher recurrence rates were reported reaching 40% and 10% in the first and second month, respectively.

Cancer patients with a diagnosis of incidental VTE observed on routine imaging are therapeutically challenging. The standardization committee of the International Society on Thrombosis and Haemostasis issued a guidance statement recommending and addressing this issue from both the diagnostic and therapeutic perspective [19]. Incidental VTE was reported to be ranging between 33% and 50% [20, 21].

1. Careful review of history to exclude symptomatic VTE.
2. In patients with incidental PE involving the main, lobar, segmental, or multiple subsegmental pulmonary arteries, no further testing is required to confirm the diagnosis.
3. In patients with isolated SSPE, a careful review of the images by radiologists and compression ultrasonography of the lower limbs are required to detect concomitant incidental DVT.
4. In patients with incidental iliofemoral DVT on CT of the abdomen and pelvis, confirming the diagnosis with Doppler ultrasonography of the pelvis and compression ultrasonography of the lower limbs is needed.

Furthermore, breakthrough thrombosis risk is amplified by a magnitude of 5 [16, 17]. The use of antiangiogenic chemotherapy combined with surgery and insertion of central lines and catheters adds to the risks of clotting and to the challenges.

The cross-talk between cancer and thrombosis is triggered by activation of platelets with a reciprocal interaction, whereby platelets fuel cancer growth with subsequent microparticle formation and activation of coagulation [22–25].

Therapeutic Approach to CAT

Prophylaxis of CAT

In Ambulatory Patients

Thromboprophylaxis should not be used routinely in outpatients with cancer but might be considered in individuals at very high thrombotic risk.

Identification of these high-risk patients can be aided by the use of risk assessment scores, such as that developed by Khorana et al. [26, 27] which identifies as higher-risk patients based on:

- Type of cancer with stomach, pancreas, lung, gynecological, bladder, testicular cancer, or lymphoma as high-risk
- The presence of a platelet count >350 × 109/L
- The presence of hemoglobin concentration <100 g/L
- The presence of leucocyte count pre-chemotherapy >11 × 109/L
- A body mass index of >35 kg/m^2

Alternatively, an international practice guideline, while also not recommending routine prophylaxis, suggests consideration in patients with locally advanced or metastatic pancreatic and lung cancer who are not deemed at excessive risk for bleeding.

The clinical benefit of all risk scores remains uncertain since they have not been thoroughly evaluated in randomized controlled trials of risk-adapted thromboprophylaxis.

Therefore, it seems reasonable to consider the following approach for prophylaxis for cancer patients not in hospital:

LMWH

(a) In outpatients with cancer who have no additional risk factors for VTE, we suggest against routine prophylaxis with LMWH, low-dose UFH, or vitamin K antagonists.

(b) In outpatients with solid tumors who have additional risk factors for VTE and who are at low risk of bleeding, prophylactic dose LMWH or low-dose UH should be considered.

Additional risk factors for venous thrombosis in cancer outpatients:
- Previous venous thrombosis
- Immobilization
- Angiogenesis inhibitors (e.g., bevacizumab (Avastin®))
- Regimens containing thalidomide, lenalidomide, or pomalidomide
- Metastatic pancreatic cancer
- Metastatic lung cancer
- Hormonal therapy (?)

DOACs as Thromboprophylaxis Agents in the Ambulatory Setting

Rivaroxaban

In high-risk ambulatory patients with cancer (Khorana score of ≥ 2) [CASSINI trial], treatment with rivaroxaban at a dose of 10 mg daily for a duration of 180 days did not result in a significantly lower incidence of VTE or VTE-related death. In a pre-specified supportive analysis involving the same population, the same endpoint was assessed during the intervention period (first receipt of trial agent to last dose plus 2 days).During the intervention period, rivaroxaban led to a substantially lower incidence of such events, with a low incidence of major bleeding as the primary endpoint occurred in 25 of 420 patients (6.0%) in the rivaroxaban group and in 37 of 421 (8.8%) in the placebo group (hazard ratio, 0.66; 95% confidence interval [CI], 0.40–1.09; $P = 0.10$) in the period up to day 180 whereas in the pre-specified intervention-period analysis, VTE occurred in 11 patients (2.6%) in the rivaroxaban group and in 27 (6.4%) in the placebo group (hazard ratio, 0.40; 95% CI, 0.20–0.80). Major bleeding occurred in 8 of 405 patients (2.0%) in the rivaroxaban group and in 4 of 404 (1.0%) in the placebo group (hazard ratio, 1.96; 95% CI, 0.59–6.49) [28].

Apixaban

In the AVERT trial, apixaban therapy at a dose of 2.5 mg twice daily resulted in a significantly lower rate of VTE than did placebo among intermediate-to-high-risk ambulatory patients with cancer who were starting chemotherapy. The rate of major bleeding episodes was higher with apixaban than with placebo. VTE occurred in 12 of 288 patients (4.2%) in the apixaban group and in 28 of 275 patients (10.2%) in the placebo group (hazard ratio, 0.41; 95% confidence interval [CI], 0.26–0.65; $P < 0.001$) [29].

> Among intermediate-to-high-risk ambulatory patients with cancer who were starting chemotherapy.
> Rivaroxaban at a dose of 10 mg daily for a duration of 180 days did not result in a significantly lower incidence of VTE or VTE-related death.
> Apixaban therapy at a dose of 2.5 mg twice daily resulted in a significantly lower rate of VTE than did placebo.

Prophylaxis in Hospitalized Patients with Cancer

Large randomized control trials have demonstrated reduced rates of VTE in acutely ill medical patients with the use of prophylactic LMWH or fondaparinux [30–32].

(a) Patients with active or recent cancer admitted to hospital should receive thromboprophylaxis throughout their admission unless contraindicated (2C).
(b) Either LMWH or UFH can be used at prophylactic doses.
(c) Thromboprophylaxis should be reviewed in patients with thrombocytopenia. A platelet count of $<50 \times 109/L$ is a relative contraindication to pharmacological prophylaxis (1C).
(d) Dose modification should be considered in renal insufficiency and extremes of body weight.

For these purposes, active cancer should be considered to include a diagnosis of cancer, other than basal cell or squamous cell carcinoma of the skin, within the previous 6-month period, and any treatment for cancer within the previous 6-month period or recurrent or metastatic cancer.

Compliance to thromboprophylaxis guidelines, however, remains an important obstacle to its success [33].

Prophylaxis of Cancer Patients During Chemotherapy

In the setting of certain hematological malignancies, notably multiple myeloma (MM), VTE risk increases dramatically due to the multi-agent regimen used to treat the malignancy, especially if it contains thalidomide, lenalidomide, or pomalidomide. The role of thromboprophylaxis in this setting has been reviewed in two BCSH guidelines, which recommend risk assessment and treatment with low-dose aspirin if low risk and LMWH or dose-adjusted warfarin if non-low risk. Thromboprophylaxis should be continued until disease control is achieved [34, 35]. The International Myeloma Working Group (IMWG) developed a VTE risk assessment tool for patients with multiple myeloma receiving immunomodulatory drugs. The tool consists of a list of 17; patients, myeloma, and treatment specific risk factors. If no or any one of the risk factors is present in a patient receiving thalidomide, lenalidomide, or pomalidomide, aspirin once daily is recommended. If two or more risk factors are present, a prophylactic dose of low-molecular-weight heparin or warfarin targeted at an INR of 2–3 is recommended. The IMWG risk score is based on expert opinion without any validation studies and should therefore not be regarded as a firm guideline.

Patients without a history of VTE receiving adjuvant hormonal therapies for cancer should not routinely receive thromboprophylaxis.

Patients with essential thrombocytosis and polycythemia vera should receive aspirin as prophylaxis in case of cardiovascular risk, above the age of 60 years or previous thrombosis.

Postsurgical VTE Prevention

Cancer surgery patients remain at elevated risk for VTE for an extended period of time following hospital discharge. Randomized control trials have shown that extending prophylaxis up to 4 weeks is effective and safe in reducing postoperative VTE [36–38].

Guidelines recommend patients receive preoperative subcutaneous heparin, followed by continuous administration of anticoagulation starting 12–24 hours after surgery. Antithrombotic prophylaxis should be continued for at least 7–10 days postoperatively. A Cochrane review that included cancer patients undergoing abdominal, pelvic, or thoracic surgery showed that extended prophylaxis following cancer surgery reduced the rate of DVT by over 50% and that of proximal DVT by 75% compared with prophylaxis given for 7–10 days [39]. A recent Cochrane review found no difference between perioperative thromboprophylaxis with LMWH versus UFH and LMWH compared with fondaparinux in their effects on mortality, thromboembolic outcomes, major bleeding, or minor bleeding in people with cancer. There was a lower incidence of wound hematoma with LMWH compared to UFH [40].

In response to this, several guidelines now recommend extended prophylaxis for all patients undergoing elective cancer surgery, although some, such as ASCO, recommend extended prophylaxis only for cancer patients at high thrombotic risk who are undergoing major abdominal or pelvic surgery.

Both ASCO and NCCN guidelines recommend that all "high-risk" cancer patients undergoing major abdominopelvic surgery be considered for extended VTE prophylaxis. In the NCCN guidelines, high-risk features in this setting include surgery for gastrointestinal malignancies, prior history of VTE, anesthesia time >2 h, bed rest >4 days, advanced stage, and age >60 years.

Therefore:

(a) Use of LMWH once a day or a low dose of UFH three times a day is recommended. There is no data allowing conclusions regarding the superiority of one type of LMWH over others.

(b) Prophylaxis should be started 12–24 h postoperatively and continued for duration of hospitalization.

(c) Extended prophylaxis (4 weeks) to prevent postoperative VTE after major laparotomy in cancer patients should be considered in patients with a high VTE risk and low bleeding risk.

(d) The use of LMWH for the prevention of VTE in cancer patients undergoing laparoscopic surgery may be recommended in the same way as for laparotomy.

(e) Mechanical methods alone are not recommended except when pharmacological methods are contraindicated.

In patients receiving pharmacological anticoagulation for the treatment of CAT and undergoing surgery, please refer to Chap. 15.

Treatment of CAT

Initial Treatment of VTE in Cancer Patients

Heparin and Low-Molecular-Weight Heparins

Options for the initial treatment of cancer-associated thrombosis include LMWH, unfractionated heparin (UFH), and fondaparinux.

All major guidelines continue to recommend monotherapy with low-molecular-weight heparins (LMWHs) as the preferred treatment strategy for cancer-associated thrombosis.

These recommendations were based on results from three randomized controlled trials (RCTs) in which one of three different LMWHs, dalteparin, enoxaparin, and tinzaparin, was compared with warfarin in patients with symptomatic proximal deep vein thrombosis (DVT) or pulmonary embolism (PE).

In the CLOT (Randomized Comparison of Low-Molecular- Weight Heparin versus Oral Anticoagulant Therapy for the Prevention of Recurrent Venous Thromboembolism in Patients with Cancer) trial, dalteparin was given at a daily dose of 200 IU/kg for the first month, followed by 75%–83% of the same dose for 5 months [38]. In CLOT, dalteparin reduced the risk of symptomatic recurrent thrombosis by 52% relative to warfarin, and there was no difference in major bleeding between the two treatment arms.

In the other two studies, the LMWH was given for only 3 months. All of these trials consistently showed that a LMWH is better than warfarin in reducing the risk of recurrent VTE [41, 42].

A Cochrane review combining results of these controlled trials found a 53% reduction in the incidence of VTE in cancer patients virtually identical to what was shown in the CLOT trial [43]. There are no direct comparisons of 3 months vs. 6 months of treatment.

UFH can be used in those with severe renal impairment (creatinine clearance [CrCl], 30 mL/min) given its shorter half-life, reversibility with protamine sulfate, and dependence on hepatic clearance. Fondaparinux is a reasonable choice in patients with a history of HIT.

Therefore, LMWHs are recommended for the initial treatment of established VTE in cancer patients who have no contraindication to anticoagulation whereas the use of vitamin K antagonists is not recommended due to inferior efficacy. Therapeutic dosing varies depending on the specific LMWH. Dalteparin only has a regulatory indication in Canada for extended treatment of CAT; the other LMWHs, however, have been used successfully. Based on Thrombosis Canada Guidelines:

1. Baseline CBC and renal function should be checked prior to starting LMWH.
2. For specific dosing for each LMWH, please refer to Chap. 1, and it should be capped to the nearest prefilled syringe and also should be capped at actual body weight.
3. Caution is advised for patients with active bleeding or severe thrombocytopenia (platelet count $<50 \times 109/L$) in whom anticoagulation can be dangerous; urgent referral to a hematologist or thrombosis expert for management is recommended.
4. In patients with severe renal insufficiency (creatinine clearance [CrCl] <30 mL/min), LMWH is generally avoided because of its dependence on renal clearance. However, the following options may be considered if appropriate in the specific case:
   • It is possible to use LMWH if anti-Xa level measurement is available to guide dose adjustment. Some experts suggest that a dose reduction should be considered if the trough anti-Xa level is >0.4 IU/mL; however, good data showing a correlation between these levels and poor clinical outcomes is lacking.
   • For tinzaparin, the available evidence demonstrates no accumulation in patients with CrCl levels down to 20 mL/min. There are limited data available in patients with an estimated CrCl <20 mL/min.
5. If none of the above criteria is satisfied, then warfarin can be considered.
6. In patients who have a history of heparin-induced thrombocytopenia (HIT) or are suspected to have HIT, fondaparinux can be used for the initial treatment of established VTE.

DOACs for the Treatment of CAT Patients

The role of the new oral anticoagulants, edoxaban, rivaroxaban, and apixaban, VTE in cancer patients is becoming somehow clearer, whereas the role of dabigatran remains yet to be determined.

Two RCTs have recently been reported, comparing a DOAC with LMWH in the treatment of CAT. The SELECT-D pilot study compared rivaroxaban with dalteparin for the treatment of CAT. Over 400 patients were recruited. The VTE recurrence rate at 6 months was 11% (95% CI 7–17%) for patients on dalteparin and 4% (95% CI 2–9%) for patients on rivaroxaban. Major bleeds were similar across trial arms. There were more clinically relevant nonmajor bleeds (CRNMBs) on the rivaroxaban arm [20]. In a retrospective study on 641 patients, rivaroxaban was comparable to dalteparin in the prevention of VTE recurrence while having no significant differences with major or minor bleeding [44]. Observational data and data from Korean registry as well as a meta-analysis of published data on rivaroxaban pointed to its efficacy [45–48].

An ongoing trial COSIMO will provide information on outcomes associated with switching from LMWH or VKA therapy to rivaroxaban for the treatment or secondary prevention of cancer-associated thrombosis in a real-life setting [49].

The HOKUSAI VTE Cancer Study compared 5 days of LMWH followed by edoxaban 60 mg once daily with dalteparin at a dose of 200 IU/kg for 1 month followed by dalteparin 150 IU/kg in cancer patients with VTE. The primary outcome was a composite of recurrent VTE and major bleeding. 1046 patients were recruited. Edoxaban demonstrated non-inferiority with dalteparin with a primary-outcome event in 67 of the 522 patients (12.8%) in the edoxaban group with 71 of the 524 patients (13.5%) in the dalteparin group (hazard ratio, 0.97; 95% confidence interval [CI], 0.70–1.36; $P = 0.006$ for non-inferiority; $P = 0.87$ for superiority). It appears that edoxaban results in fewer recurrent VTE events, at the expense of more major bleeding episodes. Recurrent VTE occurred in 41 patients (7.9%) in the edoxaban group and in 59 patients (11.3%) in the dalteparin group (difference in risk, −3.4 percentage points; 95% CI, −7.0 to 0.2). Major bleeding occurred in 36 patients (6.9%) in the edoxaban group and in 21 patients (4.0%) in the dalteparin group [20].

ADAM VTE Trial on Apixaban 10 mg twice daily for 7 days followed by 5 mg twice daily was presented in an abstract form. Major bleeding occurred in none of the apixaban-treated patients compared with 3 of 2.1% in patients treated with LMWH, whereas recurrence occurred only in 3.4% compared to 14.1% in the LMWH-treated group [50].

Major bleeding was higher in gastrointestinal (13.1%) and urothelial (7.9%) cancers and it would seem unreasonable to use DOACs to manage CAT in such cancers [20, 21].

A final issue worthy of consideration lies with the potential for drug-drug interactions. DOACs, while subject to fewer interactions than warfarin, are particularly sensitive to medicines, which inhibit P-glycoprotein or cytochrome P450 3A4 (CYP3A4). These include chemotherapies and supportive care medicines commonly used in oncology. Nevertheless, if patients are unable to take a LMWH, DOACs may be a better choice than warfarin. However, patients need to be aware of the limitations of data and the possible risks should they choose to take DOACs for the treatment of CAT.

In a recent Cochrane review, it was concluded that DOACs appeared superior in reducing recurrent VTE in patients with CAT compared to LMWH and VKAs, but an increased risk of major bleeding versus LMWH cannot be ruled out [50].

Therefore, the recommendations of Thrombosis Canada and the recent ASH data are to consider DOACs only in patients:
1. Who have a non-GI active cancer.
2. Do not have a high risk of GI bleeding.
3. Do not have relevant drug-drug interactions.
4. Both edoxaban after a minimum of 5 days of LMWH and rivaroxaban can be used if the patient declines injections and accepts a higher risk of bleeding.
5. Recently data on apixaban is also emerging in CAT.
6. The use of other DOACs (dabigatran) is discouraged.
7. Monitoring of renal function, body weight, and drug-drug interactions is essential during treatment with a DOAC.

The doses of both DOACs are discussed in detail in Chap. 1.

- Edoxaban: is only given after an initial 5-day treatment with therapeutic LMWH, edoxaban 60 mg once daily is given. The dose is reduced to 30 mg once daily in those who have creatinine clearance between 30 and 50 mL/min, weigh 60 kg or less or are taking potent P-glycoprotein inhibitors (such as erythromycin, cyclosporine, dronedarone, quinidine, or ketoconazole). Evidence for edoxaban is stronger than for rivaroxaban in this patient population and edoxaban is the preferred DOAC for CAT treatment.
- Rivaroxaban: Initial LMWH is not required. Dosing is as usual at 15 mg twice daily for 3 weeks followed by a daily dose of 20 mg.
- For patients with cancer on DOACs and undergoing surgery or invasive procedures please refer to Chap. 12 for the approach to bridging.
- Data of the ADAM VTE Trial on Apixaban 10 mg twice daily for 7 days followed by 5 mg twice daily have been recently published in an abstract form. Major bleeding occurred in 0 of the 142 (0%) in apixaban-treated patients compared with 3 of the 145 patients (2.1%) treated with LMWH, whereas recurrence occurred in 5 patients (3.4%) in the apixaban group and 20 patients (14.1%) treated with LMWH [50].

Duration of Therapy in Cancer-Related Thrombosis

The optimal duration of anticoagulant therapy in cancer-associated thrombosis is not known. Expert guidelines indicate that physicians should continue therapy for 3–6 months and for as long as the cancer is active and patients are receiving chemotherapy. Beyond this period, "indefinite" therapy is recommended in patients with known metastases because of their high VTE risk.

1. In patients with cancer-associated thrombosis initial treatment should be with LMWH for 6 months, if tolerated (1A).
2. Indefinite anticoagulation in patients with active cancer or persistent risk factors.

Treatment of Incidental VTE

Given the absence of randomized studies of anticoagulant therapy in cancer patients with incidental venous thrombosis, optimal management remains unknown. However, the low-quality evidence available suggests that, in cancer patients, incidental PE and DVT are indicative of a generalized prothrombotic state and can be associated with a significant risk of early recurrent thrombosis and similarly poor survival rate as symptomatic thrombosis. Current American College of Chest Physicians guidance favors anticoagulant therapy for incidental venous thrombosis where the diagnosis is secure [51]. The one exception may be patients with isolated subsegmental PE, which may have a more benign natural history [52], but there is no clear consensus on this at present [53]. The merits of anticoagulation for symptomatic abdominal vein thrombosis require individual risk assessment [54], and it is recommended that cancer patients with incidental abdominal vein thrombosis are considered similarly.

> Cancer patients with incidental pulmonary embolus or DVT should be therapeutically anticoagulated as for symptomatic disease (1C).

Recurrent CAT and Breakthrough Thrombosis

Patients with cancer-associated VTE have a higher risk of recurrence on treatment than those without cancer [16]. If recurrence occurs in patients taking warfarin, they should be managed by a switch to LWMH.

If patients are using LMWH at approximately 75% of the normal therapeutic dose after the first month of treatment, they should increase to the full weight-based therapeutic dose.

For those already receiving full-dose LMWH, there is some evidence to support further increasing the dose of LMWH by 20–25% and/or splitting the dose for the OD formulations [54]. The benefit of dividing higher doses is uncertain but in the only comparative trial, there was a trend in the cancer subgroup for lower recurrence using twice daily compared to once daily enoxaparin with no significant increase in bleeding [55].

If there is continued evidence of clot extension, then an option is to increase the LMWH dose guided by anti-Xa measurement. A suggested regimen is to aim for a peak anti-Xa level of 1.6–2.0 u/mL for once-daily LMWH and 0.8–1.0 u/mL peak for twice-daily treatment [56, 57].

Therefore, for patients with recurrence or breakthrough thrombosis despite being on anticoagulation, the following recommendations may apply:

1. Those who develop recurrence on warfarin or DOACs should be switched to LMWH.
2. Insertion of vena cava filters is not recommended for recurrent thrombosis alone.
3. HIT has to be excluded and adherence to therapy confirmed.
4. Increasing the dose of LMWH by 25% had been shown to be effective.
5. Thrombolysis should be restricted to patients with life- or limb-threatening thromboembolic events (ASCO) or in those with massive or submassive PE with moderate to severe right ventricular enlargement or dysfunction (NCCN).

Prevention and Treatment of Catheter-Related Thrombosis (CRT)

Central venous catheter (CVC) placement increases the risk of thrombosis in people with cancer. Thrombosis often necessitates the removal of the CVC, resulting in treatment delays and thrombosis-related morbidity and mortality [58].

Thromboprophylaxis

Routine use of anticoagulants at a prophylactic or therapeutic dose to prevent catheter-related thrombosis in cancer patients is not recommended. Thromboprophylaxis may be only considered:

- In higher-risk cancer patients when the perceived risk of thrombosis outweighs the risk of bleeding and the burden of anticoagulation (e.g. in those with prior venous thrombosis).
- If a patient has a history of a catheter-associated DVT and now has a new indwelling catheter, Thrombosis Canada suggested to provide them with higher than usual doses of LMWH thromboprophylaxis.
- Warfarin targeted at INR 2–3 is effective but is associated with more bleeding.

Treatment of Catheter-Related Thrombosis CRT

The goals of treatment for CAT are:

- To improve acute symptoms
- To decrease long-term morbidity
- To prolong patency and survival of the catheter
- To prevent embolization and recurrent thrombosis

The usual approach includes the following:

1. CVC can be kept in place if it is functional, well positioned, and not infected.
2. After an initial 3–5 days of heparin or LMWH, long-term anticoagulation may involve the continuation of LMWH alone, conversion to warfarin, or DOACS such as apixaban, edoxaban, or rivaroxaban.
3. If LMWH is transitioned to warfarin, there should be an overlap for a minimum of 5 days and until the international normalized ratio (INR) is therapeutic; an initial 5–7 days of LMWH is also required prior to starting dabigatran or edoxaban.
4. Close surveillance for resolution of symptoms is recommended; if symptoms persist despite appropriate treatment, the CVC may require removal.

5. The duration of anticoagulation following line removal in patients without other ongoing thrombotic risk factors is again controversial due to a lack of good quality data. Some physicians continue to anticoagulate for 3 months, while others shorten the duration. The decision-making process should include thorough consideration of other potential risks for thrombosis, the size of the clot, and the extent to which it occludes the vessel. Duration of 6 weeks' anticoagulation may be appropriate if there are no risk factors and the clot is small and nonocclusive.
6. It may be appropriate to extend anticoagulation beyond 3 months in the absence of recanalization and in the context of progressive disease.
7. The evidence, however, is not conclusive for the effect of LMWH on mortality, the effect of VKA on mortality and catheter-related VTE, and the effect of LMWH compared to VKA on mortality and catheter-related VTE. LMWH reduces catheter-related VTE compared to no LMWH. People with cancer with CVCs considering anticoagulation should balance the possible benefit of reduced thromboembolic complications with the possible harms and burden of anticoagulants [56].

CAT and Thrombocytopenia

It is usually recommended to proceed with full anticoagulation as long as the platelets are above 50×10^9/L.

In the presence of high thrombotic risks with platelets dropping below 50×10^9/L, it is suggested to proceed with anticoagulation with platelet transfusion support to maintain a level between 40 and 50×10^9/L.

If the thrombotic risks are low with low risk of progression, dose reduction by 50% for LMWH or deescalating to a prophylactic dose may be accepted as long as the platelets are between 25 and 50×10^9/L.

If on the other hand the platelets drop below 25×10^9/L, stopping anticoagulation is justified as long as it is resumed in full dose once the target of 50×10^9/L is reached [59].

References

1. Merli GJ, Weitz HH. Venous thrombosis and cancer: what would Dr. trousseau teach today? Ann Intern Med. 2017;167(6):440–1.
2. Varki A. Trousseau's syndrome: multiple definitions and multiple mechanisms. Blood. 2007;110:1723–9.
3. Khorana AA. Malignancy, thrombosis and trousseau: the case for an eponym. J Thromb Haemost. 2003;1(12):2463–5.
4. Lee AY. Management of thrombosis in cancer: primary prevention and secondary prophylaxis. Br J Haematol. 2005;128(3):291–302.

5. Khorana AA, Francis CW, Culakova E, Kuderer NM, Lyman GH. Thromboembolism is a leading cause of death in cancer patients receiving outpatient chemotherapy. J Thromb Haemost. 2007;5(3):632–4.
6. Blom JW, Doggen CJ, Osanto S, Rosendaal FR. Malignancies, prothrombotic mutations, and the risk of venous thrombosis. JAMA. 2005;293:715–22.
7. Horsted F, West J, Grainge MJ. Risk of venous thromboembolism in patients with cancer: a systematic review and meta-analysis. PLoS Med. 2012;9(7):e1001275.
8. Prandoni P, Lensing AW, Cogo A, et al. The long-term clinical course of acute deep venous thrombosis. Ann Intern Med. 1996;125:1–7.
9. Carson JL, Kelley MA, Duff A, et al. The clinical course of pulmonary embolism. N Engl J Med. 1992;326:1240–5.
10. Sørensen HT, Mellemkj'r L, Olsen JH, et al. Prognosis of cancers associated with venous thromboembolism. N Engl J Med. 2000;343:1846–50.
11. Sorensen HT, et al. The risk of a diagnosis of cancer after primary deep venous thrombosis or pulmonary embolism. N Engl J Med. 1998;338:1169–73.
12. White RH, et al. Incidence of venous thromboembolism in the year before the diagnosis of cancer in 528,693 adults. Arch Intern Med. 2005;165:1782–7.
13. Carrier M, et al. Systematic review: the Trousseau syndrome revisited: should we screen extensively for cancer in patients with venous thromboembolism? Ann Intern Med. 2008;149:323–33.
14. Van Es N, et al. Screening for occult cancer in patients with unprovoked venous thromboembolism: a systematic review and meta-analysis of individual patients. Ann Intern Med. 2017;167(6):410–7.
15. Gheshmy A, Carrier M. Venous thromboembolism and occult cancer: impact on clinical practice. Thromb Res. 2016;140(Suppl 1):S8–11.
16. Jara-Palomares L, van Es N, Praena-Fernandez JM, Le Gal G, Otten HM, Robin P, Piccioli A, Lecumberri R, Religa P, Rieu V, Rondina M, Beckers M, Prandoni P, Salaun PY, Di Nisio M, Bossuyt PM, Kraaijpoel N, Büller HR, Carrier M. Relationship between type of unprovoked venous thromboembolism and cancer location: an individual patient data meta-analysis. Thromb Res. 2019;176:79–84.
17. Prandoni P, Lensing AW, Piccioli A, Bernardi E, Simioni P, Girolami B, Marchiori A, Sabbion P, Prins MH, Noventa F, Girolami A. Recurrent venous thromboembolism and bleeding complications during anticoagulant treatment in patients with cancer and venous thrombosis. Blood. 2002;100(10):3484–8.
18. Kearon C, Akl EA. Duration of anticoagulant therapy for deep vein thrombosis and pulmonary embolism. Blood. 2014;123(12):1794–801.
19. Di Nisio M, Lee AY, Carrier M, Liebman HA, Khorana AA, Subcommittee on Haemostasis and Malignancy. Diagnosis and treatment of incidental venous thromboembolism in cancer patients: guidance from the SSC of the ISTH. J Thromb Haemost. 2015;13(5):880–3.
20. Raskob GE, van Es N, Verhamme P, Carrier M, Di Nisio M, Garcia D, Grosso MA, Kakkar AK, Kovacs MJ, Mercuri MF, Meyer G, Segers A, Shi M, Wang TF, Yeo E, Zhang G, Zwicker JI, Weitz JI, Büller HR, Hokusai VTE Cancer Investigators. Edoxaban for the treatment of cancer-associated venous thromboembolism. N Engl J Med. 2018;378(7):615–24.
21. Young AM, Marshall A, Thirlwall J, Chapman O, Lokare A, Hill C, Hale D, Dunn JA, Lyman GH, Hutchinson C, MacCallum P, Kakkar A, Hobbs FDR, Petrou S, Dale J, Poole CJ, Maraveyas A, Levine M. Comparison of an oral factor Xa inhibitor with low molecular weight heparin in patients with cancer with venous thromboembolism: results of a randomized trial (SELECT-D). J Clin Oncol. 2018;36(20):2017–23.
22. Goubran HA, Burnouf T, Radosevich M, El-Ekiaby M. The platelet-cancer loop. Eur J Intern Med. 2013;24:393–400.
23. Goubran H, Stakiw J, Radosevich M, Burnouf T. Platelets effects on tumor growth. Semin Oncol. 2014;41(3):359–69.
24. Goubran H, Sabry W, Kotb R, Seghatchian J, Burnouf T. Platelet microparticles and cancer: an intimate cross-talk. Transfus Apher Sci. 2015;53(2):168–72.

25. Goubran H, Stakiw J, Radosevic M, Burnouf T. Cancer and thrombosis – an update. -platelet-cancer interactions. Semin Thromb Hemost. 2014;40:296–304.
26. Khorana AA, Kuderer NM, Culakova E, Lyman GH, Francis CW. Development and validation of a predictive model for chemotherapy-associated thrombosis. Blood. 2008;111(10):4902–7.
27. Khorana AA, Francis CW. Risk prediction of cancer-associated thrombosis: appraising the first decade and developing the future. Thromb Res. 2018;164(Suppl 1):S70–6.
28. Khorana AA, Soff GA, Kakkar AK, Vadhan-Raj S, Riess H, Wun T, Streiff MB, Garcia DA, Liebman HA, Belani CP, O'Reilly EM, Patel JN, Yimer HA, Wildgoose P, Burton P, Vijapurkar U, Kaul S, Eikelboom J, McBane R, Bauer KA, Kuderer NM, Lyman GH, CASSINI Investigators. Rivaroxaban for thromboprophylaxis in high-risk ambulatory patients with cancer. N Engl J Med. 2019;380(8):720–8.
29. Carrier M, Abou-Nassar K, Mallick R, Tagalakis V, Shivakumar S, Schattner A, Kuruvilla P, Hill D, Spadafora S, Marquis K, Trinkaus M, Tomiak A, Lee AYY, Gross PL, Lazo-Langner A, El-Maraghi R, Goss G, Le Gal G, Stewart D, Ramsay T, Rodger M, Witham D, Wells PS, AVERT Investigators. Apixaban to prevent venous thromboembolism in patients with cancer. N Engl J Med. 2019;380(8):711–9.
30. Samama MM, Cohen AT, Darmon JY, Desjardins L, Eldor A, Janbon C, Leizorovicz A, Nguyen H, Olsson CG, Turpie AG, Weisslinger N. A comparison of enoxaparin with placebo for the prevention of venous thromboembolism in acutely ill medical patients. Prophylaxis in Medical Patients with Enoxaparin Study Group. N Engl J Med. 1999;341(11):793–800.
31. McGarry LJ, Stokes ME, Thompson D. Outcomes of thromboprophylaxis with enoxaparin vs. unfractionated heparin in medical inpatients. Thromb J. 2006;4:17.
32. Cohen AT, Gurwith MM, Dobromirski M. Thromboprophylaxis in non-surgical cancer patients. Thromb Res. 2012;129(Suppl 1):S137–45.
33. Chin PK, Beckert LE, Gunningham S, Edwards AL, Robinson BA. Audit of anticoagulant thromboprophylaxis in hospitalized oncology patients. Intern Med J. 2009;39(12):819–25.
34. Bird JM, Owen RG, D'Sa S, Snowden JA, Pratt G, Ashcroft J, Yong K, Cook G, Feyler S, Davies F, Morgan G, Cavenagh J, Low E, Behrens J, Haemato-oncology Task Force of British Committee for Standards in Haematology (BCSH) and UK Myeloma Forum. Guidelines for the diagnosis and management of multiple myeloma 2011. Br J Haematol. 2011;154(1):32–75.
35. Snowden JA, Ahmedzai SH, Ashcroft J, D'Sa S, Littlewood T, Low E, Lucraft H, Maclean R, Feyler S, Pratt G, Bird JM, Haemato-oncology Task Force of British Committee for Standards in Haematology and UK Myeloma Forum. Guidelines for supportive care in multiple myeloma 2011. Br J Haematol. 2011;154(1):76–103.
36. Fagarasanu A, Alotaibi GS, Hrimiuc R, Lee AY, Wu C. Role of extended thromboprophylaxis after abdominal and pelvic surgery in cancer patients: a systematic review and meta-analysis. Ann Surg Oncol. 2016;23(5):1422–30.
37. Serra R, de Franciscis S. The importance of extended thromboprophylaxis in patients undergoing major surgery for cancer. Thromb Res. 2014;133(6):965–6.
38. Guo Q, Huang B, Zhao J, Ma Y, Yuan D, Yang Y, Du X. Perioperative pharmacological thromboprophylaxis in patients with cancer: a systematic review and meta-analysis. Ann Surg. 2017;265(6):1087–93.
39. Rasmussen MS, Jørgensen LN, Wille-Jørgensen P. Prolonged thromboprophylaxis with low molecular weight heparin for abdominal or pelvic surgery. Cochrane Database Syst Rev. 2009;(1):CD004318.
40. Matar CF, Kahale LA, Hakoum MB, Tsolakian IG, Etxeandia-Ikobaltzeta I, Yosuico VE, Terrenato I, Sperati F, Barba M, Schünemann H, Akl EA. Anticoagulation for perioperative thromboprophylaxis in people with cancer. Cochrane Database Syst Rev. 2018;7:CD009447.
41. Lee AY, Levine MN, Baker RI, Bowden C, Kakkar AK, Prins M, Rickles FR, Julian JA, Haley S, Kovacs MJ, Gent M, Randomized Comparison of Low-Molecular-Weight Heparin versus Oral Anticoagulant Therapy for the Prevention of Recurrent Venous Thromboembolism in Patients with Cancer (CLOT) Investigators. Low-molecular-weight heparin versus a coumarin

for the prevention of recurrent venous thromboembolism in patients with cancer. N Engl J Med. 2003;349(2):146–53.

42. Lee AYY, Kamphuisen PW, Meyer G, Bauersachs R, Janas MS, Jarner MF, Khorana AA, CATCH Investigators. Tinzaparin vs warfarin for treatment of acute venous thromboembolism in patients with active cancer: a randomized clinical trial. JAMA. 2015;314(7):677–86.

43. Francis CW, Kessler CM, Goldhaber SZ, Kovacs MJ, Monreal M, Huisman MV, Bergqvist D, Turpie AG, Ortel TL, Spyropoulos AC, Pabinger I, Kakkar AK. Treatment of venous thromboembolism in cancer patients with dalteparin for up to 12 months: the DALTECAN Study. J Thromb Haemost. 2015;13(6):1028–35.

44. Hakoum MB, Kahale LA, Tsolakian IG, Matar CF, Yosuico VE, Terrenato I, Sperati F, Barba M, Schünemann H, Akl EA. Anticoagulation for the initial treatment of venous thromboembolism in people with cancer. Cochrane Database Syst Rev. 2018;1:CD006649.

45. Chaudhury A, Balakrishnan A, Thai C, Holmstrom B, Nanjappa S, Ma Z, Jaglal MV. The efficacy and safety of rivaroxaban and dalteparin in the treatment of cancer associated venous thrombosis. Indian J Hematol Blood Transfus. 2018;34(3):530–4.

46. Kohn CG, Lyman GH, Beyer-Westendorf J, Spyropoulos AC, Bunz TJ, Baker WL, Eriksson D, Meinecke AK, Coleman CI. Effectiveness and safety of rivaroxaban in patients with cancer-associated venous thrombosis. J Natl Compr Cancer Netw. 2018;16(5):491–7.

47. Yhim HY, Choi WI, Kim SH, Nam SH, Kim KH, Mun YC, Oh D, Hwang HG, Lee KW, Song EK, Kwon YS, Bang SM. Long-term rivaroxaban for the treatment of acute venous thromboembolism in patients with active cancer in a prospective multicenter trial. Korean J Intern Med. 2018; https://doi.org/10.3904/kjim.2018.097.

48. Xing J, Yin X, Chen D. Rivaroxaban versus enoxaparin for the prevention of recurrent venous thromboembolism in patients with cancer: a meta-analysis. Medicine (Baltimore). 2018;97(31):e11384.

49. Cohen AT, Maraveyas A, Beyer-Westendorf J, Lee AYY, Mantovani LG, Bach M, COSIMO Investigators. COSIMO – patients with active cancer changing to rivaroxaban for the treatment and prevention of recurrent venous thromboembolism: a non-interventional study. Thromb J. 2018;16:21.

50. McBane RD, Wysokinski WE, Le-Rademacher J, Ashrani AA, Tafur AJ, Gundabolu K, Perez-Botero J, Perepu U, Anderson DM, Kuzma C, Leon Ferre R, Henkin S, Lenz C, Loprinzi C. Apixaban, dalteparin, in active cancer associated venous thromboembolism, the ADAM VTE Trial. St Diego: American Society of Hematology; 2018.

51. Sobieraj DM, Baker WL, Smith E, Sasiela K, Trexler SE, Kim O, Coleman CI. Anticoagulation for the treatment of cancer-associated thrombosis: a systematic review and network meta-analysis of randomized trials. Clin Appl Thromb Hemost. 2018;24:1076029618800792.

52. Kearon C, Akl EA, Comerota AJ, Prandoni P, Bounameaux H, Goldhaber SZ, Nelson ME, Wells PS, Gould MK, Dentali F, Crowther M, Kahn SR. Antithrombotic therapy for VTE disease: Antithrombotic Therapy and Prevention of Thrombosis, 9th ed: American College of Chest Physicians Evidence-Based Clinical Practice Guidelines. Chest. 2012;141(2 Suppl):e419S–96S. https://doi.org/10.1378/chest.11-2301.

53. Eyer BA, Goodman LR, Washington L. Clinicians' response to radiologists' reports of isolated subsegmental pulmonary embolism or inconclusive interpretation of pulmonary embolism using MDCT. AJR Am J Roentgenol. 2005;184(2):623–8.

54. den Exter PL, Kroft LJ, van der Hulle T, Klok FA, Jiménez D, Huisman MV. Embolic burden of incidental pulmonary embolism diagnosed on routinely performed contrast-enhanced computed tomography imaging in cancer patients. J Thromb Haemost. 2013;11(8):1620–2.

55. Lee AY. Treatment of established thrombotic events in patients with cancer. Thromb Res. 2012;129(Suppl 1):S146–53.

56. Tait C, Baglin T, Watson H, Laffan M, Makris M, Perry D, Keeling D, British Committee for Standards in Haematology. Guidelines on the investigation and management of venous thrombosis at unusual sites. Br J Haematol. 2012;159(1):28–38.

57. Carrier M, Lee AY. Prophylactic and therapeutic anticoagulation for thrombosis: major issues in oncology. Nat Clin Pract Oncol. 2009;6(2):74–84.
58. Merli GJ, Vanscoy GJ, Rihn TL, Groce JB 3rd, McCormick W. Applying scientific criteria to therapeutic interchange: a balanced analysis of low-molecular-weight heparins. J Thromb Thrombolysis. 2001;11(3):247–59.
59. Samuelson Bannow BT, Lee A, Khorana AA, Zwicker JI, Noble S, Ay C, Carrier M. Management of cancer-associated thrombosis in patients with thrombocytopenia: guidance from the SSC of the ISTH. J Thromb Haemost. 2018;16(6):1246–9.

Chapter 6
Anticoagulation in Pregnancy and Lactation

Otto Moodley, Derek Pearson, and Hadi Goubran

Abbreviations

ART	Assisted reproductive technology
ASH	American Society of Hematology
BMI	Body mass index
CTPA	Computerized tomography pulmonary arteriography
DOACs	Direct oral anticoagulants
DVT	Deep vein thrombosis
HIT	Heparin-induced thrombocytopenia
IBD	Inflammatory bowel disease
IVF	In vitro fertilization
LMWH	Low-molecular-weight heparin
OHSS	Ovarian hyper-stimulation syndrome
PE	Pulmonary embolism
RCOG	Royal College of Obstetricians and Gynaecologists
SC	Subcutaneous
SLE	Systemic lupus erythematosus
SOGC	Society of Obstetricians and Gynaecologists of Canada
UFH	Unfractionated heparin
V/Q scan	Ventilation/perfusion scan
VTE	Venous thromboembolism

O. Moodley (✉) · D. Pearson · H. Goubran
Saskatoon Cancer Centre, College of Medicine, University of Saskatchewan, Saskatoon, SK, Canada
e-mail: Otto.moodley@saskcancer.ca; Derek.pearson@saskcancer.ca; Hadi.goubranmessiha@saskcancer.ca

© Springer Nature Switzerland AG 2020
H. Goubran et al. (eds.), *Precision Anticoagulation Medicine*,
https://doi.org/10.1007/978-3-030-25782-8_6

Introduction

Pregnant women have a fourfold to fivefold increased risk of thromboembolism compared with non-pregnant women during pregnancy and 15- to 35 fold increased risk early after delivery. Approximately 80% of thromboembolic events in pregnancy are venous with a prevalence of 0.5–2.0 per 1000 VTE, which represents one of the leading causes of maternal mortality in the United States, accounting for 9.3% of all maternal deaths [1].

Thromboprophylaxis

The risk of pregnancy-related VTE in thrombophilic women with a positive family history appears to be 2–4 times greater than that in thrombophilic women without a positive family history of VTE.

The Royal College of Obstetricians and Gynaecologists (RCOG) of the United Kingdom suggested that all women should undergo a documented assessment of risk factors for VTE in early pregnancy or pre-pregnancy. That risk assessment should be repeated if the woman is admitted to hospital for any reason or develops other intercurrent problems and should be repeated again intrapartum or immediately postpartum. Figure 6.1 illustrates the risk stratification algorithm suggested by the RCOG [2]:

Low-molecular-weight heparins [LMWHs] are the agents of choice for antenatal and postnatal thromboprophylaxis and are safe in breastfeeding. Figures 6.2 and 6.3 illustrate the antenatal and postnatal assessment and thromboprophylaxis management strategies.

Prophylactic doses of the LMWHs are:

- Dalteparin 5000 U SC once daily
- Enoxaparin 40 mg SC once daily
- Nadroparin 2850 U SC daily
- Tinzaparin 4500 U SC once daily

Monitoring of anti-Xa levels is not required when LMWH is used for low-dose thromboprophylaxis.

For patients with previous VTE or those with high-risk thrombophilia including antiphospholipid syndrome, factor V Leiden mutation, antithrombin deficiency [3], or prothrombin gene mutation [4] intermediate doses of LMWH could be offered or weight-based dose adjustment may be used [3–5].

For women who have no family history of VTE but have antithrombin deficiency or are homozygous for the prothrombin gene mutation, the American Society of Hematology [ASH] guideline panel suggests against using antepartum antithrombotic prophylaxis to prevent a first venous thromboembolic event [3].

Risk factors for venous thromboembolism in pregnancy and puerperium		
Pre-existing	Previous VTE	
	Thrombophilia	*Congenital* Antithrombin deficiency Protein C deficiency Protein S deficiency Factor V Leiden mutation Prothrombin gene mutation
		Acquired Antiphospholipid antibodies Persistent lupus anticoagulant and/or persistent moderate-/high-titer anticardiolipin antibodies and/or β2-glycoprotein 1 antibodies
	Medical comorbidities, e.g., cancer; heart failure; active SLE, inflammatory polyarthropathy, or IBD; nephrotic syndrome; type I diabetes mellitus with nephropathy; sickle cell disease; current intravenous drug users	
	Age >35 years	
	Obesity (BMI ≥ 30 kg/m²) either pre-pregnancy or in early pregnancy	
	Parity ≥ 3 (a woman becomes para 3 after her third delivery)	
	Smoking	
	Gross varicose veins (symptomatic or above knee or with associated phlebitis, edema/skin changes)	
	Paraplegia	
Obstetric risk factors	Multiple pregnancy Current preeclampsia Caesarean section Prolonged labor (>24 hours) Mid-cavity or rotational operative delivery Stillbirth Preterm birth Postpartum hemorrhage >1 L/requiring transfusion	
New onset/transient *These risk factors are potentially reversible and may develop at later stages in gestation than the initial risk assessment or may resolve and therefore what is important is an ongoing individual risk assessment*	Any surgical procedure in pregnancy or puerperium except immediate repair of the perineum, e.g., appendectomy, postpartum sterilization Bone fracture	
	Hyperemesis, dehydration Ovarian hyper stimulation syndrome (first trimester only) Assisted reproductive technology (ART), and in vitro fertilization (IVF) Admission or immobility (≥3 days' bed rest) e.g. pelvic girdle pain restricting mobility Current systemic infection (requiring intravenous antibiotics or admission to hospital) e.g. pneumonia, pyelonephritis, postpartum wound infection Long-distance travel (>4 hours)	

Fig. 6.1 Risk factors for venous thromboembolism in pregnancy and the puerperium

**Antenatal assessment and management
(at booking and if patient admitted)**

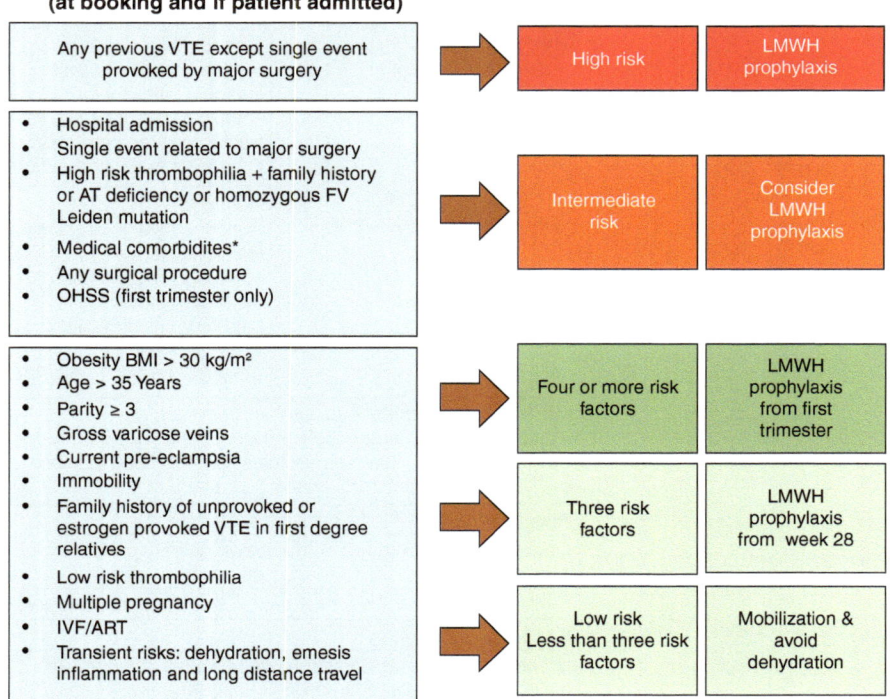

Fig. 6.2 Therapeutic algorithm for thromboprophylaxis in the antenatal period modified from the RCOG UK guidelines [2]. ART assisted reproductive technology, IVF in vitro fertilization, OHSS ovarian hyper-stimulation syndrome. *Cancer, heart failure, active systemic lupus, inflammatory bowel disease, inflammatory polyarthritis, nephrotic syndrome, type I diabetes with nephropathy, sickle cells, or current intravenous drug use

The guideline *suggests against* antepartum anticoagulant prophylaxis in women not already receiving long-term anticoagulant therapy who have a history of prior VTE associated with a nonhormonal temporary provoking risk factor and no other risk factors [3].

For thromboprophylaxis the booking or most recent weight can be used to guide dosing.

It is only necessary to monitor the platelet count if the woman has had prior exposure to unfractionated heparin (UFH).

Doses of LMWH should be reduced in women with renal impairment.

Intermediate doses of the LMWHs are (for detailed dosage please refer to Chap. 1):

- Dalteparin 5000 U SC twice daily or 10,000 U SC once daily
- Enoxaparin 40 mg SC twice daily or 80 mg SC once daily

Post-natal assessment and management

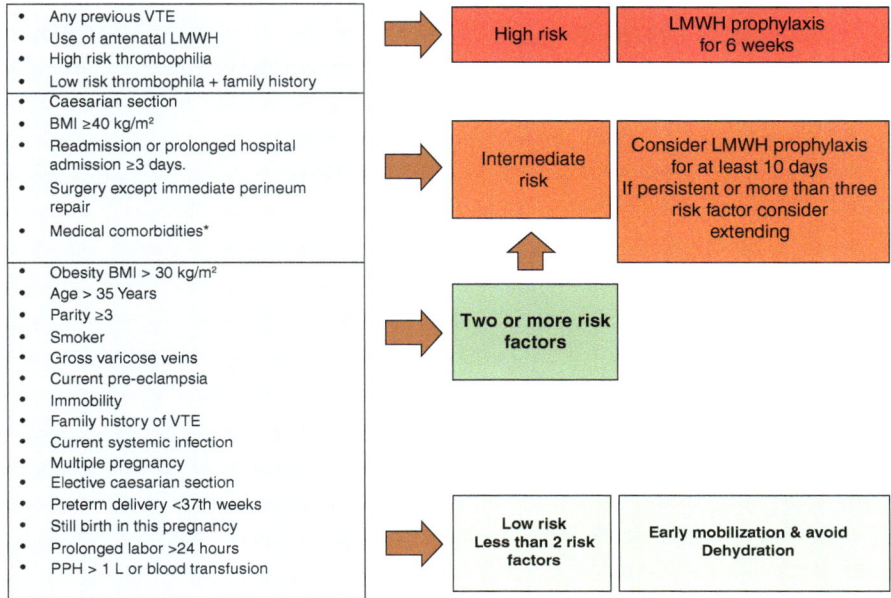

Fig. 6.3 Approach to thromboprophylaxis in the postnatal period modified from the suggested algorithm of the RCOG UK [2]. PPH postpartum hemorrhage. *Cancer, heart failure, active systemic lupus, inflammatory bowel disease, inflammatory polyarthritis, nephrotic syndrome, type I diabetes with nephropathy, sickle cells, or current intravenous drug use

- Nadroparin 2850 U SC twice daily or 5700 U SC once daily
- Tinzaparin 10,000 U SC once daily
- Any LMWH adjusted to peak anti-Xa levels of 0.2–0.6 U/mL [4]

Warfarin crosses the placenta and can lead to teratogenicity and should be avoided. At present, direct oral anticoagulants (DOACs) should not be used during pregnancy.

Timing of initiation, discontinuation during labor, and duration of therapy: Antepartum thromboprophylaxis should be initiated as early as possible.

To reduce the risk of maternal hemorrhage and epidural hematoma at the time of delivery, planned delivery and discontinuation of prophylaxis when spontaneous labor commences are needed.

In certain centers where thromboprophylaxis is continued beyond 32 weeks, the dose of LMWH should be given more than 12 hours prior to epidural placement and 24 hours for higher LMWH doses.

In anticipation of a spontaneous delivery, some obstetricians opt to use UFH from week 34 to 35 of gestation.

If prophylactic UFH is substituted for LMWH close to term, practice guidelines do not require a delay in epidural placement following up to 10,000 units of UFH daily.

Resumption of prophylaxis should be delayed until adequate hemostasis guaranteed and generally at least 12 hours post-delivery or epidural removal.

The duration of postpartum prophylaxis is usually 6 weeks.

Diagnosis

Symptoms that mimic VTE, such as leg swelling, groin discomfort, and dyspnea, are common in normal pregnancy. Therefore, the majority of pregnant women investigated for VTE (>90%) will not have VTE [5].

The diagnosis, therefore, rests on imaging as most of the decision tools were not validated in pregnancy and D-dimer could be elevated [3, 4].

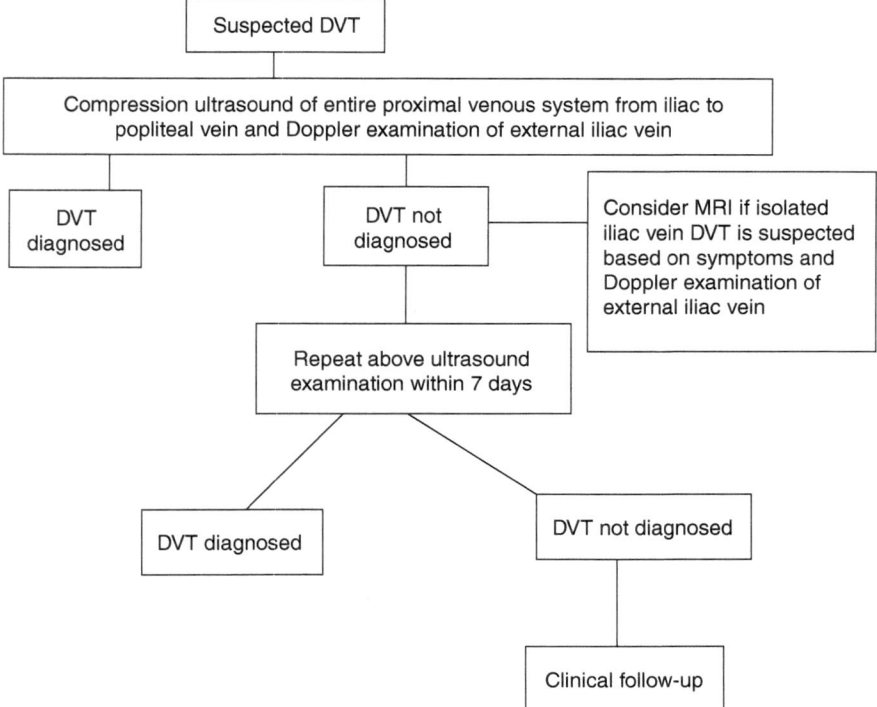

Fig. 6.4 Adapted from Society of Obstetricians and Gynaecologists of Canada (SOGC) algorithm for investigation of suspected DVT in pregnant patients from Chan et al. [6] (with permission)

Fig. 6.5 Adapted from Society of Obstetricians and Gynaecologists of Canada (SOGC) algorithm for investigation of suspected PE in pregnant patients from Chan et al. [6] (with permission)

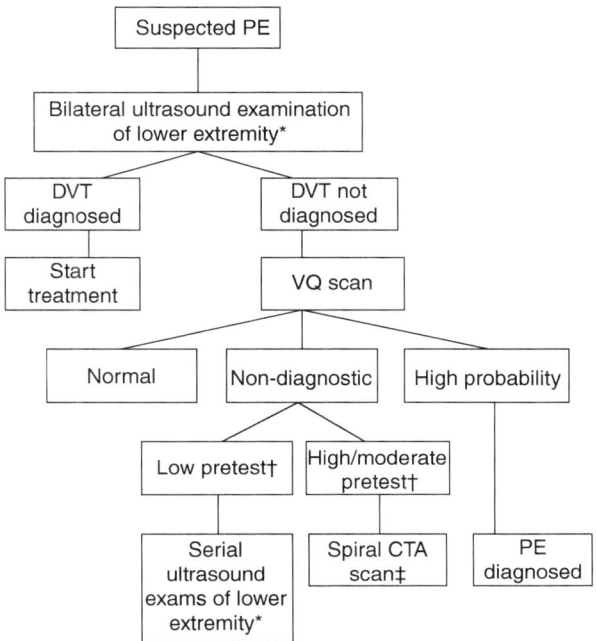

Thrombosis Canada suggested the following algorithms for the diagnosis of DVT and PE, respectively (Figs. 6.4 and 6.5):

Treatment of VTE in Pregnancy, Postpartum Period, and During Breastfeeding

UFH and LMWH do not cross the placenta and, therefore, are safe for the fetus.

Warfarin crosses the placenta and may cause teratogenicity as well as pregnancy loss and fetal bleeding and is therefore contraindicated for the treatment of VTE in pregnancy.

Direct oral anticoagulants (including apixaban, dabigatran, edoxaban, and rivaroxaban) which are likely to cross the placenta, and the human reproductive risks of these medications are unknown. They should also be avoided in pregnancy [3, 4, 6, 7].

In the initial management of DVT, the leg should be elevated and a graduated elastic compression stocking applied to reduce edema. Mobilization with graduated elastic compression stockings should be encouraged.

Anticoagulant Regimen

For pregnant women with acute VTE, the ASH guideline panel recommends LMWH over UFH [3], whereas the ASH guideline panel *suggests against* the addition of catheter-directed thrombolysis therapy to anticoagulation [3].

Low-molecular-weight heparin: Weight-based doses given subcutaneously once or twice daily.

- Dalteparin: 100 U/kg twice daily or 200 U/kg daily
- Enoxaparin: 1 mg/kg twice daily or 1.5 mg/kg once daily
- Tinzaparin: 175 U/kg once daily

Routine measurement of peak anti-Xa activity for patients on LMWH for treatment of acute VTE in pregnancy or postpartum is not recommended except in women at extremes of body weight (less than 50 and 90 kg or more) or with other complicating factors (e.g., with renal impairment or recurrent VTE). Routine platelet count monitoring should not be carried out [7].

Women should be taught to self-inject LMWH and arrangements made to allow safe disposal of needles and syringes. Outpatient follow-up should include clinical assessment and advice with monitoring of peak anti-Xa levels if appropriate [7].

The dose of LMWH should be adjusted over the course of pregnancy; however, this remains controversial. In the absence of robust data, three options can be considered:

1. No further dose adjustment after initial dosing
2. Dose adjustment guided by changes in weight
3. Dose adjustment guided by peak anti-factor Xa LMWH levels (samples obtained 2–4 hours after a dose) to maintain anti-factor Xa levels of 0.6–1.0 units/mL if a twice-daily regimen is used and slightly higher levels if a once-daily regimen is chosen [7]

Unfractionated heparin: Continuous infusion of intravenous heparin adjusted to maintain a therapeutic aPTT or subcutaneous heparin every 12 hours in doses adjusted to prolong the aPTT 6 hours after injection into the therapeutic range (usually 333 IU/Kg as loading dose followed by 250 IU/Kg/SC q 12 hours) [8].

Obstetric patients who are postoperative and receiving UFH should have platelet count monitoring performed every 2–3 days from days 4 to 14 or until heparin is stopped [7].

Any woman who is considered to be at high risk of hemorrhage and in whom continued heparin treatment is considered essential should be managed with intravenous unfractionated heparin until the risk factors for hemorrhage have resolved [4].

Labor and delivery: The risks of anticoagulant-related maternal hemorrhage and epidural hematoma in women using anticoagulants at the time of delivery can be minimized with careful planning.

Women receiving therapeutic subcutaneous UFH or LMWH should generally have a planned delivery. Twice-daily therapeutic doses of subcutaneous UFH or LMWH should be discontinued 24 hours before induction of labor or caesarean section, while patients taking once-daily therapeutic doses of LMWH should take only 50% of their dose on the morning of the day prior to delivery [3, 4, 7].

Pregnant women receiving LMWH or UFH should be instructed to withhold their injection at the early signs of spontaneous labor and neuraxial anesthesia should not be used [3, 4, 6, 7].

In patients receiving therapeutic doses of LMWH, wound drains (abdominal and rectus sheath) should be considered at caesarean section and the skin incision should be closed with interrupted sutures to allow drainage of any hematoma and those considered to be at high risk of hemorrhage and, in whom continued heparin treatment is considered essential, should be managed with intravenous unfractionated heparin until the risk factors for hemorrhage have resolved [7].

Postpartum anticoagulation: Postpartum LMWH or UFH therapy should be restarted as soon as it is safe to do so – usually within 6–24 hours of delivery, after ensuring adequate hemostasis. Full-dose LMWH or UFH should generally be delayed 24 hours following epidural catheter removal.

Postpartum warfarin is usually started after 5 days. If no bleeding concerns, it can be initiated at the same time as LMWH or UFH. Heparin or LMWH is continued after an overlap of at least 5 days and until an INR ≥ 2.0 is reached and maintained for at least 24 hours.

Although vitamin K antagonists cross the placenta and can lead to teratogenicity, warfarin is safe for the breastfed infant when administered to the nursing mother (usually after the 5th day of delivery to avoid postpartum bleeding). LMWH, UFH, acenocoumarol, fondaparinux, and danaparoid are also safe options [3].

DOACs are contraindicated [3, 4, 7].

Duration of anticoagulation: Should be continued at least 6–12 weeks postpartum or at least 3 months of full anticoagulation has been administered and the total duration is dependent on the initial indication of anticoagulation.

Special Considerations

Superficial Thrombophlebitis
For pregnant women with proven acute superficial vein thrombosis, the ASH guideline panel suggests using LMWH over not using any anticoagulant [3].

Heparin-induced thrombocytopenia (HIT):
Pregnant women who develop heparin-induced thrombocytopenia or have heparin allergy and require continuing anticoagulant therapy should be managed with an alternative anticoagulant under specialist advice.

Consideration should be given to the use of newer anticoagulants (fondaparinux, argatroban, or r-hirudin) in pregnant women who are unable to tolerate heparin (LMWH or unfractionated heparin) or danaparoid and who require continuing anticoagulant therapy [4].

Pulmonary embolism (PE) and massive PE
In pregnant women, if PE is suspected, V/Q lung scanning is preferable over CT pulmonary angiography [4, 9].

For treatment of massive PE, intravenous UFH is the preferred, initial treatment in massive PE and right ventricular dysfunction in the absence of hemodynamic instability; the ASH guideline panel *suggests against* the addition of systemic thrombolytic therapy to anticoagulation compared with anticoagulation alone [3]. For pregnant women, on the other hand, with acute pulmonary embolism and life-threatening hemodynamic instability, the ASH guideline panel as well as Guidelines of the Royal College of Obstetricians and Gynaecologists of the United Kingdom *suggests* that thrombolytic therapy should be considered [7].

One regimen for the administration of intravenous UFH is:
- Loading dose of 80 units/kg, followed by a continuous intravenous infusion of 18 units/kg/hour.
- If a patient has received thrombolysis (see below), the loading dose of heparin should be omitted and an infusion started at 18 units/kg/hour with APTT level at 4–6 hours to keep the ratio at 1.5–2.5 average laboratory control value.

Inferior vena cava (IVC) filter use:
Placement of a temporary IVC filter in obstetric practice could be considered when recurrent thromboembolism occurs despite adequate anticoagulation or when anticoagulation is contraindicated due to active bleeding. IVC filters should be removed once the contraindication to anticoagulation has been corrected [7].

There was a strong recommendation for low-molecular-weight heparin (LWMH) over unfractionated heparin for acute VTE. Most recommendations were conditional, including those for either twice-per-day or once-per-day LMWH dosing for the treatment of acute VTE and initial outpatient therapy over hospital admission with low-risk acute VTE, as well as against routine anti-factor Xa (FXa) monitoring to guide dosing with LMWH for VTE treatment. There was a strong recommendation (low certainty in evidence) for antepartum anticoagulant prophylaxis with a history of unprovoked or hormonally associated VTE and a conditional recommendation against antepartum anticoagulant prophylaxis with prior VTE associated with a resolved nonhormonal provoking risk factor [5].

References

1. ACOG Practice Bulletin No. 196: Thromboembolism in pregnancy. Obstet Gynecol. 2018;132(1):e1–e17. https://doi.org/10.1097/AOG.0000000000002706.
2. Royal College of Obstetricians and Gynaecologists. Reducing the risk of venous thromboembolism during pregnancy and the puerperium. Green-top guideline no. 37a, Guidelines of the Royal College of Obstetricians and Gynaecologists of the UK, April 2015. p. 1–40.
3. Bates SM, Rajasekhar A, Middeldorp S, McLintock C, Rodger MA, James AH, et al. American Society of Hematology 2018 guidelines for management of venous thromboembolism: venous thromboembolism in the context of pregnancy. Blood Adv. 2018;2:3317–59.
4. Pregnancy: thromboprophylaxis. Thrombosis Canada Guidelines, 2017.
5. Akinshina S, Makatsariya A, Bitsadze V, Khizroeva J, Khamani N. Thromboprophylaxis in pregnant women with thrombophilia and a history of thrombosis. J Perinat Med. 2018;46(8):893–9. https://doi.org/10.1515/jpm-2017-0329.
6. Chan WS, Rey E, Kent NE, VTE in Pregnancy Guideline Working Group, Chan WS, Kent NE, Rey E, Corbett T, David M, Douglas MJ, Gibson PS, Magee L, Rodger M, Smith RE, Society of Obstetricians and Gynecologists of Canada. Venous thromboembolism and antithrombotic therapy in pregnancy: SOGC Clinical Practice Guideline. J Obstet Gynaecol Can. 2014;36(6):527–53.
7. Royal College of Obstetricians and Gynaecologists. Thromboembolic disease in pregnancy and the puerperium: acute management. Green-top guideline no. 37b, Guidelines of the Royal College of Obstetricians and Gynaecologists of the UK, April 2015. p. 1–32.
8. Cushman M, Wendy Lim W, Zakai N. 2011 Clinical practice guide on anticoagulant dosing and management of anticoagulant associated bleeding complications in adults. Presented by the American Society of Hematology, adapted in part from the: American College of Chest Physicians Evidence-Based Clinical Practice Guideline on Antithrombotic and Thrombolytic Therapy. Quick Reference, 2011.
9. van Mens TE, Scheres LJ, de Jong PG, Leeflang MM, Nijkeuter M, Middeldorp S. Imaging for the exclusion of pulmonary embolism in pregnancy. Cochrane Database Syst Rev. 2017;1:CD011053.

Chapter 7
Anticoagulation in Autoimmune Rheumatic Diseases

Gaafar Ragab, Mohamed Tharwat Hegazy, Veronica Codullo, Mervat Mattar, and Jérôme Avouac

Abbreviations

AAV	ANCA-associated vasculitis
ANCA	Antineutrophil cytoplasmic antibody
aPL	Antiphospholipid
APS	Antiphospholipid syndrome
AS	Ankylosing spondylitis
AT III	Antithrombin III
BD	Behçet's disease
CI	Confidence interval
CVA	Cerebrovascular accident
DM	Dermatomyositis
DVT	Deep vein thrombosis
ECP	Eosinophil cationic protein
EGPA	Eosinophilic granulomatosis with polyangiitis
EPO	Eosinophil peroxidase
EULAR	European league against rheumatism
GCA	Giant cell arteritis
GPA	Granulomatosis with polyangiitis
HDL-C	High-density lipoprotein cholesterol

G. Ragab (✉) · M. T. Hegazy
Internal Medicine Department, Rheumatology and Clinical Immunology Unit,
Faculty of Medicine, Cairo University, Giza, Egypt
e-mail: gragab@kasralainy.edu.eg

V. Codullo · J. Avouac
Université Paris Descartes, Service de Rhumatologie, Hôpital Cochin, Paris, France
e-mail: veronica.codullo@aphp.fr

M. Mattar
Internal Medicine and Hematology, Cairo University, Giza, Egypt

© Springer Nature Switzerland AG 2020
H. Goubran et al. (eds.), *Precision Anticoagulation Medicine*,
https://doi.org/10.1007/978-3-030-25782-8_7

HR	Hazard ratio
IBD	Inflammatory bowel disease
IL	Interleukin
IPH	Idiopathic pulmonary hypertension
LDL-C	Low-density lipoprotein cholesterol
LVV	Large vessel vasculitis
MBP	Major basic protein
MI	Myocardial infarction
MPA	Microscopic polyangiitis
NOACs	New oral anticoagulants
PAI-1	Plasminogen activator inhibitor-1
PAN	Polyarteritis nodosa
PH	Pulmonary hypertension
PM	Polymyositis
PR3	Proteinase 3
PsA	Psoriatic arthritis
Pso	Psoriasis
pSS	Primary Sjögren syndrome
PTE	Pulmonary thromboembolism
Ptn C	Protein C
Ptn S	Protein S
PVD	Peripheral vascular disease
RA	Rheumatoid arthritis
SLE	Systemic lupus erythematosus
SS	Sjögren syndrome
SSc	Systemic sclerosis
TA	Takayasu's arteritis
TNF-α	Tumor necrosis factor alpha
tsDMARDs	Targeted synthetic disease-modifying antirheumatic drugs
VTE	Venous thromboembolism

Introduction

Autoimmune rheumatic diseases are characterized by common features, including systemic involvement, polypharmacy, and the presence of comorbidities. Recent large epidemiological studies shed light on their role as risk factors for thromboembolic complications. Different mechanisms were hypothesized to account for this increased risk. The decision regarding anticoagulation in the context of this group of diseases needs to be individualized based on many factors. In this chapter we will try to address this issue.

Epidemiology

Recent large-scale epidemiological studies (in hospitalized patients) have highlighted systemic autoimmune diseases as a risk factor for venous thromboembolism (VTE) [1–3].

Fig. 7.1 Risk of VTE among patients with systemic rheumatologic diseases

Disease	Risk of VTE (%)
Rheumatoid arthritis	1.17–1.91
Ankylosing spondylitis	1.16–1.93
Systemic lupus erythematosus	1.23–3.71
Systemic sclerosis	1.61–1.97
Polymyositis/dermatomyositis	3.04–3.36
Sjögren syndrome	2.02–2.19
Polymyalgia	1.91
Polyarteritis nodosa	2.57–3.53
Behçet disease	1.68

Adapted from Tamaki et al. [4]

These studies recommended to consider autoimmune disease as a hypercoagulable state and assumed that there may be a role for thromboprophylaxis in hospitalized patients with certain autoimmune diseases, especially if associated with other risk factors; this will be discussed later in this chapter.

Autoimmune rheumatic diseases such as rheumatoid arthritis (RA), systemic lupus erythematosus (SLE), inflammatory bowel disease (IBD), and Behçet's disease (BD) have been linked to an increased risk of venous thromboembolism (VTE) (Fig. 7.1) [4].

Pathogenesis

Inflammation is an important feature in most of autoimmune and immune-mediated disorders [5].

Systemic inflammation affects thrombotic responses by suppressing fibrinolysis, downregulating anticoagulants, and upregulating procoagulants (Fig. 7.2). Inflammation appears to change the hemostatic balance in a thrombogenic direction [6].

Proposed Mechanisms for the Increased VTE with Inflammation

1. *Factors increasing hypercoagulability*:
   - Increased tissue factor expression (through inflammation in an interleukin(IL)-6-mediated mechanism [8] or proteinase 3, PR3 ANCA) [9, 10].
   - Increased microparticles: In systemic autoimmune conditions such as RA, SLE, systemic sclerosis, and vasculitis, levels of platelet-derived microparticles are elevated [11].

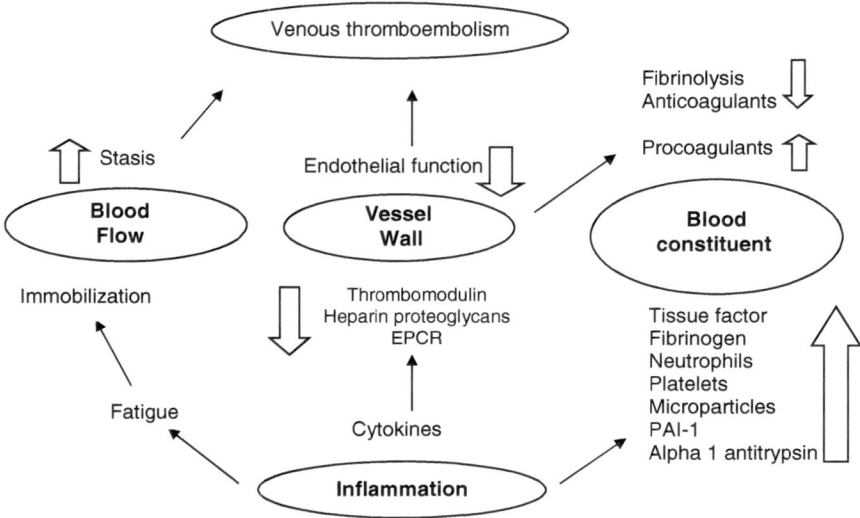

EPCR: endothelial protein c receptor.   PAI-1: Plasminogen activator inhibitor 1.

Fig. 7.2 Proposed mechanisms for the increased VTE with inflammation (Adapted from Zöller et al. [7])

- Platelet activation: The autoimmune reactions and the production of anti-platelet antibodies are suggested to contribute to platelet activation, release of vasoactive and thrombogenic agents, and accelerated atherosclerosis in many autoimmune diseases [12]. In SLE, immune complexes activate platelets by interacting with Fc receptors. In RA, the platelet is a well-known source of prostaglandins within the inflamed synovium [13]. In EGPA: through EPO (eosinophil peroxidase) and MBP (major basic protein) [14].
- Increased fibrinogen level through inflammation [15].
- NETosis has been implicated in the pathogenesis of SLE [16] and AAV and hypercoagulability via complement activation and the interaction with coagulation factors [17, 18].

2. *Lack of inhibitors* (through inflammation):
   - Reduced thrombomodulin (through tumor necrosis factor alpha (TNF-α), IL-1) [19].
   - Increased plasminogen activator inhibitor-1 (PAI-1). In patients with RA and ankylosing spondylitis, TNF-α inhibition causes reduced PAI-1. This means that TNF-α is likely involved in inhibition of the fibrinolytic system among patients with chronic inflammation [20].

3. *Other risk factors*:
   - Age, sex, and other comorbidities frequently associated with autoimmune disorders: diabetes mellitus, hypertension, and dyslipidemia [7].
   - Hospitalization and decreased mobilization [21].
   - Nephrotic-range proteinuria [7].
   - Drugs: steroids and immunosuppressive drugs [4] will be discussed later in this chapter.

In this chapter we will discuss the following:

1. Vasculitis:
   (A) Behçet's disease
   (B) ANCA-associated vasculitis
   (C) Large vessel vasculitis (LVV)
2. Systemic lupus erythematosus (SLE)
3. Systemic sclerosis (SSc)
4. Miscellaneous:
   - Rheumatoid arthritis, psoriasis (Pso), and psoriatic arthritis (PsA)
   - Ankylosing spondylitis (AS)
   - Sjögren syndrome (SS)
   - Sarcoidosis
5. Other autoimmune diseases as antiphospholipid syndrome will be not discussed in this chapter

1. *Vasculitis*:
   (A) *Behçet's Disease*

Behçet's disease (BD) is a multi-systemic auto-inflammatory disorder with variable vessel vasculitis that involves the skin, mucosa, joints, eyes, arteries, veins, nervous system, and gastrointestinal system.

Vascular BD is considered one of the main factors responsible of the overall mortality in BD patients [22]. The frequency of vascular involvement in BD in various studies ranges from 7% to 57% of BD patients depending on the geographic location. Venous involvement in BD is more common and makes up to 75% of all vascular complications [23].

It can manifest by deep vein thrombosis (DVT), superficial thrombophlebitis, cerebral venous sinus thrombosis, vena cava thrombosis, or Budd–Chiari syndrome [24].Thrombosis in BD is suggested to be as a result of vasculitis rather than hypercoagulable state [25]. Arterial involvement is present between in 1% and 7% of the patients [24]. The most characteristic arterial manifestations in BD patients are aneurysms, typically of the pulmonary artery and its major branches, whereas arterial thrombosis is less common [26]. These complications may remain asymptomatic or result in life- or organ-threatening infarctions such as acute myocardial infarction, stroke, intestinal infarction, intermittent claudication, or gangrene of the lower extremities [25]. Arterial occlusions and venous thromboses sometimes coexist in the same patient and maybe associated with aneurysms [27]. Thus, the coexistence of thrombosis and aneurysms is a characteristic feature of BD [28].

Management

The use of anticoagulation in BD cases with thrombotic events is debatable. DVT in BD is thought to be as a result of vasculitis rather than hypercoagulability. The European League Against Rheumatism (EULAR) guidelines [29] recommended the use of glucocorticoids and immunosuppressive agents such as cyclophosphamide, azathioprine, or cyclosporine A in acute DVT related to BD.

A meta-analysis performed by Hatemi and his colleagues [29] included three retrospective studies and reported efficacy of immunosuppressive drugs and/or anti-coagulants for preventing recurrences of DVT in patients with BD [30–32]. However, they found no statistically significant difference in the rate of thrombosis relapse between anticoagulants and immunosuppressive agents compared with immunosuppressives alone.

The use of immunosuppressive medications reduced the risk of recurrent thrombosis (hazard ratio [HR] 0.27 [95% CI 0.14–0.52], $P < 0.0001$). Glucocorticoid use also showed a trend toward prevention of recurrence, but this did not reach statistical significance (HR 0.71 [95% CI 0.14–1.07], $P = 0.099$) [29].

The EULAR task force also concluded that there are no data to support the role of anticoagulation in BD [29]. A counterargument was raised in another retrospective study that suggested that not adding anticoagulant may increase the risk of postthrombotic syndrome [33].

Cerebral venous thrombosis should be treated with high doses of corticosteroids followed by tapering. Methylprednisolone should be given as daily parenteral pulses of 1000 mg for 3–5 days followed by oral prednisone starting at 1 mg/kg daily. Maintenance oral corticosteroids should be tapered over 2–3 months. Anticoagulants may be added for a short duration [29].

Suggestions based on recent evidence:

A. Treatment of venous involvement includes the combination of immunosuppressive drugs and anticoagulation in certain situations [29].
B. The use of anticoagulation should be considered after the exclusion of pulmonary artery aneurysm and assessment of the risk of bleeding, and it is especially recommended for:
   1. Recurrent or refractory thrombosis in spite of receiving proper immunosuppressive drugs [34]
   2. Association with other causes of thrombophilia, Factor V Leiden, prothrombin gene mutation; protein C (Ptn C), protein S (Ptn S), and antithrombin III (AT III) deficiencies; and antiphospholipid (aPL) antibodies [35]
      • The levels of Ptn C, Ptn S, AT III, and aPL antibodies may be low in the presence of acute thrombus. Therefore, to reach reliable conclusions, the levels of anticoagulant proteins and other prothrombotic conditions should be evaluated when the acute period has subsided [35].
   3. Thrombosis in atypical places, e.g., cerebral venous thrombosis and Budd–Chiari syndrome [29, 35]

(B) *ANCA-Associated Vasculitis (AAV)*

Fig. 7.3 Percent of VTE in AAV from the French Vasculitis Study Group cohort [37]

ANCA-associated vasculitis	Percent of VTE (%)
EGPA	8.2
GPA	8
MPA	7.6

EGPA Eosinophilic granulomatosis with polyangiitis, *GPA* Granulomatosis with polyangiitis, *MPA* Microscopic polyangiitis

Patients with active antineutrophil cytoplasmic antibody (ANCA)-associated vasculitis are in hypercoagulable states and have a very high risk of VTE. This risk probably remains elevated, although to a much lower degree, during remission [36].

The French Vasculitis Study Group cohort included 1130 patients with AAV reported cases who experienced VTE during a mean follow-up period of 58.4 months (Fig. 7.3) [37].

This is to compare with polyarteritis nodosa (PAN) where VTE percentage was only 2.5%.

A meta-analysis by Ames and his colleagues reported increased risk of venous thrombosis in patients with EGPA, ranging between 5.8% and 30% [38]. Eosinophil-specific proteins including major basic protein (MBP), eosinophil peroxidase (EPO), and eosinophil cationic protein (ECP) were implicated as participating in thrombo-embolic diathesis. MBP and EPO can stimulate platelet activation [14].These proteins inhibit the capacity of endothelial cells to produce activated Ptn C [39].

There is increased risk of VTE especially in active cases of AAV; this may be attributed to the increased inflammation, decreased mobility, nephrotic-range proteinuria [4], and the use of more immunosuppressive drugs as corticosteroids [40, 41] and cyclophosphamide. Indeed, regimens containing cyclophosphamide were suspected to increase the risk of VTE in patients with cancer [42]. However, this role was not studied in this group of vasculitic diseases in particular.

Patients with AAV may experience symptoms mimicking or masking VTE like peripheral edema, for many different reasons including high-dose glucocorticoids, chronic kidney disease, or medications such as calcium channel inhibitors. However, clinicians should maintain high suspicion of VTE, especially of lower extremity DVT [43].

There are no recommendations for the use of antiplatelets or anticoagulation as a prophylaxis in cases with AAV. However, vigorous use of other preventive strategies is critical. This includes standard preventive measures in hospitalized patients and patient education about DVT prevention in the setting of car or airplane travel. Employing a low threshold for screening cases with AAV with signs or symptoms of VTE can detect these important events that can be associated with morbidity and even mortality [21].

No specific guidelines are available for VTEs and/or pulmonary embolism treatment in AAV patients [44]. The European Society of Cardiology recommends 3–6 months of anticoagulation after a VTE [45] (for anticoagulation options, see Chap. 2).

The use of anticoagulation in cases with VTE is a challenging issue with no consensus. As previously mentioned, there is increased risk of VTE in active cases with AAV. Such cases have also increased bleeding tendency specifically those with severe lung manifestations (diffuse alveolar hemorrhage, large cavitary lesions), renal failure, or pulmonary-renal syndrome [46]. For this reason, acute management of thrombotic events as well as duration of anticoagulation therapy is particularly challenging, and treatment should be tailored in each case after a thorough assessment of the bleeding risk and the extent of thrombosis.

Insertion of vena cava filter is recommended in patients with absolute contraindications for anticoagulation therapy [47]. In cases with intra-alveolar hemorrhage with DVT or VTE, vena cava filter and plasmapheresis are the salvage therapies besides mechanical ventilation if needed.

(C) Large Vessel Vasculitis (LVV)

LVV usually includes giant cell arteritis (GCA) and Takayasu's arteritis (TA).

- *Giant cell arteritis (GCA)*

This chronic granulomatous vasculitis of large and medium sized arteries is the most frequent form of vasculitis affecting persons over 50 years of age. Women are affected more frequently than men (3:1 to 5:1).

Increased risk of VTE, both DVT and pulmonary thromboembolism (PTE), in particular during the first year after diagnosis has been observed. The relative risk for DVT and PTE in GCA patients was 2.4 and 3.1, respectively [48].

GCA was studied in Spain to investigate thrombophilic risk factors. There was no correlation between ischemic manifestations and thrombotic risk factors such as aPL antibodies, Ptn C deficiency, Ptn S deficiency, AT III deficiency, Factor V Leiden mutation, or prothrombin gene G20210A mutation [49].

A recent cohort study evaluating nearly 3500 patients with GCA reported an increased risk of myocardial infarction (MI), cerebrovascular accident (CVA), and peripheral vascular disease (PVD), especially in the first month after the diagnosis [50]. Another Spanish study on 287 GCA patients reported a 3% incidence of stroke, mostly within 1 month of diagnosis, with permanent visual loss being the best predictor of stroke occurrence [51].

Antiplatelet/anticoagulant therapy prior to the diagnosis of GCA was not associated with reduction in severe ischemic complications. However, antiplatelet/anticoagulant therapy demonstrated a marginal benefit when used together with corticosteroid therapy in patients with established GCA without associated bleeding risk [52].

- *Takayasu's Arteritis (TA)*

TA is a granulomatous panarteritis of the aorta and its major branches resulting in localized stenoses, vascular occlusion, and aneurysm formation. It affects people younger than 50 years.

In a Korean retrospective study on TA, 21 of 190 (11%) patients, almost all of them were young females with mean age < 40 years, presented with stroke [53].

In TA the use of antiplatelet treatment appears to have a protective effect against ischemic events, while neither anticoagulants nor corticosteroids/immunosuppressive drugs seem to be able to prevent cardiovascular events [54].

It is important to treat the associated renovascular hypertension of Takayasu's arteritis with angiotensin II receptor antagonists. Concomitant therapies include low-dose aspirin and statins even in normolipidemic patients [55]. Statins have many benefits other than lipid lowering, as they have anti-inflammatory [56] and anti-oxidant properties. They also improve endothelial function [57].

2. *Systemic Lupus Erythematosus*

SLE is an independent risk factor for developing both arterial and venous thrombotic events. Thrombosis has been reported in about 10–26% of patients with SLE in different studies [58–60]. In one study, the risk of VTE was highest during the first 30 days after diagnosis of SLE [61]. However, in another study, the risk of thrombosis remained elevated throughout the course of the disease [60]. The risk may further increase when associated with other risk factors, or in the presence of inherited or acquired prothrombotic abnormalities, or triggering events, particularly, associated aPL antibodies. The presence of aPLs has been described in about 40% of SLE patients [62], while about 20% of antiphospholipid syndrome (APS) patients have SLE [63] (see Chap. 8). In SLE cases with aPL seropositivity, a meta-analysis supported the use of low-dose aspirin for thrombosis prophylaxis [64]. Bleeding risk should, however, be considered [65]. It is not clear whether to apply this approach in all cases with aPL seropositivity or to reserve it only for cases with high-risk of thrombosis (high titers of antibodies or triple positivity) [66]. Several factors should be considered. In addition to other co-morbidities and drug-drug interactions. Such patients may also use anticoagulation during highrisk periods as pregnancy and puerperium, post-operatively or if bedridden. According to the latest EULAR recommendations for the management of SLE, treatment of cases with APS in the context of SLE should not differ from the treatment of primary APS [67]. The treatment of Neuropsychiatric SLE depends on whether the underlying cause is either inflammatory or embolic/thrombotic/ischaemic. Differentiation between the two entities may not be easy in clinical practice, and different etiologies may coexist. In the latest EULAR recommendations, a combination of immunosuppression and anticoagulation/thrombolytic therapy may be considered in these patients [67].

A challenging topic is the possible procoagulant hemostatic effect of glucocorticoids. Whether glucocorticoid use contributes to a hypercoagulable state, and thereby increases the thrombotic risk, is controversial [41]. A recent study showed increased Factor VIII activity after use of IV pulses of methylprednisolone. In patients with additional risk factors of VTE and needing pulse methylprednisolone, anticoagulation prophylaxis should be considered [40].

The use of NSAIDs may increase cardiovascular risk as a class effect: ibuprofen is associated with a higher risk of stroke, diclofenac with higher cardiovascular toxicity, and naproxen seems to be the least harmful. On the other hand, NSAIDs interact synergistically with warfarin and increase the risk of GIT bleeding, their association being contraindicated [68, 69].

Serositis in SLE

Acute pericarditis could be the first manifestation of systemic lupus erythematosus. The possible prevalence of serositis in patients with SLE was 17.9% [70]. Serositis is highly associated with active lupus disease, fever (≥38 °C), and high D-dimer. This suggests that higher disease activity and hypercoagulability may both contribute to the generation and development of serositis in SLE [70].

NSAIDs are the mainstay of the therapy of inflammatory pericarditis [71].

In contrast to antiplatelet therapies, concomitant use of heparin and full anticoagulant is often perceived as a possible risk factor for the development of hemorrhagic pericardial effusion that may result in cardiac tamponade [72].

On the other hand, a study of 274 patients with acute pericarditis or myopericarditis, of different etiologies, reported that the use of heparin or other anticoagulants was not associated with an increased risk of cardiac tamponade [73].

The use of anticoagulant therapy has also been considered a possible poor prognostic predictor in the setting of acute pericarditis; however a multivariate analysis of about 500 cases of acute pericarditis did not confirm this suspicion [74].

3. *Systemic Sclerosis (SSc)*

A large cohort study performed on 1181 cases with SSc over 47 years showed that the risk of VTE in SSc is comparable to the general population [75]. Another study done in British Columbia, Canada, on 1245 cases with SSc showed that SSc patients are at a substantially increased risk of VTE, especially within the first year after SSc diagnosis [76]. In this study, the incidence rates of PE, DVT, and VTE were 3.47, 3.48, and 6.56 per 1000 person-years, respectively, whereas the corresponding rates in 12,670 non-SSc individuals, who were age and sex matched, were 0.78, 0.76, and 1.37 per 1000 person-years. Compared with non-SSc individuals, the multivariable HRs among SSc patients were 3.73 (95% confidence interval [95% CI] 1.98–7.04), 2.96 (95% CI 1.54–5.69), and 3.47 (95% CI 2.14–5.64) for PE, DVT, and VTE, respectively. The age-, sex-, and entry time-matched HRs for PE, DVT, and VTE were highest during the first year after SSc diagnosis (32.77 [95% CI 6.60–162.75], 8.50 [95% CI 3.13–23.04], and 12.03 [95% CI 5.27–27.45], respectively).

Additional studies in different geographic regions and other ethnic groups are needed.

The presence of pulmonary hypertension (PH), peripheral arterial disease, positive anti-Scl-70, and aPL antibodies are risk factors for VTE. VTE does not independently predict SSc survival [75].

The role of anticoagulation in the treatment of pulmonary hypertension remains uncertain and sometimes contradictory. Anticoagulation in treatment of PH associated with connective tissue disease seems to be associated with unfavorable risk to benefit ratio due to an increased rate of bleeding from the gastrointestinal tract. Anticoagulation is not indicated in scleroderma-associated PH or in severe Raynaud's or digital ulcers. However, conditions with increased thrombophilia (as with aPL antibodies) favor anticoagulation in SSc [77].

It is however not encountered to such extent in the experience of our two centers.

A review of 1138 charts identified 275 patients with SSc-PH ($n = 78$; 28% treated with warfarin) and 155 patients with idiopathic pulmonary hypertension (IPH) ($n = 91$; 59% treated with warfarin). The probability that warfarin improved median survival by 6 months or more was 23.5% in SSc-PH and 27.7% in IPH. Conversely, there was a >70% probability that warfarin provided no significant benefit or was harmful.

There is a low probability that warfarin improves survival in SSc-PH and IPH. Given the availability of other PH therapies with demonstrable benefits, there is no strong rationale to use warfarin to improve survival of these patients [78].

SSc can also cause arrhythmias, either ventricular or supraventricular arrhythmias [79]. For management in cardiology, see Chap. 3.

4. Miscellaneous

- Rheumatoid arthritis, psoriasis (Pso), and psoriatic arthritis (PsA)

In our paper assessing the mortality profile of patients with RA, pulmonary embolism was the third cause of cardiovascular death when RA was listed as the underlying cause of death (8.3%) [80].

Other studies reported that patients with RA have a 1.5- to 6-fold increased risk of VTE, compared to non-RA patients [81–83].

There was a bias in these results as most of the studies identified their RA cohort from admitted cases in hospitals who had severe RA, more immobilization, and more aggressive medications, in comparison with typical RA patients seen in the outpatient clinics [2, 82]. Some reports showed that the new targeted synthetic disease-modifying antirheumatic drugs (tsDMARDs) in particular with Jak1/Jak2 inhibitors showed a higher incidence of VTE. There are limited peer-reviewed publications summarizing trial data about the thromboembolic risks with baricitinib in RA [84].

In a recently published study, no association was found between using baricitinib in treating RA patients and major adverse cardiovascular events, arterial thrombotic events, or congestive heart failure. However, despite an imbalance in occurrence of VTE between baricitinib- and placebo-treated patients in the placebo-controlled study periods, the overall incidence rate for VTE in baricitinib-treated patients falls within the reported range for patients with RA [85].

Regarding the use of tofacitinib, in spite of the increased levels of cholesterol, low-density lipoprotein cholesterol (LDL-C) and high-density lipoprotein cholesterol (HDL-C), after using it, the atherogenic index did not appear to change. Also, the rate of CV events was found to be low, comparable to that of placebo and methotrexate [86].

Patients with PsA, RA, and Pso had an elevated incidence of VTE compared with patients without these common inflammatory disorders after adjusting for age and sex. The age- and sex-adjusted risk for PTE was significantly elevated compared with controls except for patients with mild psoriasis, who fell within the same risk for those who do not have the aforementioned disease [87].

- *Ankylosing Spondylitis (AS)*

A meta-analysis demonstrated a significant association between AS and VTE with an overall 1.6-fold (95% CI, 1.05–2.44) increased risk compared with non-AS participants of matched age and sex [88]. The pathogenesis of increased VTE in AS is not well understood, but it may be attributed to the higher inflammatory burden; increased inflammatory cytokines as IL-6, IL-8, and TNF-α that can promote the coagulation cascade inhibit the anticoagulation pathway and impair fibrinolysis [89]. Also, chronic inflammation can lead to endothelial dysfunction [90]. Moreover, cases with AS have arthritis with limited mobility rendering them at a higher risk of venous stasis [88].

- *Polymyositis (PM) and Dermatomyositis (DM)*

A recent meta-analysis demonstrated that both PM and DM are associated with an elevated risk of VTE. The increased systemic inflammation associated with PM/DM may cause hypercoagulability by upregulating procoagulants, downregulating anticoagulants, and suppressing fibrinolysis. Also, the possibility of associated malignancy may be a cause of the hypercoagulable state [91].

These mechanisms suggest that patients with PM/DM should be carefully monitored for the development of these conditions and suggest that physicians should carefully monitor patients with PM and DM for VTE, particularly those with other conventional risk factors [92].

- *Sjögren Syndrome (SS)*

Among 1175 of primary Sjögren syndrome (pSS) cases (mean age 56.7 years, 87.6% women), the incidence of PTE, DVT, and VTE was 3.9, 2.8, and 5.2 per 1000 person-years, respectively. These findings also provide population-based evidence that patients with pSS have a substantially increased risk of VTE, especially within the first year after SS diagnosis [93]. This may be due to the increased inflammation at the time of diagnosis with its sequelae on the hypercoagulable state as previously discussed.

- *Sarcoidosis*

The cumulative incidence of VTE among patients with sarcoidosis at 10 years was 4.0%, which corresponded to an approximately threefold increased risk of incident VTE adjusted for age, sex, and calendar year. Significantly elevated risk was observed in both DVT and PTE [94, 95].

Prophylactic Anticoagulation for Cases with Increased Thrombosis Risk

Based on our previous discussion, almost all autoimmune diseases are associated with hypercoagulable state manifesting in increased incidence of DVT and VTE. This raises the issue of whether or not there is a need for prophylactic anticoagulation in hospitalized cases with autoimmune diseases especially when associated with other risk factors as diabetes mellitus, hypertension, dyslipidemia,

Baseline features	Score
Active cancer (patients with local or distant metastases and/or in whom chemotherapy or radiotheraphy had been performed in the previous 6 months)	3
Previous VTE (with the exclusion of superficial vein thrmobosis)	3
Reduced mobility	3
Already known thrombophilic condition	3
Recent (≤1 month) trauma and/or surgery	2
Elderly age (≥70 years)	1
Heart and/or respiratory failure	1
Acute myocardial infarction or ischemic stroke	1
Acute infection and/or *rheumatologic disorder*	1
Obesity (BMI ≥30)	1
Ongoing hormonal treatment	1

Fig. 7.4   Padua risk score [97]

immobilization, peripheral edema, and medications. The decision of anticoagulation depends on the estimated risk of thrombosis in acutely ill hospitalized medical patients. Prophylactic anticoagulation is recommended in cases with increased risk of thrombosis, but in patients at low risk of thrombosis, no recommendation for resorting to anticoagulation [96].

The *Padua* Prediction Score is a *risk assessment model* for the identification of patients at risk of VTE. It identifies admitted patients who may be at high risk for VTE and would benefit from thromboprophylaxis. Patients with higher Padua risk score ≥ 4 have a high incidence of VTE [97] (Fig. 7.4).

Strategies to Improve VTE Prophylaxis in Different Rheumatic Diseases

1. Early mobilization in hospitalized cases [21].
2. Early suspicion of DVT (any new limb swelling) [21].
3. Pulmonary embolism should be suspected in any case with rheumatological condition presenting with new onset dyspnea [98].
4. Control of active diseases and induction of remission: treating inflammation in autoimmune diseases is probably the most important way of preventing VTE [99].
5. Prophylactic anticoagulation in high risk hospitalized patients especially in cases with active diseases [99].
6. Bleeding risk should be assessed and the benefits from anticoagulation should be weighed against the risk of thrombosis [47].
7. Drug interactions should be considered [100].

VTE prophylaxis measures should be decided within 24 hours of hospital admission, otherwise, a risk assessment and contraindications for prophylaxis [98].

Recommendations for Joint and Soft Tissue Injections

Local injection of joints and soft tissue is a fundamental tool in the practice of rheumatology. Many cases are anticoagulated and need local injection in daily practice.

A retrospective study was done in the USA on 640 arthrocentesis and joint injection procedures performed in 514 anticoagulated patients between 2001 and 2009. They further compared the incidence of bleeding in 456 procedures performed in patients with an international normalized ratio 2.0 or greater and 184 procedures performed in patients with an international normalized ratio less than 2.0. Only one procedure (0.2%) resulted in early, significant, clinical bleeding in the fully anticoagulated group. There was no statistically significant difference in early and late complications between patients who had procedures performed with an international normalized ratio 2.0 or greater and those whose anticoagulation was adjusted to an international normalized ratio less than 2.0 [101].

Another Irish study was done on patients receiving warfarin. Patients were divided into two groups. In the first group of patients in whom warfarin was withheld, 32 injections were performed in 18 patients (13 RA, 11 osteoarthritis, 5 spondyloarthropathy, and 1 each of adhesive capsulitis, rotator cuff tendinopathy, and trochanteric bursitis). In patients who continued warfarin, 32 injections were performed in 21 patients (11 RA, 7 osteoarthritis, 6 crystal arthritis, 4 rotator cuff tendinopathy, 2 spondyloarthropathy, 1 adhesive capsulitis, and 1 carpal tunnel syndrome). There were no clinical hemarthroses or complications in either group. They concluded that joint and soft tissue injections appear to be safe in patients receiving warfarin anticoagulation with an INR <3 [102].

From the previous two studies, we conclude that for patients taking warfarin, provided the INR is within the therapeutic range, i.e., less than 3, the risk of significant hemorrhage following joint or soft tissue injection appears to be very low [101, 102]. However, these recommendations may differ between countries and according to type of joint as there will be a higher bleeding risk with injection of hip joints or spine.

In a retrospective medical record review of 1050 arthrocentesis and joint injection procedures performed in consecutive adult patients in Mayo Clinic in Rochester, Minnesota, over 6 years, in patients taking NOACs, there were no bleeding complications and no need to withhold anticoagulation treatment before the procedure [103].

These agents have a shorter half-life than warfarin; consideration should be given to avoid interventional procedures during peak drug activity. According to the Guidelines from the American Society of Regional Anesthesia and Pain Medicine, the European Society of Regional Anaesthesia and Pain Therapy, the American Academy of Pain Medicine, the International Neuromodulation Society, the North American Neuromodulation Society, and the World Institute of Pain, for low-risk procedures, stoppage of rivaroxaban, apixaban, and dabigatran for two half-life intervals may be considered. A 24-hour interval after interventional pain procedures before their resumption may be considered [104].

If bleeding should occur in patients taking NOACs, it can be managed by withholding the NOAC and providing supportive care [105]. For the reversal of NOACs, see Chap. 12.

It appears to be safe to do the procedure without stoppage of anticoagulation; however, caution should be given to assess the bleeding risk especially with supratherapeutic levels of INR (>3), thrombocytopenia, usage of aspirin, and associated comorbidities [101]. In this context the authors recommend postinjection observation.

Drug Interactions

The pharmacological armamentarium employed by rheumatologists encompasses many drug groups that interact with currently used anticoagulants mainly warfarin and NOACs. The long list includes NSAIDs and many other drugs, either potentiating their effects or decreasing it. For a comprehensive discussion, see Chap. 1.

Paracetamol is the gold standard analgesic and antipyretic therapy for patients receiving warfarin; clinicians may not recognize the potential interaction between the two medications [106].

Paracetamol increases the anticoagulant effect of warfarin, even at a recommended therapeutic dosing regimen, i.e., 2 g/day, thus requiring close INR monitoring [107]. The dose–effect relationship, i.e., the relationship between the dose of harm-producing substances and the severity of their effect on exposed individuals [100], of this drug–drug interaction was observed between 2 and 4 g/day [107, 108].

Conclusion

Many rheumatic diseases are associated with increased risk of thrombosis. Attention to this potentially serious complication can't be overemphasized. It requires a high index of suspicion and early detection. The decision regarding the need and choice of anticoagulation is based on the disease type and its clinical presentation, activity, severity, and comorbidities. Awareness of drug–drug interactions is mandatory.

References

1. Yusuf HR, Hooper WC, Beckman MG, Zhang QC, Tsai J, Ortel TL. Risk of venous thromboembolism among hospitalizations of adults with selected autoimmune diseases. J Thromb Thrombolysis. 2014;38(3):306–13.
2. Zoller B, Li X, Sundquist J, Sundquist K. Risk of pulmonary embolism in patients with autoimmune disorders: a nationwide follow-up study from Sweden. Lancet (London, England). 2012;379(9812):244–9.

3. Ramagopalan SV, Wotton CJ, Handel AE, Yeates D, Goldacre MJJBM. Risk of venous thromboembolism in people admitted to hospital with selected immune-mediated diseases: record-linkage study. BMC Med. 2011;9(1):1.
4. Tamaki H, Khasnis A. Venous thromboembolism in systemic autoimmune diseases: a narrative review with emphasis on primary systemic vasculitides. Vascular medicine (London, England). 2015;20(4):369–76.
5. Rahman P, Inman RD, El-Gabalawy H, Krause DO. Pathophysiology and pathogenesis of immune-mediated inflammatory diseases: commonalities and differences. J Rheumatol Suppl. 2010;85:11–26.
6. Tamaki H, Khasnis A. Venous thromboembolism in systemic autoimmune diseases: a narrative review with emphasis on primary systemic vasculitides. Vasc Med. 2015;20(4):369–76.
7. Zöller B, Li X, Sundquist J, Sundquist K. Autoimmune diseases and venous thromboembolism: a review of the literature. Am J Cardiovasc Dis. 2012;2(3):171–83.
8. Spronk HM, Govers-Riemslag JW, ten Cate H. The blood coagulation system as a molecular machine. BioEssays. 2003;25(12):1220–8.
9. Steppich BA, Seitz I, Busch G, Stein A, Ott I. Modulation of tissue factor and tissue factor pathway inhibitor-1 by neutrophil proteases. Thromb Haemost. 2008;100(6):1068–75.
10. Haubitz M, Gerlach M, Kruse HJ, Brunkhorst R. Endothelial tissue factor stimulation by proteinase 3 and elastase. Clin Exp Immunol. 2001;126(3):584–8.
11. Ardoin SP, Shanahan JC, Pisetsky DS. The role of microparticles in inflammation and thrombosis. Scand J Immunol. 2007;66(2–3):159–65.
12. Gasparyan AY, Stavropoulos-Kalinoglou A, Mikhailidis DP, Toms TE, Douglas KM, Kitas GD. The rationale for comparative studies of accelerated atherosclerosis in rheumatic diseases. Curr Vasc Pharmacol. 2010;8(4):437–49.
13. Boilard E, Blanco P, Nigrovic PA. Platelets: active players in the pathogenesis of arthritis and SLE. Nat Rev Rheumatol. 2012;8(9):534–42.
14. Rohrbach MS, Wheatley CL, Slifman NR, Gleich GJ. Activation of platelets by eosinophil granule proteins. J Exp Med. 1990;172(4):1271–4.
15. de Moerloose P, Boehlen F, Neerman-Arbez M. Fibrinogen and the risk of thrombosis. Semin Thromb Hemost. 2010;36(1):7–17.
16. Fuchs TA, Abed U, Goosmann C, Hurwitz R, Schulze I, Wahn V, et al. Novel cell death program leads to neutrophil extracellular traps. J Cell Biol. 2007;176(2):231–41.
17. Nakazawa D, Tomaru U, Suzuki A, Masuda S, Hasegawa R, Kobayashi T, et al. Abnormal conformation and impaired degradation of propylthiouracil-induced neutrophil extracellular traps: implications of disordered neutrophil extracellular traps in a rat model of myeloperoxidase antineutrophil cytoplasmic antibody-associated vasculitis. Arthritis Rheum. 2012;64(11):3779–87.
18. Kessenbrock K, Krumbholz M, Schonermarck U, Back W, Gross WL, Werb Z, et al. Netting neutrophils in autoimmune small-vessel vasculitis. Nat Med. 2009;15(6):623–5.
19. Lentz S, Tsiang M, Sadler J. Regulation of thrombomodulin by tumor necrosis factor-alpha: comparison of transcriptional and posttranscriptional mechanisms. Blood. 1991;77(3):542–50.
20. Rijken DC, Lijnen HR. New insights into the molecular mechanisms of the fibrinolytic system. J Thromb Haemost. 2009;7(1):4–13.
21. Abdel-Razeq H. Venous thromboembolism prophylaxis for hospitalized medical patients, current status and strategies to improve. Annals of thoracic medicine. 2010;5(4):195–200.
22. Kalko Y, Basaran M, Aydin U, Kafa U, Basaranoglu G, Yasar T. The surgical treatment of arterial aneurysms in Behcet disease: a report of 16 patients. J Vasc Surg. 2005;42(4):673–7.
23. Saadoun D, Wechsler B. Behcet's disease. Orphanet J Rare Dis. 2012;7:20.
24. Calamia KT, Schirmer M, Melikoglu M. Major vessel involvement in Behcet's disease: an update. Curr Opin Rheumatol. 2011;23(1):24–31.
25. Emmi G, Squatrito D, Silvestri E, Grassi A, Emmi L. Pathogenesis of Behçet syndrome. In: Emmi L, editor. Behçet's syndrome: from pathogenesis to treatment. Milano: Springer Milan; 2014. p. 53–66.
26. Atzeni F, Sarzi-Puttini P, Doria A, Boiardi L, Pipitone N, Salvarani C. Behcet's disease and cardiovascular involvement. Lupus. 2005;14(9):723–6.

27. Duzgun N, Ates A, Aydintug OT, Demir O, Olmez U. Characteristics of vascular involvement in Behcet's disease. Scand J Rheumatol. 2006;35(1):65–8.
28. Ceyran H, Akçali Y, Kahraman C. Surgical treatment of vasculo-Behçet's disease. A review of patients with concomitant multiple aneurysms and venous lesions. VASA Zeitschrift fur Gefasskrankheiten. 2003;32(3):149–53.
29. Hatemi G, Christensen R, Bang D, Bodaghi B, Celik AF, Fortune F, et al. 2018 update of the EULAR recommendations for the management of Behcet's syndrome. Ann Rheum Dis. 2018;77(6):808–18.
30. Ahn JK, Lee YS, Jeon CH, Koh EM, Cha HS. Treatment of venous thrombosis associated with Behcet's disease: immunosuppressive therapy alone versus immunosuppressive therapy plus anticoagulation. Clin Rheumatol. 2008;27(2):201–5.
31. Desbois AC, Wechsler B, Resche-Rigon M, Piette JC, Huong Dle T, Amoura Z, et al. Immunosuppressants reduce venous thrombosis relapse in Behcet's disease. Arthritis Rheum. 2012;64(8):2753–60.
32. Alibaz-Oner F, Karadeniz A, Ylmaz S, Balkarl A, Kimyon G, Yazc A, et al. Behcet disease with vascular involvement: effects of different therapeutic regimens on the incidence of new relapses. Medicine. 2015;94(6):e494.
33. Seyahi E, Cakmak OS, Tutar B, Arslan C, Dikici AS, Sut N, et al. Clinical and ultrasono-graphic evaluation of lower-extremity Vein Thrombosis in Behcet syndrome: an observa-tional study. Medicine. 2015;94(44):e1899-e.
34. Güngen AC, Çoban H, Aydemir Y, Düzenli H. Consider Behcet's disease in young patients with deep vein thrombosis. Respiratory medicine case reports. 2016;18:41–4.
35. Korkmaz C. Is anticoagulation unnecessary in Behcet's disease with deep venous thrombo-sis? Clin Rheumatol. 2008;27(3):405–6.
36. Ma TT, Huang YM, Wang C, Zhao MH, Chen M. Coagulation and fibrinolysis index profile in patients with ANCA-associated vasculitis. PLoS One. 2014;9(5):e97843.
37. Allenbach Y, Seror R, Pagnoux C, Teixeira L, Guilpain P, Guillevin L. High frequency of venous thromboembolic events in Churg-Strauss syndrome, Wegener's granulomatosis and microscopic polyangiitis but not polyarteritis nodosa: a systematic retrospective study on 1130 patients. Ann Rheum Dis. 2009;68(4):564–7.
38. Ames PRJ, Margaglione M, Mackie S, Alves JD. Eosinophilia and thrombophilia in churg strauss syndrome: a clinical and pathogenetic overview. Clin Appl Thromb Hemost. 2010;16(6):628–36.
39. Slungaard A, Vercellotti GM, Tran T, Gleich GJ, Key NS. Eosinophil cationic granule pro-teins impair thrombomodulin function. A potential mechanism for thromboembolism in hypereosinophilic heart disease. J Clin Invest. 1993;91(4):1721–30.
40. Miskiewicz P, Milczarek-Banach J, Rutkowska-Hinc B, Kondracka A, Bednarczuk T. High-dose intravenous methylprednisolone therapy in patients with Graves' orbitopathy is associ-ated with the increased activity of factor VIII. J Endocrinol Invest. 2018;42(2):217–25.
41. van Zaane B, Nur E, Squizzato A, Gerdes VE, Buller HR, Dekkers OM, et al. Systematic review on the effect of glucocorticoid use on procoagulant, anti-coagulant and fibrinolytic factors. Journal of thrombosis and haemostasis : JTH. 2010;8(11):2483–93.
42. Levine MN. Prevention of thrombotic disorders in cancer patients undergoing chemotherapy. Thromb Haemost. 1997;78(1):133–6.
43. Monach PA. ANCA-associated vasculitis: a prothrombotic state even in remission? J Rheumatol. 2013;40(12):1935–7.
44. Groh M, Pagnoux C, Baldini C, Bel E, Bottero P, Cottin V, et al. Eosinophilic granulomato-sis with polyangiitis (Churg-Strauss) (EGPA) Consensus Task Force recommendations for evaluation and management. Eur J Intern Med. 2015;26(7):545–53.
45. Torbicki A, Perrier A, Konstantinides S, Agnelli G, Galie N, Pruszczyk P, et al. Guidelines on the diagnosis and management of acute pulmonary embolism: the Task Force for the Diagnosis and Management of Acute Pulmonary Embolism of the European Society of Cardiology (ESC). Eur Heart J. 2008;29(18):2276–315.
46. Emmi G, Silvestri E, Squatrito D, Amedei A, Niccolai E, D'Elios MM, et al. Thrombosis in vasculitis: from pathogenesis to treatment. Thrombosis journal. 2015;13:15.

47. Jaff MR, McMurtry MS, Archer SL, Cushman M, Goldenberg N, Goldhaber SZ, et al. Management of massive and submassive pulmonary embolism, iliofemoral deep vein thrombosis, and chronic thromboembolic pulmonary hypertension: a scientific statement from the American Heart Association. Circulation. 2011;123(16):1788–830.
48. Avina-Zubieta JA, Bhole VM, Amiri N, Sayre EC, Choi HK. The risk of deep venous thrombosis and pulmonary embolism in giant cell arteritis: a general population-based study. Ann Rheum Dis. 2016;75(1):148–54.
49. Manna R, Latteri M, Cristiano G, Todaro L, Scuderi F, Gasbarrini G. Anticardiolipin antibodies in giant cell arteritis and polymyalgia rheumatica: a study of 40 cases. Br J Rheumatol. 1998;37(2):208–10.
50. Tomasson G, Peloquin C, Mohammad A, Love TJ, Zhang Y, Choi HK, et al. Risk for cardiovascular disease early and late after a diagnosis of giant-cell arteritis: a cohort study. Ann Intern Med. 2014;160(2):73–80.
51. Gonzalez-Gay MA, Vazquez-Rodriguez TR, Gomez-Acebo I, Pego-Reigosa R, Lopez-Diaz MJ, Vazquez-Trinanes MC, et al. Strokes at time of disease diagnosis in a series of 287 patients with biopsy-proven giant cell arteritis. Medicine. 2009;88(4):227–35.
52. Martinez-Taboada VM, Lopez-Hoyos M, Narvaez J, Munoz-Cacho P. Effect of antiplatelet/anticoagulant therapy on severe ischemic complications in patients with giant cell arteritis: a cumulative meta-analysis. Autoimmun Rev. 2014;13(8):788–94.
53. Hwang J, Kim SJ, Bang OY, Chung CS, Lee KH, Kim DK, et al. Ischemic stroke in Takayasu's arteritis: lesion patterns and possible mechanisms. Journal of clinical neurology (Seoul, Korea). 2012;8(2):109–15.
54. de Souza AW, Machado NP, Pereira VM, Arraes AE, Reis Neto ET, Mariz HA, et al. Antiplatelet therapy for the prevention of arterial ischemic events in takayasu arteritis. Circ J. 2010;74(6):1236–41.
55. Berlit P. Review: diagnosis and treatment of cerebral vasculitis. Ther Adv Neurol Disord. 2010;3(1):29–42.
56. Weitz-Schmidt G, Welzenbach K, Brinkmann V, Kamata T, Kallen J, Bruns C, et al. Statins selectively inhibit leukocyte function antigen-1 by binding to a novel regulatory integrin site. Nat Med. 2001;7(6):687–92.
57. Bonetti PO, Lerman LO, Napoli C, Lerman A. Statin effects beyond lipid lowering—are they clinically relevant? Eur Heart J. 2003;24(3):225–48.
58. Burgos PI, Alarcon GS. Thrombosis in systemic lupus erythematosus: risk and protection. Expert Rev Cardiovasc Ther. 2009;7(12):1541–9.
59. Sarabi ZS, Chang E, Bobba R, Ibanez D, Gladman D, Urowitz M, et al. Incidence rates of arterial and venous thrombosis after diagnosis of systemic lupus erythematosus. Arthritis Rheum. 2005;53(4):609–12.
60. Romero-Diaz J, Garcia-Sosa I, Sanchez-Guerrero J. Thrombosis in systemic lupus erythematosus and other autoimmune diseases of recent onset. J Rheumatol. 2009;36(1):68–75.
61. Lee JJ, Pope JE. A meta-analysis of the risk of venous thromboembolism in inflammatory rheumatic diseases. Arthritis Res Ther. 2014;16(5):435.
62. Bustamante JG, Bhimji SS. Antiphospholipid syndrome (antiphospholipid antibody syndrome, APS, APLS). StatPearls. Treasure Island (FL): StatPearls Publishing StatPearls Publishing LLC; 2018.
63. Bazzan M, Vaccarino A, Marletto FJTJ. Systemic lupus erythematosus and thrombosis. Thromb J. 2015;13(1):16.
64. Arnaud L, Mathian A, Ruffatti A, Erkan D, Tektonidou M, Cervera R, Forastiero R, Pengo V, Lambert M, Martinez-Zamora MA, Balasch J, Zuily S, Wahl D, Amoura Z. Efficacy of aspirin for the primary prevention of thrombosis in patients with antiphospholipid antibodies: An international and collaborative meta-analysis. Autoimmun Rev. 2014;13(3):281–91.
65. ASCEND Study Collaborative Group, Bowman L, Mafham M, Wallendszus K, Stevens W, Buck G, Barton J, Murphy K, Aung T, Haynes R, Cox J, Murawska A, Young A, Lay M, Chen F, Sammons E, Waters E, Adler A, Bodansky J, Farmer A, McPherson R, Neil A, Simpson D,

Peto R, Baigent C, Collins R, Parish S, Armitage J. Effects of aspirin for primary prevention in persons with diabetes mellitus. N Engl J Med. 2018;379(16):1529–39.

66. Pengo V, Ruffatti A, Legnani C, Gresele P, Barcellona D, Erba N, Testa S, Marongiu F, Bison E, Denas G, Banzato A, Padayattil Jose S, Iliceto S. Clinical course of high-risk patients diagnosed with antiphospholipid syndrome. J Thromb Haemost. 2010;8(2):237–42.

67. Fanouriakis A, Kostopoulou M, Alunno A, Aringer M, Bajema I, Boletis JN, Cervera R, Doria A, Gordon C, Govoni M, Houssiau F, Jayne D, Kouloumas M, Kuhn A, Larsen JL, Lerstrøm K, Moroni G, Mosca M, Schneider M, Smolen JS, Svenungsson E, Tesar V, Tincani A, Troldborg A, van Vollenhoven R, Wenzel J, Bertsias G, Boumpas DT. 2019 update of the EULAR recommendations for the management of systemic lupus erythematosus. Ann Rheum Dis. 2019;78(6):736–45.

68. Fanelli A, Ghisi D, Aprile PL, Lapi F. Cardiovascular and cerebrovascular risk with nonsteroidal anti-inflammatory drugs and cyclooxygenase 2 inhibitors: latest evidence and clinical implications. Ther Adv Drug Saf. 2017;8(6):173–82.

69. Fanelli A, Romualdi P, Vigano R, Lora Aprile P, Gensini G, Fanelli G. Non-selective non-steroidal anti-inflammatory drugs (NSAIDs) and cardiovascular risk. Acta Biomed. 2013;84(1):5–11.

70. Liang Y, Leng R-X, Pan H-F, Ye D-QJRI. The prevalence and risk factors for serositis in patients with systemic lupus erythematosus: a cross-sectional study. Rheumatol Int. 2017;37(2):305–11.

71. Adler Y, Charron P, Imazio M, Badano L, Baron-Esquivias G, Bogaert J, et al. 2015 ESC Guidelines for the diagnosis and management of pericardial diseases: The Task Force for the Diagnosis and Management of Pericardial Diseases of the European Society of Cardiology (ESC) Endorsed by: The European Association for Cardio-Thoracic Surgery (EACTS). Eur Heart J. 2015;36(42):2921–64.

72. Imazio M, Brucato A, Spodick DH, Adler Y. Prognosis of myopericarditis as determined from previously published reports. J Cardiovasc Med (Hagerstown). 2014;15(12):835–9.

73. Imazio M, Cooper LT. Management of myopericarditis. Expert Rev Cardiovasc Ther. 2013;11(2):193–201.

74. Hohlfeld T, Saxena A, Schror K. High on treatment platelet reactivity against aspirin by non-steroidal anti-inflammatory drugs–pharmacological mechanisms and clinical relevance. Thromb Haemost. 2013;109(5):825–33.

75. Johnson SR, Hakami N, Ahmad Z, Wijeysundera DN. Venous thromboembolism in systemic sclerosis: prevalence, risk factors, and effect on survival. J Rheumatol. 2018;45(7):942–6.

76. Schoenfeld SR, Choi HK, Sayre EC, Aviña-Zubieta JA. Risk of pulmonary embolism and deep venous thrombosis in systemic sclerosis: a general population-based study. Arthritis Care Res (Hoboken). 2016;68(2):246–53.

77. Palazzini M, Manes A, Gotti E, Dardi F, Rinaldi A, Galiè N. Anticoagulant treatment in patients with pulmonary arterial hypertension associated with systemic sclerosis: more shadows than lights. J Scleroderma Relat Disord. 2018;3(1):39–42.

78. Johnson SR, Granton JT, Tomlinson GA, Grosbein HA, Le T, Lee P, et al. Warfarin in systemic sclerosis-associated and idiopathic pulmonary arterial hypertension. A Bayesian approach to evaluating treatment for uncommon disease. J Rheumatol. 2012;39(2):276–85.

79. Vacca A, Meune C, Gordon J, Chung L, Proudman S, Assassi S, et al. Cardiac arrhythmias and conduction defects in systemic sclerosis. Rheumatology (Oxford). 2014;53(7):1172–7.

80. Avouac J, Amrouche F, Meune C, Rey G, Kahan A, Allanore Y. Mortality profile of patients with rheumatoid arthritis in France and its change in 10 years. Semin Arthritis Rheum. 2017;46(5):537–43.

81. Bacani AK, Gabriel SE, Crowson CS, Heit JA, Matteson EL. Noncardiac vascular disease in rheumatoid arthritis: increase in venous thromboembolic events? Arthritis Rheum. 2012;64(1):53–61.

82. Johannesdottir SA, Schmidt M, Horvath-Puho E, Sorensen HT. Autoimmune skin and connective tissue diseases and risk of venous thromboembolism: a population-based case-control study. J Thromb Haemost. 2012;10(5):815–21.

83. Choi HK, Rho YH, Zhu Y, Cea-Soriano L, Avina-Zubieta JA, Zhang Y. The risk of pulmonary embolism and deep vein thrombosis in rheumatoid arthritis: a UK population-based outpatient cohort study. Ann Rheum Dis. 2013;72(7):1182–7.

84. Scott IC, Hider SL, Scott DL. Thromboembolism with Janus Kinase (JAK) inhibitors for rheumatoid arthritis: how real is the risk? Drug Saf. 2018;41(7):645–53.

85. Taylor PC, Weinblatt ME, Burmester GR, Rooney TP, Witt S, Walls CD, et al. Cardiovascular safety during treatment with baricitinib in rheumatoid arthritis. Arthritis Rheumatol. 2019;71(7):1042–55.

86. Kawalec P, Sladowska K, Malinowska-Lipien I, Brzostek T, Kozka M. European perspective on the management of rheumatoid arthritis: clinical utility of tofacitinib. Ther Clin Risk Manag. 2018;14:15–29.

87. Ogdie A, Kay McGill N, Shin DB, Takeshita J, Jon Love T, Noe MH, et al. Risk of venous thromboembolism in patients with psoriatic arthritis, psoriasis and rheumatoid arthritis: a general population-based cohort study. Eur Heart J. 2018;39(39):3608–14.

88. Ungprasert P, Srivali N, Kittanamongkolchai W. Ankylosing spondylitis and risk of venous thromboembolism: a systematic review and meta-analysis. Lung India. 2016;33(6):642–5.

89. Xu J, Lupu F, Esmon CT. Inflammation, innate immunity and blood coagulation. Hamostaseologie. 2010;30(1):5–6, 8–9.

90. Jezovnik MK, Poredos P. Idiopathic venous thrombosis is related to systemic inflammatory response and to increased levels of circulating markers of endothelial dysfunction. Int Angiol. 2010;29(3):226–31.

91. Khorana AA. The wacky hypercoagulable state of malignancy. Blood. 2015;126(4):430–1.

92. Li Y, Wang P, Li L, Wang F, Liu Y. Increased risk of venous thromboembolism associated with polymyositis and dermatomyositis: a meta-analysis. Ther Clin Risk Manag. 2018;14:157–65.

93. Avina-Zubieta JA, Jansz M, Sayre EC, Choi HK. The risk of deep venous thrombosis and pulmonary embolism in primary sjogren syndrome: a general population-based study. J Rheumatol. 2017;44(8):1184–9.

94. Ungprasert P, Crowson CS, Matteson EL. Association of sarcoidosis with increased risk of VTE: a population-based study, 1976 to 2013. Chest. 2017;151(2):425–30.

95. Ungprasert P, Crowson CS, Matteson EL. Epidemiology and clinical characteristics of sarcoidosis: an update from a population-based cohort study from Olmsted County, Minnesota. Reumatismo. 2017;69(1):16–22.

96. Saigal S, Sharma JP, Joshi R, Singh DK. Thrombo-prophylaxis in acutely ill medical and critically ill patients. Indian J Crit Care Med. 2014;18(6):382–91.

97. Barbar S, Noventa F, Rossetto V, Ferrari A, Brandolin B, Perlati M, et al. A risk assessment model for the identification of hospitalized medical patients at risk for venous thromboembolism: the Padua Prediction Score. J Thromb Haemost. 2010;8(11):2450–7.

98. measures TJCMfFPi. 2018. Available from: https://www.jointcommission.org/performance_measurement.aspx.

99. Esmon CT, Esmon NL. The link between vascular features and thrombosis. Annu Rev Physiol. 2011;73:503–14.

100. Holford NH, Sheiner LB. Understanding the dose-effect relationship: clinical application of pharmacokinetic-pharmacodynamic models. Clin Pharmacokinet. 1981;6(6):429–53.

101. Ahmed I, Gertner E. Safety of arthrocentesis and joint injection in patients receiving anticoagulation at therapeutic levels. Am J Med. 2012;125(3):265–9.

102. Conway R, O'Shea FD, Cunnane G, Doran MF. Safety of joint and soft tissue injections in patients on warfarin anticoagulation. Clin Rheumatol. 2013;32(12):1811–4.

103. Yui JC, Preskill C, Greenlund LS. Arthrocentesis and joint injection in patients receiving direct oral anticoagulants. Mayo Clin Proc. 2017;92(8):1223–6.

104. Narouze S, Benzon HT, Provenzano DA, Buvanendran A, De Andres J, Deer TR, et al. Interventional spine and pain procedures in patients on antiplatelet and anticoagulant medications: guidelines from the American Society of Regional Anesthesia and Pain Medicine, the European Society of Regional Anaesthesia and Pain Therapy, the American Academy of Pain

Medicine, the International Neuromodulation Society, the North American Neuromodulation Society, and the World Institute of Pain. Reg Anesth Pain Med. 2015;40(3):182–212.
105. Burnett A, Siegal D, Crowther M. Specific antidotes for bleeding associated with direct oral anticoagulants. BMJ (Clinical research ed). 2017;357:j2216.
106. Hughes GJ, Patel PN, Saxena N. Effect of acetaminophen on international normalized ratio in patients receiving warfarin therapy. Pharmacotherapy. 2011;31(6):591–7.
107. Zhang Q, Bal-dit-Sollier C, Drouet L, Simoneau G, Alvarez JC, Pruvot S, et al. Interaction between acetaminophen and warfarin in adults receiving long-term oral anticogulants: a randomized controlled trial. Eur J Clin Pharmacol. 2011;67(3):309–14.
108. Mahe I, Bertrand N, Drouet L, Bal Dit Sollier C, Simoneau G, Mazoyer E, et al. Interaction between paracetamol and warfarin in patients: a double-blind, placebo-controlled, randomized study. Haematologica. 2006;91(12):1621–7.

Chapter 8
Antiphospholipid Syndrome

Mervat Mattar, Hamdy M. A. Ahmed, and Gaafar Ragab

Abbreviations

aCL	Anticardiolipin antibodies
ADAMTS-13	A disintegrin and metalloproteinase with a thrombospondin type 1 motif member 13
ADP	Adenosine diphosphate
anti-PF4	Anti-platelet factor 4
aPL	Antiphospholipid antibodies
ApoER2	Apolipoprotein E receptor 2
APS	Antiphospholipid syndrome
ASA	Aspirin
CAPS	Catastrophic antiphospholipid syndrome
CD	Cluster of differentiation
CNS	Central nervous system
Cox	Cyclooxygenase
DIC	Disseminated intravascular clotting
ELISA	Enzyme-linked immunosorbent assay;
F	Coagulation factor
GAPSS	Global antiphospholipid syndrome score
GPL	IgG aPL units
HELLP	Hemolysis, elevated liver enzymes, and low platelet syndrome
HIT	Heparin-induced thrombocytopenia

M. Mattar (✉)
Internal Medicine and Hematology, Cairo University, Giza, Egypt

H. M. A. Ahmed
Division of Clinical Immunology and Rheumatology,
University of Alabama at Birmingham, Birmingham, USA

Rheumatology and Clinical immunology, Faculty Of Medicine Cairo University, Giza, Egypt

G. Ragab
Internal Medicine Department, Rheumatology and Clinical Immunology Unit,
Faculty of Medicine, Cairo University, Giza, Egypt
e-mail: gragab@kasralainy.edu.eg

© Springer Nature Switzerland AG 2020
H. Goubran et al. (eds.), *Precision Anticoagulation Medicine*,
https://doi.org/10.1007/978-3-030-25782-8_8

HLA	Human leucocyte antigen
HMG-Co A	β-hydroxy β-methylglutaryl-CoA
Ig	Immunoglobulin
INR	International normalized ratio
IVIG	Intravenous immunoglobulins
LMWH	Low molecular weight heparin
LRP8	Low-density lipoprotein receptor-related protein 8
MPL	IgM aPL units
mTOR	Mammalian target of rapamycin
PTT	Partial thromboplastin time
SLE	Systemic lupus erythematosus
TLR	Toll-like receptor
TTP-HUS	Thrombotic thrombocytopenic purpura–hemolytic uremic syndrome
Xa	Activated factor X

Antiphospholipid Syndrome: Definition and Epidemiology

Persistent high serum levels of antiphospholipid antibodies (aPL) can be associated with venous thromboembolism, arterial thrombosis (accelerated atherosclerosis, stroke, myocardial infarction), valvular heart disease, and obstetric accidents. It includes non-inflammatory bland thrombosis with no signs of perivascular inflammation or leukocytoclastic vasculitis [1, 2].

Studies have estimated that the prevalence of antiphospholipid antibodies in the general population ranges between 1% and 5%, but the antibody titer in most of these studies was low [3]. Antiphospholipid antibodies are found in approximately 30–40% of patients with SLE, but only about 10% have APS [4].

Although it is an uncommon disease, as much as 10% of patients with deep vein thrombosis test positive for aPL [5]. In one study, it was estimated that the incidence of antiphospholipid syndrome (APS) is ~five new cases per 100,000 individuals per year and that the prevalence is ~40–50 cases per 100,000 individuals. The prevalence of catastrophic antiphospholipid syndrome (CAPS), a rare, life-threatening form of APS, has been estimated to be <1% of all cases of APS [5].

Pathogenesis of APS

Autoantibodies are formed against plasma proteins with high affinity for anionic phospholipids especially targeting an epitope within domain I of β2 glycoprotein I, and prothrombin is responsible for the increased thrombotic risk [6]. One of the targets of anti-β2GPI antibodies is apoER2, also called LRP8, a receptor found on endothelial cells but also on platelets and monocytes. Apo ER2 targeting on endothelial cells is hypothesized to initiate signaling of inhibition of the synthesis of nitric oxide synthase through protein phosphatase 2 activation and translocation of nuclear factor kappa B [7]. Upregulation of tissue factor expression and down-regulation of thrombomodulin could also be involved in the loss of antithrombotic properties of endothelial cells. Antiphospholipid antibodies increase platelet activation and aggregation with downregulation of β2GPI/von Willebrand factor interaction increased expression of platelet membrane glycoprotein IIb/IIIa expression [8]. Thrombosis happens in the presence of a second hit ("two-hit hypothesis") [9].

APS Clinical Presentation

Clinically, APS includes cardiovascular, obstetric, neurological, hematological, cardiac, renal, ocular, skin, and other manifestations (Fig. 8.1).

Revised Classification Criteria for APS [12]

These include:

(a) Laboratory criteria:
    (i) Lupus anticoagulant present in plasma (detected according to the guide-lines of the International Society of Thrombosis and Hemostasis (Scientific Subcommittee on Lupus Anticoagulant/Phospholipid-Dependent Antibodies))
    (ii) Immunoglobulins G and/or M (IgG and/or IgM) anti-cardiolipin antibod-ies (aCL) in serum or plasma (medium/high titer ($\geq$40) GPL (IgG) or MPL (IgM) phospholipid units or $\geq$ 99th percentile) measured by standard enzyme-linked immunosorbent assay (ELISA)
    (iii) IgG and/or IgM anti-β2 glycoprotein I antibodies (β2 GP1) in serum or plasma (medium/high titer ($\geq$40) GPL (IgG) or MPL (IgM) phospholipid units or $\geq$ 99th percentile) measured by standard enzyme-linked immuno-sorbent assay (ELISA)

(b) Clinical criteria:
    (i) One or more episodes of arterial, venous, or small vessel thrombosis in any tissue or organ (confirmed by objective validated criteria (imaging study or histopathology))
    (ii) One or more unexplained deaths of a morphologically normal fetus $\geq$10th gestational week. One or more premature births ($\leq$34th gestational week) of a morphologically normal neonate because of eclampsia, severe pre-eclampsia, or placental insufficiency

Clinical manifestations of antiphospholipid syndrome (APS)	
Cardiovascular (younger ages, no other risk factor)	Arterial thrombosis Venous thrombosis (superficial and deep) Pulmonary embolism or hypertension Myocardial infarction (Libman–Sacks): Asymptomatic valve thickening, vegetation, or aortic or mitral insufficiency
Neurological	Stroke Epilepsy Migraine Vascular dementia Chorea Myelitis Guillain–Barre syndrome
Hematological	Thrombocytopenia Hemolytic anemia
Ocular	Retinal vein or artery thrombosis
Hepatic	Portal or hepatic vein thrombosis (Budd–Chiari syndrome)
Skin	Livedo reticularis Skin ulcers Purpura Splinter hemorrhage Digital gangrene
Renal	Microangiopathy Renal vein thrombosis Nephropathy
Bone	Avascular necrosis
Adrenals	Adrenal thrombosis
Obstetric	Recurrent early (<10 weeks) pregnancy loss Abortion at or after the tenth week of gestation Preeclampsia with premature birth Eclampsia Placental insufficiency Hypertension with pregnancy HELLP Neonatal APS

HELLP: hemolysis, elevated liver enzymes, and low platelet syndrome [1, 2, 10, 11]

Fig. 8.1 Clinical presentation of APS

(iii) Three or more unexplained consecutive spontaneous abortions ≤9th gestational week (maternal anatomic and hormonal abnormalities and chromosomal abnormalities excluded)

NB:

A. At least one clinical and one laboratory criterion is mandatory.
B. Autoantibodies and lupus anticoagulant have to be confirmed on two or more occasions at least 12 weeks apart.

Seronegative APS:

There is no consensus on the definition of seronegative APS. These patients have the usual vascular and pregnancy complications of APS and test negative for classic aPL [13].

Those patients usually have some of the clinical non-classification criteria: migraine, stroke, amaurosis fugax, sensorineural hearing loss, transverse myelitis, cognitive dysfunction, seizures, chorea, multiple sclerosis-like illness (pseudo-multiple sclerosis), brain MRI white matter lesions, labile hypertension, pulmonary hypertension, accelerated atherosclerosis, mitral valve disease, aortic valve disease, Budd–Chiari syndrome, Addison's disease, thrombophlebitis, superficial venous thrombosis, leg ulcers, livedo reticularis, Raynaud's, splinter hemorrhage, avascular necrosis of the bones, Evans syndrome, positive Coomb's, hemolytic anemia, and thrombocytopenia [14, 15].

Up to one-third of seronegative APS patients may test positive for non-criteria aPL including IgA aCL, IgA β2 GP1, IgG anti-β2-GPI Domain-I (DI), IgG and IgM antiphosphatidylserine/prothrombin complex (aPS/PT), IgG and IgM antiphosphatidylethanolamine antibodies (aPE), and IgG anticardiolipin/vimentin antibodies (aCL/Vim) [16].

There is some evidence that treating these patients with anticoagulation may improve their outcomes. However, physicians should keep in mind the possibility of wrong diagnosis of seronegative APS and consider benefits and harms of treatment with anticoagulation [17, 18].

APS-Associated Conditions

APS may occur in association with other conditions. It is most commonly associated with SLE. Other autoimmune conditions that can be associated with APS include Sjogren's syndrome, rheumatoid arthritis, psoriatic arthritis, polymyalgia rheumatica, Behcet's disease, autoimmune thrombocytopenic purpura, and autoimmune hemolytic anemia [19]. Antiphospholipid antibodies can be also found with some infectious diseases as hepatitis C virus, HIV, human T-cell lymphotropic virus type 1, syphilis, and bacterial sepsis [20]. Some drugs as hydralazine, sulfasalazine, procainamide, quinidine, propranolol, hydralazine, phenytoin, chlorpromazine, amoxicillin, etanercept, infliximab, adalimumab, and interferon alpha could be related to formation of aPL too [21]. Finally, solid and hematological malignancies may be associated with thrombosis and aPL antibodies [22, 23].

APS in Hispanic population can be associated with HLA DRw53 and DR7 genes. In Caucasian population, it is more associated with HLA DR4 gene [24].

Differential Diagnoses

This may include disseminated intravascular coagulation (DIC), infective endocarditis, and thrombotic thrombocytopenic purpura (TTP) [25, 26].

Risk Stratification

High Thrombotic Risk Indicators

Risk stratification for thrombotic events should take into account the presence of traditional cardiovascular factors. Clinical coexisting hypertension, dyslipidemia, diabetes mellitus, cigarette smoking, systemic inflammatory conditions (infectious or autoimmune), and inherited thrombophilia are thrombotic risk factors. The detection of autoimmune antibodies as antinuclear antibodies (ANA) and anti-double-stranded deoxyribonucleic acid antibodies (ds-DNA) may exhibit an inclination to thrombosis [1]. A previous history of thrombosis and abortions may pose as risk factors for obstetric-related APS complications with pregnancy failure. Racial factors, e.g., black race, may be a risk factor [27]. Also, the presence of high platelet volume, positive LA and aCL, and anti-beta 2-GP1 antibodies, referred to as triple positivity, is associated with more susceptibility to thrombosis. In addition, each aPL test confers a characteristic thrombotic risk, with LA being appointed as the most dangerous [28–30]. Other endothelial-related parameters including decreased plasminogen and elevated plasminogen activator inhibitor-1 levels can increase risk of thrombosis as well.

Risk factors for pregnancy failure include low complement levels, decreased platelet counts, and a previous history of thrombosis and pregnancy failure [28].

Risk Categories for aPL Positivity in APS [29]

(i) Category I: includes patients with more than one positive test in any combination
(ii) Category II: a single positive test should be classified as:
   IIa if LA-positive
   IIb if positive for antibodies against cardiolipins (aCLs)
   IIc if positive for anti-β_2GPI antibodies)

Incidental aPL finding may be associated with 1% risk of thrombosis [30–32]. As the number of positive aPL tests rises, initial thrombosis risk will reach as high as 5% per year and 37% after 10 years for triple-positive cases (LA, aCL, and aβ2GPI) [33, 34]. First thrombotic incidents are more common in asymptomatic carriers of triple positivity. Patients with triple positivity are also at highest risk for both venous and arterial thrombosis and for obstetric complications [11, 12]. Even with the use of anticoagulants, thrombosis recurrence is higher in triple positive cases.

Persistent aPL on two occasions even with D-dimer negativity following stopping anticoagulation was associated with a 13% person-year rate of recurrence [29].

The Global Antiphospholipid Syndrome Score for Thrombosis Prediction [35]

The Global Antiphospholipid Syndrome Score (GAPSS) comprises the antiphospholipid antibody profile and other cardiovascular risk factors. Points are allocated to different risk factors:

 (i) aCL (IgG) or IgM isotype): 5 points
 (ii) Anti-β2GP1 (IgG or IgM isotype): 4 points
(iii) LA: 4 points
(iv) Antiprothrombin/phosphatidylserine complex antibodies (IgG or IgM isotype): 3 points
 (v) Hyperlipidemia: 3 points
(vi) Arterial hypertension: 1 point

Patients with GAPSS values higher or equal to 11 were shown to have a higher risk of recurrences [36]. The GAPSS score was validated both in rheumatologic patients, regarding thrombosis or pregnancy morbidity, and APS and SLE patients [37–40].

Treatment of APS

Thromboprophylaxis in APS

Approximately 3–24% of APS patients develop recurrent events even during adequate treatment. Primary and secondary prophylaxes are indicated with the coexistence of SLE, during perioperative management, and in the presence of other cardiovascular factors. Primary prophylaxis includes antiplatelets, anticoagulants (both standard and direct oral). Hydroxychloroquine is indicated in cases of SLE. In secondary prophylaxis, other immunomodulators may be used (see Figs. 8.2 and 8.3).

Treatment of Active First Thrombotic Event

Full long-term anticoagulation together with lab screening is the most important treatment in APS with no known risk factors presenting with unprovoked VTE [44, 45]. Anticoagulation for 3–6 months is advised in patients with low-risk aPL profile plus a known acutely incriminated risk factor if no investigational evidence of residual thrombosis [46]. However, there is still a high risk of recurrence especially during the following 6 months [47]. International normalized ratio (INR) of moderate (2–3) to

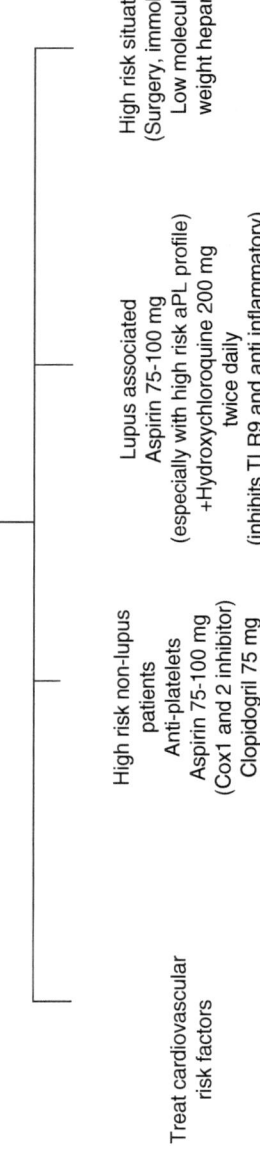

Fig. 8.2 APS primary prophylaxis [41]. Cox cyclooxygenase, TLR Toll-like receptor, aPL antiphospholipid antibodies

APS Secondary Prophylaxis

Arterial	Venous	Immunomodulators
Anticoagulants	Anticoagulants	Rituximab
Heparin in high-risk periods	Heparin in high-risk periods	(anti CD20)
Warfarin (Anti F II,VII,Ix,X)	Warfarin (Anti F II,VII,Ix,X)	Eculizumab
INR >3	INR 2-3	(Anti complement)
Or INR =2	If Warfarin allergy or failure to reach IN	Statins
+ antiplatelet	R 2-3 :	(HMG Co A inhibitors)
DOACS are not recommended	Apixaban (Anti F Xa	sirolimus
	Rivaroxaban(AntiF Xa)	mTOR inhibitor
	NB : Rivaroxiban contraindicated with	
	triple aPL positivity	

Fig. 8.3 Secondary APS prophylaxis [41–43]. DOACS direct oral anticoagulants, HMGCo A β-hydroxy β-methylglutaryl-CoA, mTOR mammalian target of rapamycin

high (3–4) intensity anticoagulation is advised both in venous and non-cerebral arterial thrombosis. If there is a stroke, the addition of low-dose aspirin to anticoagulation is advised [48]. In case of recurrent venous thrombosis despite reaching an INR of 2–3, it is advised to increase target INR 3–4, add low-dose aspirin, or shift to therapeutic dose LMWH [43].

The available DOAC data in the APS population are limited. Also recent randomized trial data show a tendency to higher incidence of thrombosis among high-risk APS patients receiving DOACs [49, 50].

Patients with APS were not excluded from the original DOAC VTE treatment trials; however, limited information is available for this patient subgroup. A small post hoc analysis of possible APS patients who received dabigatran vs VKA showed no difference in VTE recurrence rates [50].

Thus, DOAC, especially rivaroxaban, should not be used in patients with triple aPL positivity who develop venous or arterial thrombosis. DOAC use may currently be restricted to APS patients with venous thrombosis who fail to achieve target INR or with contraindication [43], allergy, or intolerance to warfarin [42].

Aspirin Allergy

In cases of aspirin allergy and especially during pregnancy, rapid oral aspirin desensitization could be held in the intensive care unit. This was reportedly successful in three patients [51]. It would be recommended for desensitization to be held before pregnancy.

Prognosis

Ten-year survival is approximately 90–94%. New event risk is remarkable after anticoagulation cessation despite aPL negativity [52] especially those with unprovoked thrombosis, thus necessitating continuation of therapy. Those with provoked thrombosis are less liable for recurrence after anticoagulant cessation [53].

Management of APS in Special Situations

Management of Pregnancy with APS (Fig. 8.4)

Aspirin, hydroxychloroquine, and low-molecular-weight heparin (LMWH) may be used to decrease the risk of thrombosis, aspirin to start preferably before pregnancy.

Combining LMWH and low-dose aspirin (ASA) may be beneficial for pregnant aPL-positive women.

Oral anticoagulation can be given after delivery as warfarin can be safely used with lactation [54].

Libman–Sacks Endocarditis (Nonbacterial Thrombotic Endocarditis)

It comprises asymptomatic 3 mm or more thickening of the proximal or middle portions of the valve leaflet with irregular nodules on the atrial aspect of the mitral valve or the vascular surface of the aortic valve, and/or moderate-to-severe valvular regurgitation or stenosis. It can affect 15% and 30% of patients with APS with an incidence rate of 5% over a 10-year period [61]. Criteria for inclusion include patients with no previous history of valvular heart disease or infective endocarditis. Histopathologic analysis shows vegetations to be typically less than 4 mm in size, sterile, fibrinous in nature. They may show fibroblastic organization, neorevascularization, or mononuclear inflammatory cell infiltration. These may progress into fibrous plaque formation and scarring with focal calcifications [62]. The existence of aPLs and complement on the affected valves implies aPL-mediated valvular endothelial cell activation with complement fixation [63].

Anticoagulation is mandatory in these as they might have even a much greater risk for vegetation embolization than patients with infective endocarditis [64]. Valve replacement surgery is an option when needed, but there is a greater risk for thrombotic and bleeding complications [65].

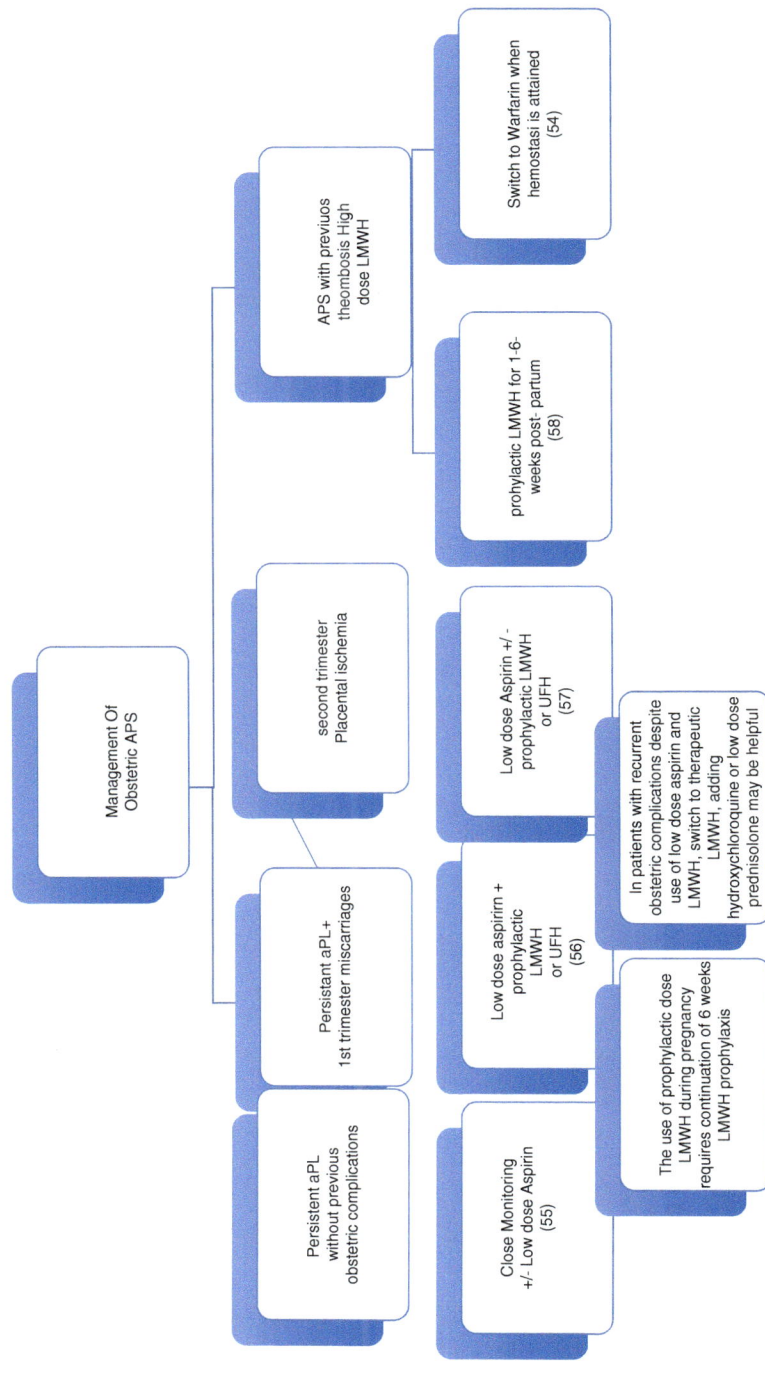

Fig. 8.4 Management of APS during pregnancy [54–58]. NB: Hydroxychloroquine [59] and pravastatin [60] have both been stated to preserve placental perfusion in some studies. APS antiphospholipid syndrome, APL antiphospholipid antibodies, LMWH low-molecular-weight heparin, UFH unfractionated heparin

CAPS

A rare, catastrophic form of APS that is associated with cytokine storm. It affects 1% of all patients with APS and can be associated with SLE in 40%. It includes very rapid (less than a week) multiple thrombotic events involving 3 or more different systems in the presence of aPL. Thrombosis could be evident radiologically or histologically. CAPS can be triggered by different factors including infections, surgery, drugs, obstetric complications, and cancer; however, there may be no triggers in some of the cases. It includes the very rapid (less than a week) involvement of 3 or more systems or tissues with the presence of aPL. Histopathology confirms small vessel occlusion [66].

Pathogenesis of CAPS

In the setting of a precipitating factor, and in the presence of aPL, molecular mimicry may provide the signal that causes the acute thrombotic state characteristic of CAPS [67]. APLs participate by activating platelets, inhibiting anticoagulants, inhibiting fibrinolysis, and activating the complement pathway. This can further cause endothelial activation and apoptosis with tissue factor release together with other prothrombotic substances [68].

Criteria for preliminary classification of CAPS include four items to be considered [66]. These include:

1. Evidence of involvement of three or more organs, systems, and/or tissues
2. Development of manifestations, either simultaneously or in less than a week
3. Confirmation by histopathology of small-vessel occlusion
4. Laboratory confirmation of the presence of aPL twice 12 weeks apart

If all four criteria are present, then this is considered as catastrophic antiphospholipid syndrome.

Probable catastrophic antiphospholipid syndrome is considered if:

(a) All four criteria, except only two organs, systems, and/or tissues involved
(b) Criteria 1, 2, and 4
(c) Criteria 1, 3, and 4, with the development of a third event more than 1 week but within 1 month of presentation, despite anticoagulation

NB: Vasculitis may coexist, but significant thrombosis must be present as well.

Differential Diagnosis of CAPS

CAPS should be differentiated from thrombotic thrombocytopenic purpura–hemolytic uremic syndrome (TTP-HUS), DIC, hemolytic elevated liver enzymes, low platelet syndrome (HELLP), and heparin-induced thrombocytopenia (HIT) [69, 70] (see Table 8.1).

Table 8.1 Differential diagnosis of CAPS [17, 71, 72]

	CAPS	TTP–HUS	DIC	HELLP	HIT	Cancer-associated thrombosis
Precipitating events/ clinical history	APS SLE Malignancy Pregnancy Infection Surgery Trauma	Malignancy Pancreatitis Surgery Infection Pregnancy	Infection Malignancy Hepatic disease Pregnancy	Pregnancy	Previous exposure to heparin	Cancer known or unknown
Type of vascular thrombosis	Microvascular Macrovascular	Microvascular	Microvascular	Microvascular Macrovascular	Macrovascular	Superficial or deep venous Arterial
Bleeding complications	Not usually present	Not present	Present	May be present	Not present	Not present
Organ failure	Present multiple organ failure	May be present (renal, CNS)	May be present (pulmonary)	May be present (renal, CNS, pulmonary)	Not present	May be present if complicated by DIC
Hemolytic anemia	May be present	Present	May be present	Present	Not present	Not present
Schistocytes	May be present	Present	May be present	May be present	Not present	Not present
Thrombocytopenia	May be present	Present ++	Present +	Present +	Present ++	Not present
Other labs	aPL	Decreased ADAMTS13	Prolonged PTT Decreased fibrinogen Increased fibrinogen degradation products Mild decreased ADAMTS13	Elevated liver enzymes	Anti-PF4	Cancer markers DIC markers

ADAMTS a disintegrin and metalloproteinase with a thrombospondin type 1 motif, member 13, *Anti- PF4* anti-Platelet factor 4, *aPL* antiphospholipid antibodies, *APS* antiphospholipid syndrome, *CAPS* catastrophic antiphospholipid syndrome, *CNS* central nervous system, *DIC* disseminated intravascular clotting, *HELLP* hemolytic elevated liver enzymes low platelet syndrome, *HIT* heparin-induced thrombocytopenia, *PTT* partial thromboplastin time, *SLE* systemic lupus erythematosus, *TTP–HUS* thrombotic thrombocytopenic purpura–hemolytic uremic syndrome

It is suggested that TTP and CAPS coexist and that CAPS is uncommon presentation of APS that results in TTP. This is supported by the fact that both occur with SLE and that it is recommended that both conditions are to be treated with plasma exchange and rituximab. This could be important to avoid delay in treatment.

Treatment of CAPS

Early and appropriate treatment of infections and maintenance of therapeutic INR level may be helpful in decreasing the incidence of CAPS [43]. In addition to antiplatelets and anticoagulation, corticosteroids, intravenous immunoglobulins (IVIG), plasma exchange using fresh frozen plasma, and immunomodulators including monoclonal antibodies can be used (Fig. 8.5).

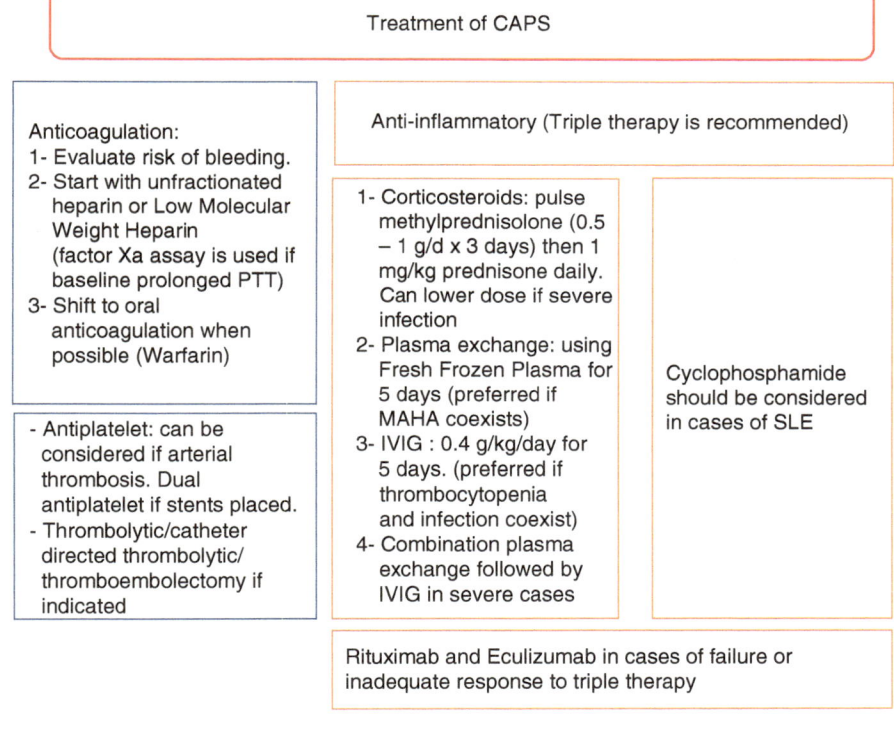

Fig. 8.5 Treatment of CAPS [26, 70, 72]. Xa activated factor X, CAPS catastrophic antiphospholipid syndrome, IVIG intravenous immunoglobulins, MAHA microangiopathic hemolytic anemia, PTT partial thromboplastin time

The 14th International Congress on Antiphospholipid Antibodies Task Force Report on Catastrophic Antiphospholipid Syndrome recommendations [71]:

(i) Think of CAPS in front of a patient with severe multi-organ involvement with thrombotic microangiopathic anemia findings.
(ii) The possible interplay in different pathogenic pathways between the different microangiopathic syndromes should be kept in mind.
(iii) High titers of aPL may be a useful hallmark for the differential diagnosis, but the full clinical picture must be taken into account.
(iv) Testing for antibodies against HP4, fibrinogen, ADAMTS-13 activity, and ADAMTS-13 autoantibody is encouraged.
(v) The performance of a biopsy is not required for diagnostic purposes although it is highly recommended.
(vi) Regarding treatment for CAPS, the following levels of evidence and grades of recommendations were found:
  • CAPS should not be left untreated: grade of recommendation B.
  • Anticoagulation or glucocorticoids should not be used alone: grade of recommendation B.
  • Anticoagulation + glucocorticoids should be the backbone of therapy: grade of recommendation B.
  • Triple therapy (anticoagulation + plasma exchange and/or IVIG: grade of recommendation B.

• If infection is ongoing with CAPS, IVIG should be used: grade of recommendation D.
• Tetra-therapy (anticoagulation + plasma exchange and/or IVIG + cyclophosphamide) to patients with SLE or other autoimmune disease that could benefit from extra immunosuppression: grade of recommendation D.
• Although cyclophosphamide is used more, there is no enough evidence to suggest that it is better than other immunosuppressant medications: Grade of recommendation D.
• Rituximab, anti-CD 20 recombinant monoclonal antibody, may have a role as an initial adjuvant therapy in high-risk patients, especially those with microangiopathic hemolytic anemia (MAHA), a potential marker for relapsing cases.
• Rituximab may have a role as a second-line therapy in patients with disease refractory to standard triple therapy.
• Rituximab may be an alternative adjuvant therapy in CAPS patients in whom anticoagulation is a contraindication.

NB:

1. Treatment should start as soon as possible on strong suspicion even if patient does not meet classification criteria [72].
2. Anticoagulation by intravenous unfractionated heparin should be started in the acute setting. Direct oral anticoagulant use data are sparse [73].

3. Triple combination therapy with anticoagulants, steroids, and plasma exchange and/or IVIG is reported to lower mortality rate to 28% [74], and thus it is now recommended over any of them alone [43]. The use of both plasma exchange concomitant with IVIG has been reported with 100% survival [75]. Replacement by fresh frozen plasma replaces natural anticoagulants as antithrombin and proteins C and S but also contains clotting factors [76]. Albumin has been used successfully as replacement fluid for plasma exchange [77].

   Plasma exchange is preferred if there is MAHA association [78].
4. IVIG may be preferred if there is associated immune thrombocytopenia [72].
5. The experience of use of Rituximab and Ecluzumab is currently restricted to only a small number of reports [78–80] and is recommended if failure or no adequate response to triple therapy [43].

Risk Factors for CAPS Relapse

Refractory cases are those that do not respond to triple therapy (or those with recurrence). Relapsing cases are those that develop CAPS after 30 days of remission. Higher relapses are noted in the presence of concomitant SLE, age above 36 years old, pulmonary and renal involvement, lupus anticoagulant positivity and associated MAHA [81].

Travel with APS

Both hypoxia and prolonged immobility might increase thrombotic tendency during air flights [82–84].

   Air-traveling patients with APS are risk-stratified according to duration of flights, aPL profile, age, associated autoimmune disorder, and cardiovascular disease [85]. Low-risk includes persons with no medical conditions who are travelling for less than 8 hours or fewer than 5000 kilometers. Air-traveling patients are advised to avoid tight clothes, have ample hydration, and have frequent calf muscle exercises. Patients with additional risk factors, e.g., smoking, obesity, pregnancy, hormone replacement, or oral contraceptives, especially with longer travel times and distances, are considered moderate-risk. High-risk patients are those with previous thromboembolism, known hypercoagulability, had had a recent operation, or suffer a current malignancy [86]. The addition of below-the-knee graduated compression stockings (grade 2C) or a single dose of LMWH prior to flight (grade 2C) is advised [82]. An additional booster enoxaparin dose of 1 mg/kg 2–4 hours prior to flights may be advisable, especially so if duration of flight is more than 8 hours [87]. Protection by single-agent ASA is not documented [88].

References

1. Corban MT, Duarte-Garcia A, McBane RD, Matteson EL, Lerman LO, Lerman A. Antiphospholipid syndrome. Role of vascular endothelial cells and implications for risk stratification and targeted therapeutics. J Am Coll Cardiol. 2017;69(18):2317–30.
2. Chighizola CB, Andreoli L, Gerosa M, Tincani A, Ruffatti A, Meroni PL. The treatment of anti-phospholipid syndrome: a comprehensive clinical approach. J Autoimmun. 2018a;90:1–27. https://doi.org/10.1016/j.jaut.2018.02.003.
3. Gómez-Puerta JA, Cervera R. Diagnosis and classification of the antiphospholipid syndrome. J Autoimmun. 2014;48–49:20–5.
4. Lockshin MD. Update on antiphospholipid syndrome. Bull NYU Hosp Jt Dis. 2008;66(3):195–7.
5. Durcan L, Petri M. Epidemiology of the antiphospholipid syndrome. In Handbook of systemic autoimmune diseases. Vol. 12. Elsevier Ltd. 2016; p. 17–30. (Handbook of systemic autoimmune diseases) https://doi.org/10.1016/B978-0-444-63655-3.00002-8.
6. Meroni PL, Borghi MO, Raschi E, Tedesco F. Pathogenesis of antiphospholipid syndrome: understanding the antibodies. Nat Rev Rheumatol. 2011;7(6):330–9.
7. Sacharidou A, Chambliss KL, Ulrich V, Salmon JE, Shen YM, Herz J, et al. Antiphospholipid antibodies induce thrombosis by PP2A activation via apoER2-Dab2-SHC1 complex formation in endothelium. Blood. 2018;131(19):2097–110.
8. Chighizola CB, Ubiali T, Meroni PL. Treatment of thrombotic antiphospholipid syndrome: the rationale of current management—an insight into future approaches. J Immunol Res. 2015a;2015:Article ID 951424.
9. Groot PG, Meijers JC. β(2)-glycoprotein I: evolution, structure and function. J Thromb Haemost. 2011;9(7):1275–84.
10. Meroni PL, Chighizola CB, Rovelli F, Gerosa M. Antiphospholipid syndrome in 2014: more clinical manifestations, novel pathogenic players and emerging biomarkers. Arthritis Res Ther. 2014;16:209.
11. Movva S (Chief ed. Diamond, HS). Antiphosphopholipid syndrome Medscape. https://emedicine.medscape.com/article/333221-clinical. 2017.
12. Miyakis S, Lockshin MD, Atsumi T, , Branch DW, Brey RL, Cervera R et al 2006. International consensus statement on an update of the classification criteria for definite antiphospholipid syndrome (APS). J Thromb Haemost 2006, (4):295–306.
13. Hughes GR, Khamashta MA. Seronegative antiphospholipid syndrome. Ann Rheum Dis. 2003;62(12):1127.
14. Rodriguez-Garcia JL, Bertolaccini ML, Cuadrado MJ, Sanna G, Ateka-Barrutia O, Khamashta MA. Clinical manifestations of antiphospholipid syndrome (APS) with and without antiphospholipid antibodies (the so-called 'seronegative APS'). Ann Rheum Dis. 2012;71(2):242–4.
15. Sciascia S, Amigo MC, Roccatello D, Khamashta M. Diagnosing antiphospholipid syndrome: 'extra-criteria' manifestations and technical advances. Nat Rev Rheumatol. 2017;13(9):548.
16. Zohoury N, Bertolaccini ML, Rodriguez-Garcia JL, Shums Z, Ateka-Barrutia O, Sorice M, Norman GL, Khamashta M. Closing the serological gap in the antiphospholipid syndrome: the value of "non-criteria" antiphospholipid antibodies. J Rheumatol. 2017;44(11):1597–602.
17. Uthman I, Noureldine MH, Ruiz-Irastorza G, Khamashta M. Management of antiphospholipid syndrome. Ann Rheum Dis. 2019;78(2):155–61.
18. Hughes GR, Khamashta MA. 'Seronegative antiphospholipid syndrome': an update. Lupus. 2019;28(3):273–4. https://doi.org/10.1177/0961203319826358.
19. Cohen D, Berger SP, Steup-Beekman GM, Bloemenkamp KWM, Bajema IM. Diagnosis and management of the antiphospholipid syndrome. BMJ. 2010;340:c2541.
20. Mendoza-Pinto C, García-Carrasco M, Cervera R. Role of infectious diseases in the antiphospholipid syndrome (including its catastrophic variant). Curr Rheumatol Rep. 2018;20(10):62.
21. Dlott JS, Roubey RA. Drug-induced lupus anticoagulants and antiphospholipid antibodies. Curr Rheumatol Rep. 2012;14(1):71–8.

22. Vassalo J, Spector N, de Meis E, Rabello LS, Rosolem MM, do Brasil PE, et al. Antiphospholipid antibodies in critically ill patients with cancer: a prospective cohort study. J Crit Care. 2014;29:533–8.
23. Gómez-Puerta JA, Espinosa G, Cervera R. Antiphospholipid antibodies. From general concepts to its relation with malignancies. Antibodies. 2016;5:18. https://doi.org/10.3390/antib5030018.
24. Sebastiani Domenico G, Minisola G, Galeazzi M. HLA class II alleles and genetic predisposition to the antiphospholipid syndrome. Autoimmun Rev. 2003;2(6):387–94.
25. Musio F, Bohen EM, Yuan CM, Welch PG. Review of thrombotic thrombocytopenic purpura in the setting of systemic lupus erythematosus. Semin Arthritis Rheum. 1998;28:1–19.
26. Ortel TL, Erkan D, Kitchens CS. How I treat catastrophic thrombotic syndromes. Blood. 2015;126:1285–93.
27. Abu-Zeinah G, Oromendia C, De Sancho MT. Thrombotic risk factors, antithrombotic therapy, and outcomes of asymptomatic carriers of antiphospholipid antibodies and patients with antiphospholipid syndrome. Blood. 2017;130:3710.
28. Chighizola CB, Andreoli L, de Jesus GR, Banzato A, Benanzato A, Pons-Estel GJ, Erkan D, APS ACTION. The association between antiphospholipid antibodies and pregnancy morbidity, stroke, myocardial infarction, and deep vein thrombosis: a critical review of the literature. Lupus. 2015b;24(9):980–4.
29. Pengo V, Ruffatti A, Legnani C, Testa S, Fierro T, Marongiu F, et al. Incidence of a first thromboembolic event in asymptomatic carriers of high-risk antiphospholipid antibody profile: a multicenter prospective study. Blood. 2011;118:4714–8.
30. Ruffatti A, Tonello M, Visentin MS, Bontadi A, Hoxha A, De Carolis S, et al. Risk factors for pregnancy failure in patients with anti-phospholipid syndrome treated with conventional therapies: a multicentre case–control study. Rheumatology. 2011;50:1684–9.
31. Forastiero R. Multiple antiphospholipid antibodies positivity and antiphospholipid syndrome criteria re-evaluation. Lupus. 2014;23(12):1252–4.
32. Giron-Gonzalez JA, Garcıa del Rıo E, Rodrıguez C, Rodrıguez-Martorell J, Serrano A. Antiphospholipid syndrome and asymptomatic carriers of antiphospholipid antibody: prospective ~analysis of 404 individuals. J Rheumatol. 2004;31(8):1560–7.
33. Mustonen P, Lehtonen KV, Javela K, Puurunen M. Persistent anti- phospholipid antibody (aPL) in asymptomatic carriers as a risk factor for future thrombotic events: a nationwide prospective study. Lupus. 2014;23(14):1468–76.
34. Pengo V, Testa S, Martinelli I, Ghirarduzzi A, Legnani C, Gresele P, et al. Incidence of a first thromboembolic event in carriers of isolated lupus anticoagulant. Thromb Res. 2015;135(1):46–9.
35. Galli M, Borrelli G, Jacobsen EM, Marfisi RM, Finazzi G, Marchioli R, et al. Clinical significance of different antiphospholipid antibodies in the WAPS (warfarin in the anti- phospholipid syndrome) study. Blood. 2007;110(4):1178–83.
36. Kearon C, Parpia S, Spencer FA, Baglin T, Stevens SM, Bauer KA, et al. Antiphospholipid antibodies and recurrent thrombosis after a first unprovoked venous thromboembolism. Blood. 2018;131(19):2151–60.
37. Sciascia S, Sanna G, Murru V, Roccatello D, Khamashta MA, Bertolaccini ML. GAPSS: the global anti-phospholipid syndrome score. Rheumatology (Oxford). 2013a;52:1397403.
38. Sciascia S, Bertolaccini ML, Roccatello D, Khamashta MA. Independent validation of the antiphospholipid score for the diagnosis of antiphospholipid syndrome. Ann Rheum Dis. 2013b;72:142–3.
39. Sciascia S, Baldovino S, Schreiber K, Solfietti L, Radin M, Cuadrado MJ, Menegatti E, Erkan D, Roccatello D. Thrombotic risk assessment in antiphospholipid syndrome: the role of new antibody specificities and thrombin generation assay. Clin Mol Allergy. 2016a;14:6.
40. Oku K, Amengual O, Bohgaki T, Horita T, Yasuda S, Atsumi T. An independent validation of the global anti-phospholipid syndrome score in a Japanese cohort of patients with autoimmune diseases. Lupus. 2015;24:774–5.

41. Zuily S, de Laat B, Mohamed S, Kelchtermans H, Shums Z, Albesa R, et al. Validity of the global anti-phospholipid syndrome score to predict thrombosis: a prospective multicentre cohort study. Rheumatology. 2015;54(11):2071–5.
42. Islam A, Alam F, Wong KK, Kamal MA, Gan SH. Thrombotic management of antiphospholipid syndrome: towards novel targeted therapies. Curr Vasc Pharmacol. 2017;15(4):313–26.
43. Tektonidou MG, Andreoli L, Limper M, Amoura Z, Cervera R, Costedoat-Chalumeau N, et al. EULAR recommendations for the management of antiphospholipid syndrome in adults. Ann Rheum Dis. 2019:1–9. https://doi.org/10.1136/annrheumdis-2019-215213.
44. Skeith L. Anticoagulating patients with high-risk acquired thombophilias. Blood. 2018;132:439–49.
45. Kearon C, Iorio A, Palareti G, Subcommittee on Control of Anti-coagulation of the SSC of the ISTH. Risk of recurrent venous thromboembolism after stopping treatment in cohort studies: recommendation for acceptable rates and standardized reporting. J Thromb Haemost. 2010;8(10):2313–5.
46. Carrier M, Le Gal G, Wells PS, Rodger MA. Systematic review: case-fatality rates of recurrent venous thromboembolism and major bleeding events among patients treated for venous thromboembolism. Ann Intern Med. 2010;152(9):578–89.
47. Kearon C, Akl EA, Comerota AJ, Prandoni P, Bounameaux H, Goldhaber SZ, et al. Antithrombotic therapy for VTE disease: antithrombotic therapy and prevention of thrombosis, 9th ed: American College of Chest Physicians Evidence- Based Clinical Practice Guidelines. Chest. 2012;141:e419S–94S.
48. Khamashta MA, Cuadrado MJ, Mujic F, Taub NA, Hunt BJ, Hughes GR. The management of thrombosis in the antiphospholipid-antibody syndrome. N Engl J Med. 1995;332(15):993–7.
49. Pengo V, Denas G, Zoppellaro G, Jose SP, Hoxha A, Ruffatti A, et al. Rivaroxaban vs warfarin in high-risk patients with antiphospholipid syndrome. Blood. 2018;132(13):1365–71.
50. Goldhaber SZ, Eriksson H, Kakkar A, Schellong S, Feuring M, Fraessdorf M, et al. Efficacy of dabigatran versus warfarin in patients with acute venous thromboembolism in the presence of thrombophilia: findings from RE-COVER®, RE- COVERII, and RE-MEDY. Vasc Med. 2016;21(6):506–14.
51. Alijotas-Reig J, Miguel-Moncín MS, Cisteró-Bahíma A. Aspirin desensitization in the treatment of antiphospholipid syndrome during pregnancy in ASA-sensitive patients. Am J Reprod Immunol. 2006 Jan;55(1):45–50.
52. Comarmond C, Jego P, Veyssier-Belot C, Marie I, Mekinian A, Elmaleh-Sachs A, et al. Cessation of oral anticoagulants in antiphospholipid syndrome. Lupus. 2017;26(12):1291–6. https://doi.org/10.1177/0961203317699285.
53. Garcia D, Erkan D. Diagnosis and management of anti-phospholipid syndrome. NEJM. 2018;378(21):2010–21.
54. Chighizola CB, Shoenfeld Y, Meroni PL. Therapy for antiphospholipid miscarriages: throwing the baby out with the bathwater? Am J Reprod Immunol. 2018b;79(3):e12792.
55. Schreiber K, Sciascia S, de Groot PG, Devreese K, Jacobsen S, Ruiz-Irastorza G, et al. Antiphospholipid syndrome. Nat Rev Dis Primers. 2018;4:Article number: 17103.
56. Laskin CA, Spitzer KA, Clark CA, Crowther MR, Ginsberg JS, Hawker GA, et al. Low molecular weight heparin and aspirin for recurrent pregnancy loss: results from the randomized, controlled HepASA trial. J Rheumatol. 2009;36(2):279–87. https://doi.org/10.3899/jrheum.080763.
57. Rey E, Garneau P, David M, Gauthier R, Leduc L, Michon N, et al. Dalteparin for the prevention of recurrence of placental-mediated complications of pregnancy in women without thrombophilia: a pilot randomized controlled trial. J Thromb Haemost. 2009;7:58–64.
58. Fischer-Betz R, Specker C, Brinks R, Schneider M. Pregnancy outcome in patients with antiphospholipid syndrome after cerebral ischaemic events: an observational study. Lupus. 2012;21:1183–9.
59. Sciascia S, Hunt BJ, Talavera-Garcia E, Lliso G, Khamashta MA, Cuadrado MJ. The impact of hydroxychloroquine treatment on pregnancy outcome in women with antiphospholipid antibodies. Am J Obstet Gynecol. 2016b;214(2):273.e1–8.

60. Lefkou E, Mamopoulos A, Dagklis T, Vosnakis C, Rousso D, Girardi G. Pravastatin improves pregnancy outcomes in obstetric antiphospholipid syndrome refractory to antithrombotic therapy. J Clin Invest. 2016;126(8):2933–40. https://doi.org/10.1172/JCI86957.
61. Cervera R, Serrano R, Pons-Estel GJ, Ceberio-Hualde L, Shoenfeld Y, de Ramón E, Euro-Phospholipid Project Group (European Forum on Antiphospholipid Antibodies), et al. Morbidity and mortality in the antiphospholipid syndrome during a 10-year period: a multicentre prospective study of 1000 patients. Ann Rheum Dis. 2015;74:1011–8.
62. Zuily S, Regnault V, Selton-Suty C, Eschwège V, Bruntz JF, Bode-Dotto E, et al. Increased risk for heart valve disease associated with antiphospholipid antibodies in patients with systemic lupus erythematosus: meta-analysis of echocardiographic studies. Circulation. 2011;124:215–24.
63. Ziporen L, Goldberg I, Arad M, Hojnik M, Ordi-Ros J, Afek A, et al. Libman-Sacks endocarditis in the antiphospholipid syndrome: immunopathologic findings in deformed heart valves. Lupus. 1996;5:196–205.
64. Zuily S, Huttin O, Mohamed S, Marie PY, Selton-Suty C, Wahl D. Valvular heart disease in antiphospholipid syndrome. Curr Rheumatol Rep. 2013;15:320.
65. Roldan CA, Sibbitt WL, Qualls CR, Jung RE, Greene ER, Gasparovic CM, et al. Libman-Sacks endocarditis and embolic cerebrovascular disease. J Am Coll Cardiol Img. 2013;6:973.
66. Asherson R, Cervera R, de Groot P, Erkan D, Boffa MC, Piette JC, et al. Catastrophic antiphospholipid syndrome: international consensus statement on classification criteria and treatment guidelines. Lupus. 2003;12(7):530–4.
67. Cusick MF, Libbey JE, Fujinami RS. Molecular mimicry as a mechanism of autoimmune disease. Clin Rev Allergy Immunol. 2012;42(1):102–11.
68. Barratt-Due A, Fløisand Y, Orrem HL, Kvam AK, Holme PA, Bergseth G, et al. Complement activation is a crucial pathogenic factor in catastrophic antiphospholipid syndrome. Rheumatology (Oxford). 2016;55(7):1337–9.
69. George JN, Chen Q, Deford CC, Al-Nouri Z. Ten patient stories illustrating the extraordinarily diverse clinical features of patients with thrombotic thrombocytopenic purpura and severe ADAMTS13 deficiency. J Clin Apher. 2012;27:302–11.
70. Cervera R, Rodríguez-Pintó I, Espinosa G. The diagnosis and clinical management of the catastrophic antiphospholipid syndrome: a comprehensive review. J Autoimmun. 2018;92:1–11.
71. Cervera R, Rodríguez-Pintó I, Colafrancesco S, Conti F, Valesini G, Rosário C, et al. 14th international congress on antiphospholipid antibodies task force report on catastrophic antiphospholipid syndrome. Autoimmun Rev. 2014;13(7):699–707.
72. Gansner JM, Berliner N. The rheumatology/hematology interface: CAPS and MAS diagnosis and management. Hematology. 2018;2018:313–7.
73. Crowley MP, Cuadrado MJ, Hunt BJ. Catastrophic antiphospholipid syndrome on switching from warfarin to rivaroxaban. Thromb Res. 2017;153:37–9.
74. Rodríguez-Pintó I, Espinosa G, Erkan D, Shoenfeld Y, Cervera R, CAPS Registry Project Group. The effect of triple therapy on the mortality of catastrophic anti-phospholipid syndrome patients. Rheumatology. 2018;57:1264–70.
75. Ruffatti A, De Silvestro G, Marson P, Tonello M, Calligaro A, Favaro M, et al. Catastrophic antiphospholipid syndrome: lessons from 14 cases successfully treated in a single center. A narrative report. J Autoimmun. 2018;93:124–30.
76. Zanatta E, Cozzi M, Marson P, Cozzi F. The role of plasma exchange in the management of autoimmune disorders. Br J Hematol. 2019; https://doi.org/10.1111/bjh.15903.
77. Marson P, Monti G, Montani F, Riva A, Mascia MT, Castelnovo L, et al. Apheresis treatment of cryoglobulinemic vasculitis: a multicentre cohort study of 159 patients. Transfus Apher Sci. 2018;57:639–45.
78. Rodrıguez-Pinto I, Moitinho M, Santacreu I, Shoenfeld Y, Erkan D, Espinosa G, CAPS Registry Project Group (European Forum on Antiphospholipid Antibodies), et al. Catastrophic antiphospholipid syndrome (CAPS): descriptive analysis of 500 patients from the International CAPS Registry. Autoimmun Rev. 2016;15(12):1120–4.

79. Sukara G, Baresic M, Sentic M, Brcic L, Anic B. Catastrophic anti- phospholipid syndrome associated with systemic lupus erythematosus treated with rituximab: case report and a review of the literature. Acta Reumatol Port. 2015;40(2):169–75.
80. Dogru A, Ugan Y, Şahin M, Karahan N, Tunç ŞE. Catastrophic anti- phospholipid syndrome treated with rituximab: a case report. Eur J Rheumatol. 2017;4(2):145–7.
81. Rymarz A, Niemczyk S. The complex treatment including rituximab in the Management of Catastrophic Antiphospholid Syndrome with renal involvement. BMC Nephrol. 2018;19:132.
82. Yan SF, Mackman N, Kisiel W, Stern DM, Pinsky DJ. Hypoxia/hypoxemia-induced activation of the procoagulant pathways and the pathogenesis of ischemia-associated thrombosis. Arterioscler Thromb Vasc Biol. 1999;19(2):2029–35.
83. Schobersberger W, Fries D, Mittermayr M, Innerhofer P, Sumann G, Schobersberger B, et al. Changes of biochemical markers and functional tests for clot formation during long-haul flights. Thromb Res. 2002;108(1):19–24.
84. Aldington S, Pritchard A, Perrin K, James K, Wijesinghe M, Beasley R. Prolonged seated immobility at work is a common risk factor for venous thromboembolism leading to hospital admission. Int Med J. 2008;38(2):133–5.
85. Silverman D, Gendreau M. Medical issues associated with commercial flights. Lancet. 2009;373(9680):2067–77.
86. Geerts WH, Bergqvist D, Pineo GF, James K, Wijesinghe M, Beasley R, et al. Prevention of venous thromboembolism: American College of Chest Physicians Evidence-Based Clinical Practice Guidelines (8th edition). Chest. 2008;133(6 Suppl):381S–453S.
87. Cesarone MR, Becaro G, Nicolaides AN, Incandela L, De S, Geroulakos G, et al. Venous thrombosis from air travel: the LONGFLIT3 study—prevention with aspirin vs low-molecular-weight heparin (LMWH) in high-risk subjects: a randomized trial. Angiology. 2002;53(1):1–6.
88. Sandhu VK, Teves K. Antiphospholipid syndrome: the risk of travel at high altitudes. Rheumatologist. 2018;. www.the-rheumatologist.org/article/antiphospholipid-syndrome-the-risk-of-travel-at-high-altitudes.

Chapter 9
Anticoagulation in Patients with Renal Insufficiency

Rashad S. Barsoum, Hanaa Wanas, and Tamer Shehab

Abbreviations

ABMR	Antibody-mediated rejection
ADP	Adenosine diphosphate
ACS	Acute coronary syndrome
AF	Atrial fibrillation
CKD	Chronic kidney disease
DVT	Deep vein thrombosis
GFR	Glomerular filtration rate
LMWH	Low-molecular-weight heparin
NSTEMI	Non-ST segment elevation myocardial infarction
PAI	Plasminogen activator inhibitor
PAF	Platelet-activating factor
PAR	Protease-activated receptor
PCI	Percutaneous intervention
PDGF	Platelet-derived growth factor

R. S. Barsoum (✉)
The Cairo Kidney Center, Cairo, Egypt

Department of Internal Medicine and Nephrology, Kasr-El-Aini Medical School,
Cairo University, Cairo, Egypt

H. Wanas
The Cairo Kidney Center, Cairo, Egypt

Department of Pharmacology, Kasr-El-Aini Medical School, Cairo University, Cairo, Egypt
e-mail: hanaa_wanas@daad-alumni.de

T. Shehab
The Cairo Kidney Center, Cairo, Egypt

Department of Nephrology, Sahel Teaching Hospital, Ministry of Health, Cairo, Egypt

© Springer Nature Switzerland AG 2020
H. Goubran et al. (eds.), *Precision Anticoagulation Medicine*,
https://doi.org/10.1007/978-3-030-25782-8_9

PE   Pulmonary embolism
RAAS   Renin-angiotensin-aldosterone system
ROS   Reactive oxygen species
RVT   Renal vein thrombosis
STEMI   ST segment elevation myocardial infarction
TMA   Thrombotic microangiopathy
TNF   Tumor necrosis factor
tPA   Tissue plasminogen activator
vWF   von Willebrand factor

Introduction

Anticoagulants were used in nephrology many decades before the specialty was born. The first reported use was in the simple Celloidin (Collodion) dialysis tubes designed by Abel, Rowntree, and Turner in 1912. They used hirudin, extracted from leaches, to anticoagulate the blood of cats in the earliest ex vivo dialysis experiments [1]. Hirudin was also used in early experimental dialysis in humans by Haas in 1924 [2], yet it was soon replaced by heparin in 1930, contemporary to its clinical evaluation at the Karolinska Institute in Sweden. Heparin remains the time-honored anticoagulant in dialysis, throughout subsequent evolution in concepts and technology.

Heparin was also used in the prevention or amelioration of experimental nephritis in the mid-1950s [3]. Initial observations were confirmed in several subsequent experimental studies from Europe during the 1960s, which showed reduction of glomerular crescent formation, reversal of acute renal failure, and modulation of subsequent glomerulosclerosis in rats [4, 5]. The heparin benefit was attributed to its anticoagulant effect since similar results were subsequently obtained by oral anticoagulants [6], fibrinolytic agents [7], and platelet inhibitors [8]. Later studies, however, showed that the beneficial effect of heparin may extend beyond anticoagulation, including neutralization of complement, enhancement of fibrinolysis [9], inhibition of glomerular cell apoptosis [10], and suppression of mesangial expansion in experimental mesangioproliferative glomerulonephritis in rats [11].

Based on the early experimental observations, and the finding of thrombotic lesions in the glomeruli of untreated patients with various forms of glomerular and vascular diseases, anticoagulants were used clinically by many leading authorities in Europe, the USA, and Australia with impressive results [12–14]. Anticoagulants were even claimed to be of benefit in chronic kidney disease in an occasional publication [15]. However, subsequent controlled trials failed to confirm a significant benefit of this strategy; hence fell out of routine use in the era of evidence-based medicine.

Nevertheless, there is definite room for using anticoagulants in modern clinical nephrology. The conditions where anticoagulants may be considered in patients with kidney insufficiency may be classified into 3 categories: a) anticoagulation for extrarenal conditions in patients with kidney disease; b) anticoagulation for the treatment of primary or secondary renal disorders; and c) anticoagulation for extracorporeal treatment.

Blood Coagulation in Kidney Insufficiency

Kidney disease is common, affecting over 10% of the population worldwide. Many of those people may need anticoagulant therapy for diverse conditions that may or may not be related to their renal disease. Both acute and chronic impairment of kidney function may be associated with either procoagulant (Fig. 9.1) or anticoagulant (Fig. 9.2) scenarios. It is important to understand each patient's dominating setting before making the decision to anticoagulate, choosing an appropriate agent, and designing the respective follow-up protocol in order to minimize complications.

Thrombophilia in Chronic Kidney Disease (CKD)

In addition to the traditional cardiovascular risk factors dominating in CKD as diabetes, hypertension, and hyperlipidemia, CKD is a significant risk factor by its own right. This is largely attributed to a prothrombotic/procoagulant tendency caused by the following:

a) *Platelet hyperactivity*, related to the increased expression of P-selectin and PAC-1 (Fibrinogen-activated GP llb/llla) on the platelet surface membrane with subsequent enhancement of platelet/granulocyte aggregation and release of ROS (reactive oxygen species) [16, 17].

b) *Increased production of coagulation factors,* as vWF (von Willebrand factor), factor VII, and factor VIII, with significant decrease in antithrombin III activity which is essential for stopping clot formation [18–20].

c) *Overproduction of Tissue Factor,* that activates platelets and stimulates PAR-1 on platelet and endothelial surface, thereby inducing intracellular inflammatory pathways and accelerating the atherosclerosis process [21–23].

d) *Elevated homocysteine levels,* that leads to decreased throbomodulin-dependent activated protein C with permanent activation of thrombin and increased fibrin formation. It also interferes with tissue plasminogen activator (t-PA) release resulting in a hypofibrinolytic state [21, 24, 25].

e) *Activation of the renin-angiotensin-aldosterone system,* which is associated with increased levels of plasma fibrinogen and plasminogen activator inhibitor-1 (PAI-1) which inhibits activation of the fibrinolytic system by inhibiting t-PA and urokinase [26, 27].

f) *Alternation of the intraglomerular coagulation/fibrinolysis system*: Macrophages release inflammatory mediators mainly Iinterleukin-1 (IL-1) and tumor necrosis factor-alpha (TNF-α) that enhance endothelial and mesangial cells to produce

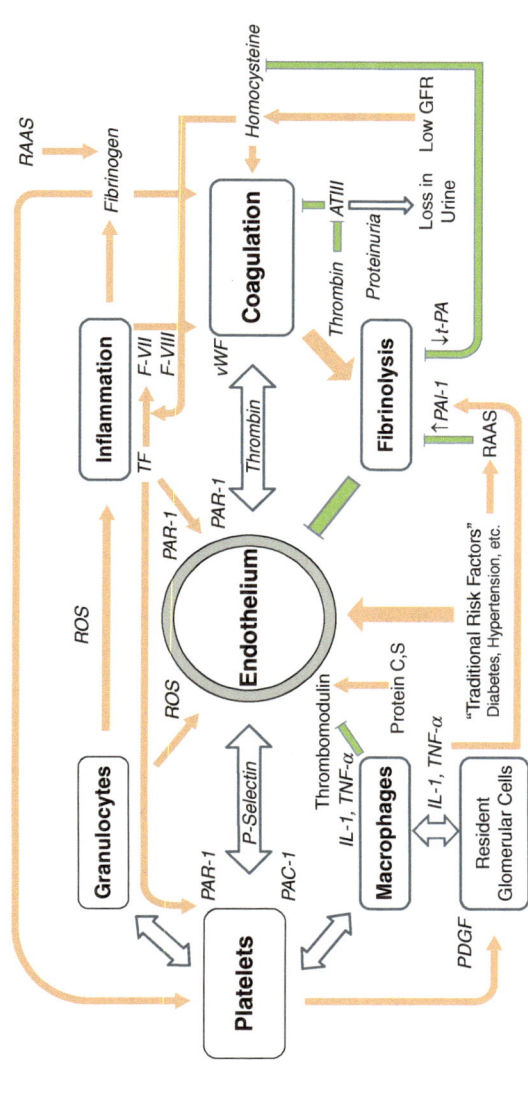

Fig. 9.1 Procoagulant mechanisms associated with chronic kidney insufficiency: *ATIII* = antithrombin III; *IL-1* = interleukin-1; *PAC-1* = fibrinogen-activated GP IIb/IIIa; *PAR-1* = protease-activated receptor-1; *PDGF* = platelet-derived growth factor; *RAAS* = renin-angiotensin-aldosterone system; *ROS* = reactive oxygen species; *TF* = tissue factor; *TNF-α* = tumor necrosis factor α; *t-PA* = tissue plasminogen activator; *vWF* = von Willebrand factor

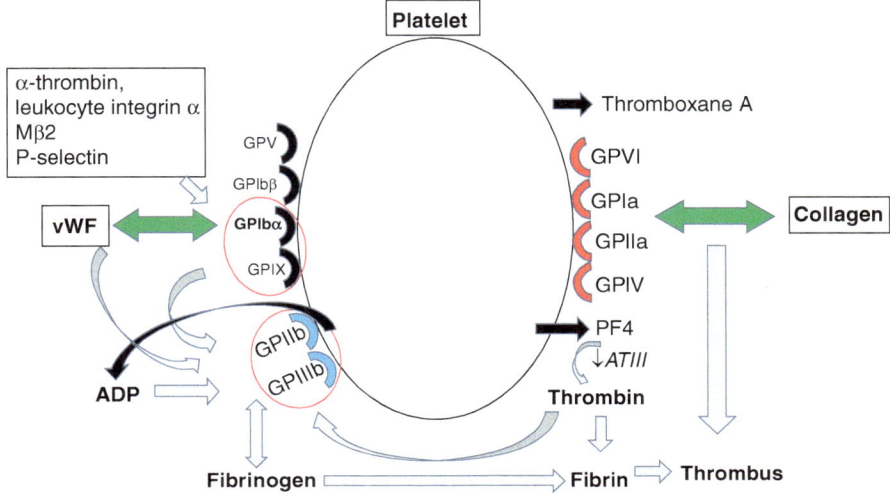

Fig. 9.2 Mechanisms of coagulopathy in advanced acute or chronic kidney impairment. The main glycoprotein platelet receptors involved in uremic coagulopathy are shown by the red circles. Explanation in text

excessive amounts of the tissue factor and reduce endothelial surface expression of thrombomodulin (a mediator of the anticoagulant effects of proteins S and C) and increase the secretion of PAI-1. These changes result in intraglomerular hypercoagulability/hypofibrinolytic state with enhancement of fibrin deposition and progression of crescent formation [28].

Uremia and the Increased Risk of Bleeding

Patients with acute or advanced chronic renal failure develop an acquired thrombocytopathy which is multifactorial in pathogenesis, affecting the all steps of platelet hemostasis. Platelets from uremic patients exhibit abnormal adhesion; reduced aggregating response to ADP, adrenaline, thrombin, and collagen; and change in the cyclooxygenase activity and arachidonic acid metabolism [29].

In uremic patients, the plasma levels of vWF and fibrinogen are increased. However, the coexisting functional defect in their interaction with glycoprotein (GP) IIb-IIIa receptors, mostly due to conformational changes of the receptors, leads to subsequent impairment of platelet aggregation. Furthermore, the interaction between vWF and thrombin-upregulated GPIb/IX receptors is impaired. This results in diminution in the intracellular processes normally responsible for expression of GPIIb-IIIa receptors and the production of thromboxane- A2 [30, 31].

Resting platelets from uremic patients exhibit a deficient assembly of cytoskeletal proteins, actin, and tropomyosin. The deficiency becomes more obvious upon platelet activation by thrombin. This explains the deficient platelet motility and secretory functions observed in uremia [32].

Deficiency of platelet storage pool of serotonin and adenosine and alternation of intra-platelet calcium mobilization play an important role in reduced platelet aggregation in uremic patients [31, 33].

Ultrafiltrate from uremic patients was found to inhibit in vitro platelet aggregation. Moreover, uremic toxins inhibit platelet-activating factor (PAF) by phagocytic leukocytes. Substances that inhibit platelet function in uremic plasma include urea, guanidinosuccinic acid, phenol and tryptophan products, small peptides containing the (Arg-Gly-Asp) sequence of amino acids, as well as parathormone. Removal of these substances with dialysis improves platelet function and aggregation. Moreover, fibrinogen fragments were found to be elevated in uremic patients and to play an important role in inhibiting platelet aggregation via competitive binding to the fibrinogen receptors [34].

Furthermore, prostacyclin and nitric oxide (NO$^{\bullet}$) production by endothelium in uremic patients is enhanced. Prostacyclin stimulates cAMP production by platelets with subsequent reduction of thromboxane A2 production. NO$^{\bullet}$ induces cGMP production that alters vascular tone interfering with vasoconstictor response to injury, platelet adhesion to the endothelium, and platelet-platelet interaction [35, 36].

Anemia, often supervening in advanced kidney disease, alters blood rheology leading to a decrease in the availability of platelets near the injured vessel. Hemoglobin reduction also leads to a decline in the NO$^{\bullet}$-scavenging capacity of injured tissues. Correction of anemia can partially correct the prolongation in the bleeding time in uremic patients.

Uremia may be associated with enhanced hyperfibrinolytic activity [37]. The augmented oxidative stress in dialysis-dependent uremic patients was shown to correlate with increased fibrinolytic activity, leading to a marked decrease in PAI-1/urokinase-type plasminogen activator (uPA) and PAI-1/tPA ratios [37, 38].

Impact of Impaired Kidney Function on the Use of Anticoagulants

Mild-to-Moderate Impairment of Kidney Function (CKD Stages I–III)

There is little concern about using anticoagulants with an estimated glomerular filtration rate (eGFR) >30ml/min/1.73sqm. Both injectable and oral anticoagulants may be used without or with minor dose modifications (Tables 9.1 and 9.2). Warfarin

Table 9.1 Dose adjustment of injectable anticoagulants for venous thromboembolism (VTE) and non-valvular atrial fibrillation (AF) with CKD

Agent	Dose adjustment according to eGFR (ml/min/1.73sqm)			Comments
	30–59	15–29	<15	
UFH	Not required	Not required	Not required	
Enoxaparin 1 mg /kg b.i.d.	Not required	Dose reduction to 1 mg/kg	Dose reduction to 1 mg/kg	Measurement of pre- and post- dose anti-Xa blood levels is essential for the use of low-molecular-weight heparin in patients with a GFR <50 mL/min to avoid supra- or sub-therapeutic anticoagulation
Dalteparin ACS (120 IU/kg BD), VTE (200 IU/kg OD)	Not required	Dose adjustment with anti-Xa level	Dose adjustment with anti-Xa level	
Tinzaparin VTE (175 IU/kg)	Not required	Dose adjustment as per anti-Xa level if GFR <20 mL/min		
Fondaparinux	Use with caution	Contraindicated	Contraindicated	
Lepirudin	CrCl (mL/min)		Dose (mg/kg/h)	Doses as low as 0.005 mg/kg/h have been used in renal failure requiring hemodialysis
	> 60		0.1–0.15	
	45–60		0.075	
	30–44		0.045	
	15–29		0.0225	
	<15		0.02 or less	
Danaparoid				Not approved for CrCl <30 mL/min
Argatroban	Renal dysfunction dose adjustment unclear. Fraction of extracorporeal clearance not clinically significant. Dose reduction of 0.1–0.6 mg/kg/min per 30 mL/min decrease in CrCl has been suggested.			Approved for CrCl <30 mL/min
Bivalirudin	HIT and VTE dosing: CrCl 60 mL/min: 0.15 mg/kg/h CrCl 30–60 mL/min: 0.08–0.1 mg/kg/h CrCl <30 mL/min or hemodialysis: 0.03–0.05 mg/kg/h			Eliminated enzymatically and renally; however, clearance relationship exists between CrCl and dose requirements
				Substantially removed during HD. Higher doses are used during cardiac interventional procedures with adjustment for renal dysfunction necessary

Table derived from References [40–42]
CrCl = Creatinine clearance, *Xa* = Activated factor X, *HIT* = Heparin-induced thrombocytopenia, *VTE* = Venous thoromboembolism, *UFH* = Unfractionated heparin

Table 9.2 Dose adjustment of warfarin and NOACs for venous thromboembolism (VTE) and non-valvular atrial fibrillation (NVAF) with CKD

Agent	Dose adjustment according to eGFR (mL/min/1.73sqm)			Renal clearance	Hemodialysis Removal (4-hour session)	Reversibility agents	Comments
	30–59	15–29	<15				
Warfarin	Not preferred	Not preferred	2.5 mg daily with frequent monitoring	<1%	<1%	Vitamin K, FFP, 4F-PCC	
Dabigatran 150 mg b.i.d.	Dose reduction to 110 mg b.i.d. if bleeding risk is high	Contraindicated	Contraindicated	80%	50–60%	Idarucizumab, FFP, or PCC may reverse *60% dialyzable*	DVT/PE: Initiate after 5 to 10 days of parental anticoagulant DI: P-glycoprotein inhibitors and inducers
Rivaroxaban 20 mg o.d	Dose reduction to 15 mg o.d.	AF: Dose reduction to 15 mg VTE: No change of initial treatment (15 mg b.i.d. for 3 weeks). Afterward dose reduction from 20mg to 15 mg o.d. if bleeding risk is high	Not recommended	36%	<1%	No specific antidote, *not* dialyzable – PCC can reverse	Must be taken with food
Apixaban 5 mg b.i.d.	No dose reduction	AF: Dose reduction to 2.5 mg b.i.d. VTE: Use with caution	*Off-label* in stage Vd 5mg b.i.d.	27%	7%	No specific antidote, *not* dialyzable	NVAF: 2.5 mg BID if ≥80 years old or ≤60 kg and sCr ≥1.5 mg/dl not recommended with prosthetic heart valve
Edoxaban 60 mg o.d.	Dose reduction to 30 mg o.d.	Dose reduction to 30 mg o.d. Use with caution	Not recommended	50%	9%	No specific antidote, *not* dialyzable	DVT/PE: Initiate after 5 to 10 days of parental anticoagulant DI: P-glycoprotein inhibitors and inducers. Short-term azithromycin use, decrease to 30 mg Qday

Table derived from References [43, 44]

AF = atrial fibrillation, DI = drug-drug interactions, DVT = deep venous thrombosis, 4F-PCC = four-factor prothrombin complex concentrate, FFP = fresh frozen plasma, NOACs = non-vitamin K dependent oral anticoagulants, NVAF = non-valvular atrial fibrillation, PE = pulmonary embolism, Stage Vd CKD = stage V on regular dialysis, VTE = venous thromboembolism and Non-Vitamin-K dependent Oral Anticoagulants (NOACs) are equally effective in reducing the incidence of stroke. Many observational studies have substantiated the safety of NOACs when used in the suggested doses, hence their preference for use in mild-to-moderate renal insufficiency (grade IB) [39].

It is noteworthy that the use of antiplatelet agents is also safe at this level of kidney function (see table 9.3)

Severe Impairment of Kidney Function (e.g. CKD Stages IV–V)

With more advanced CKD (estimated glomerular filtration rate – eGFR <30 ml/min/1.73sqm), including those on dialysis, where the risk of bleeding is augmented, the decision to anticoagulate has to be carefully weighed according to; a) the clinical indication; b) the individual CHADS2 risk score; and c) the patient's hemorrhagic risk stratification, e.g., by the HAS-BLED score.

Clinical Indications of anticoagulation in patients with kidney insufficienncy

There is a general agreement on six compelling indications where the benefit of anticoagulation usually outweighs the risk of their use, namely, (a) atrial fibrillation, (b) acute coronary syndromes, (c) status postprosthetic heart valve implantation, (d) antiphospholipid syndrome, (e) treatment and secondary prevention of severe thromboembolic events, and (f) extracorporial treatments.

There are several other clinical conditions that often require the use of antiplatelet agents in patients with kidney insufficiency as percutaneous interventions (PCI) of the coronary, renal, or peripheral arteries, scleroderma, thrombotic microangiopathy, etc. The safety and relevant pharmacokinetic features of these agents is summarized in Table 9.3.

The CHADS₂ Score

CHADS$_2$ score is helpful in estimating the risk of thrombotic events (See Chap. 3), although it ignores CKD as a risk factor. A modified score (CHA$_2$DS$_2$-VASc) improves the predictive value in mild to moderate, but not in severe, renal insufficiency [48]. Patients with CHADS2 score 0 may use antiplatelet therapy only, while oral anticoagulants are indicated with higher scores [49].

Table 9.3 Antiplatelet drugs used in patients with impaired kidney function

APD and usual recommended dose	Route of elimination	Dose adjustment with renal impairment	Reversal in bleeding	Remarks on safety/efficacy profile in renal impairment
Aspirin	Renal (pH-dependent)	None	Discontinue, platelet transfusion, and desmopressin	*HOT study*: Increased benefit with worsening kidney function, no increase in bleeding across CKD stages (increased minor bleeding compared to general population)
81–325 mg				
				UK-HARP study: No evidence of major bleeding, no worsening of renal disease; threefold risk of minor bleeding.
				The risk of GIT bleeding increases with higher doses, so a small daily long life dose 75–100 mg seems to be safe option
Clopidogrel	Renal (50%), feces (50%)	None	Discontinue, platelet transfusion, and desmopressin	*CURE study*: Beneficial effect of clopidogrel on reduction of absolute and relative primary ischemic end-points in all groups with CKD, increase in major bleeding compared to placebo but no difference in bleeding rates across eGFR groups

Table 9.3 (continued)

APD and usual recommended dose	Route of elimination	Dose adjustment with renal impairment	Reversal in bleeding	Remarks on safety/ efficacy profile in renal impairment
Loading dose: 300–600 mg				
Maintenance dose: 75 mg				
Prasugrel	Renal (60–70%)	None	Discontinue, platelet transfusion, and desmopressin	*TRITON-TIMI 38*: Reduction in MACE with and without CKD equally, bleeding risk was not assessed in CKD group
Loading dose: 60 mg				
Maintenance dose: 10 mg				*TRILOGY-ACS*: Worse primary efficacy outcome with prasugrel in patients with impaired renal function, and bleeding risk was not assessed in CKD group
Ticagrelor	Biliary	None	Discontinue	*PLATO study*: Significant reduction in primary ischemic outcome and all causes of death, no increase in major or fatal bleeding
Loading dose: 180 mg				
Maintenance dose: 90 mg PO b.i.d				
Abciximab	Spleen, RES	None	Discontinue, platelet transfusion, & desmopressin	
Loading dose: 250 µg/kg bolus				
Maintenance dose: 0.125 µg/ kg/min for 12h				
Tirofiban	Renal (40%–70%)	eGFR<30 ml/ min/1.73 m^2: 50% dose reduction	Discontinue, FFP	

(continued)

Table 9.3 (continued)

APD and usual recommended dose	Route of elimination	Dose adjustment with renal impairment	Reversal in bleeding	Remarks on safety/ efficacy profile in renal impairment
Loading dose: 0.4 µg/kg/ min 30-min bolus *Maintenane dose:* 0.1 µg/kg/ min				
Epitifibatide	Renal (50%)	eGFR<50 ml/ min/1.73 m^2: 180µg/kg/min bolus then	Discontinue, FFP	
Loading dose: 180 µg/kg bolus		1 µg/kg/min for 72h; contraindicated in patients on hemodialysis		
*Maintenance dose:*2.0 µg/kg/ min for 72h				

Table derived from References [45–47]
Relevant clinical trials: *CURE* Clopidogrel in Unstable angina to prevent Recurrent Events; *PLATO*: PLATelet inhibition and patient Outcomes; *TRILOGY-ACS* TarGeted platelet Inhibition to cLarify the Optimal strategy to manage Acute Coronary Syndromes; *TRITON-TIMI 38* TRrial to assess Improvement in Therapeutic Outcomes by optimizing platelet inhibitioN with prasug-rel-ThrombolysIs in Myocardial Infarction 38. *MACE* = Major Adverse Cardiac Events; *RES* = Reticuloendothelial system

The HAS-BLED Score

Hemorrhagic risk stratification is guided by several bleeding risk scores, preferably the HAS-BLED [49, 50]. High scores identify high-risk patients who need careful review and close follow-up, correction of modifiable risk factors like uncontrolled blood pressure, and cessation of confounding medications as aspirin and NSAIDs.

Choice of oral anticoagulants in advanced CKD; Warfarin is often preferred to NOACs in stages IV–V CKD despite weak recommendation (evidence grade 2C), owing to the relative sparsity of data on most NOACs. The recommended warfarin's starting dose is 2.5 mg daily, and the target INR should be kept between 2 and 3. Monitoring should be more frequent than usual during the first 90 days, when the risk of bleeding is highest [51].

Safety concerns have been published on the NOACs dabigatran and rivaroxaban yet not on apixaban. The latter was initially tested off-label in large studies that showed non-inferiority to warfarin and lower risk of bleeding [52]. It was recently approved by the FDA in patients with end-stage kidney disease on dialysis, without dose reduction (5 mg b.i.d.) in due consideration to the drug's dializability, unless age is ≥80 years or body weight ≤60 kg, where the dose is reduced to 2.5 mg b.i.d.

Anticoagulants In The Main Cardiac Complications of CKD

Chronic kidney disease is a major risk factor for cardiovascular disease. Clinically significant heart disease is therefore a significant comorbidity that often requires long-term anticoagulant treatment. The most common settings that impose critical decisions in this respect are atrial fibrillation, acute coronary syndromes, and coronary artery revascularization.

Atrial Fibrillation

Atrial fibrillation (AF) is the most challenging condition regarding oral anticoagulation in CKD for 2 reasons: (a) being common; and (b) being more likely to complicate than in patients with normal kidney function.

The reported annual incidence of AF in patients with CKD is more than double that in patients with normal kidney function [53]. It ranges between 17% and 24% [54], rising up to 35% per year in those on regular hemodialysis [55]. This high incidence is presumably related to the underlying cardiac pathology, oxidative stress, and the disturbed biochemical milieu supervening in CKD.

AF accelerates progression of CKD and increases the risk of thromboembolic strokes, systemic thrombosis, and myocardial infarction owing to the compromised circulatory dynamics [56].

AF is an ominous sign in hemodialysis. In a longitudinal study of 190 patients on regular hemodialysis, the 4-year mortality was 81% in patients with AF compared to 29% in those without [57]. The incidence of thromboembolic strokes in AF is more common with hemodialysis, than with peritoneal dialysis or without CKD [58, 59]. The incidence of AF, as well as its embolic complications, is more frequent during or up to 12 hours following dialysis, with a peak during the first 4 hours. This is probably attributed to rapid changes in cardiac volume and serum electrolytes and acid-base balance associated with dialysis.

In a Danish Registry study of 132,372 patients, AF also increased the risk of bleeding in patients with CKD (3587 patients), with a mean Hazzard ratio of 1.47.

It was further increased to 1.83 with hemodialysis (901 patients), apparently due to the added effects of uremia and the inevitable regular use of anticoagulants [60].

Despite these concerns, antiplatelet drugs [61] and anticoagulants [62] were shown to improve clinical outcomes including all-cause mortality, fatal stroke, fatal bleeding, and cardiac death.

Acute Coronary Syndrome (ACS)

Non-ST Elevation (NSTE) Acute Coronary Syndrome

Chronic kidney disease is present in 30–40% of patients with NSTE-ACS [63]. It is a poor prognostic factor for both early and late mortality [64]. In one study, the risk of cardiac death was 46% higher in CKD Stage II and further to 131% in stages IV and V [65].

Patients with NSTE-ACS and CKD are treated in the same way as those without renal dysfunction. Aspirin can be safely and effectively used, without dose modification [66]. The efficacy of clopidogrel in inhibiting platelet aggregation is reduced in CKD Stages I-III, even with doubling the dose [67]. On the other hand, several studies have shown that ticagrelor significantly reduces the incidence of ischemic end points and mortality in comparison to clopidogrel, without increasing the risk of major bleeding [68].

Anticoagulants may be used in reduced doses according to CKD stage (Table 9.1). Concurring with several guidelines, fondaparinux is the drug of choice in stages I–III owing to its favorable safety profile [69]. In severe kidney disease (stages IV–V), both enoxaparin and fondaparinux must be avoided, unfractionated heparin, therefore becoming the drug of choice.

Like in the general population, CKD patients with NSTE-myocardial infarction have a better one-year survival following invasive treatment by PCI. This benefit was observed in all stages of CKD yet becoming less pronounced as renal function deteriorates [70].

ST Elevation (STE) Myocardial Infarction

CKD patients with glomerular filtration rate (GFR) <70 ml/min account for 40% of STE-myocardial infarction (STE-MI) with increasing risk of serious cardiac complications such as heart failure, arrhythmias, and cardiogenic shock with deterioration of the GFR [70]. In one study, the in-hospital mortality in hemodialysis patients admitted for their first myocardial infarction was 26% where their overall first-year mortality was 59% [71].

CKD patients with STE-MI are treated according to the standard protocols for the general population. However, more aggressive treatment, particularly angioplasty, is recommended for restoration of infarct-related arterial patency. The subsequent use of antiplatelet drugs and anticoagulants is recommended as explained in NSTE-ACS.

Coronary Artery Revascularization

Dual antiplatelet therapy (DAPT) is the standard postcoronary artery stenting. Aspirin is usually combined with a P2Y12 receptor antagonist. Ticagrelor is preferred in patients with chronic kidney disease, where no dose adjustment is required as the drug and its metabolites are almost completely excreted in bile and stools.

An occasional patient may require additional anticoagulation, usually for associated AF. Since the risk of bleeding is critical in such patients particularly in Stages IV-V CKD, caution is due by weighing a prothrombotic score (as the CHADS2) against a bleeding risk score (as the HAS-BLED). Since warfarin has been associated with highest risk of bleeding in advanced CKD, its use with DAPT should be completely avoided. Unfractionated heparin may be used with the usual precautions. The direct thrombin inhibitor, Bivalirudin, has been safely used in patients with GFR <60 ml/min, with reduction of bleeding and ischemic events and a greater absolute benefit [72].

Renal Complications of Anticoagulation

Anticoagulant-related nephropathy (ARN) is an acute unexplained kidney injury with hematuria and glomerular hemorrhage in the settings of using an anticoagulant, often followed by irreversible damage to kidney and increased risk of mortality [73]. However, owing to the dearth of renal biopsies in patients receiving anticoagulants, it is sometimes disputed whether ARN is a distinct clinical entity, since other conditions as infection-related glomerulonephritis or drug induced interstitial nephritis may be underlying.

ARN was first described with warfarin and later with other anticoagulants. Warfarin-related nephropathy was first described in 1964 in patients receiving the drug on chronic basis, who developed hematuria with INR >3, yet without a linear relation to prothrombin time and concentration at higher INRs [74]. The first histological description was in 2009, showing glomerular hemorrhage, dysmorphic red cells, and obstructed tubules with red cell casts (Fig. 9.3) [75]. Electron microscopy confirmed glomerular basement disruption despite the absence of active glomerulonephritis or other inflammatory changes that could account for glomerular hemorrhage.

CKD is the strongest risk factor for ARN, with an incidence of 37%. The occurrence of ARN accelerates progression of CKD. Other risk factors include hypertension and diabetes [76].

The pathogenesis of ARN is unclear. However, it is currently presumed to result from breakdown of the glomerular endothelial barrier due to inactivation of endothelial thrombin-dependent proteinase-activated receptors (PARs) [77]. Supporting this hypothesis is that administration of PAR antagonists in animal models of CKD recapitulates some of the features of ARN. Administration of vitamin K attenuates these findings [78].

Treatment of ARN is mainly supportive, including the tight control of INR within the therapeutic range. It is unclear, though, if this will limit kidney damage, since

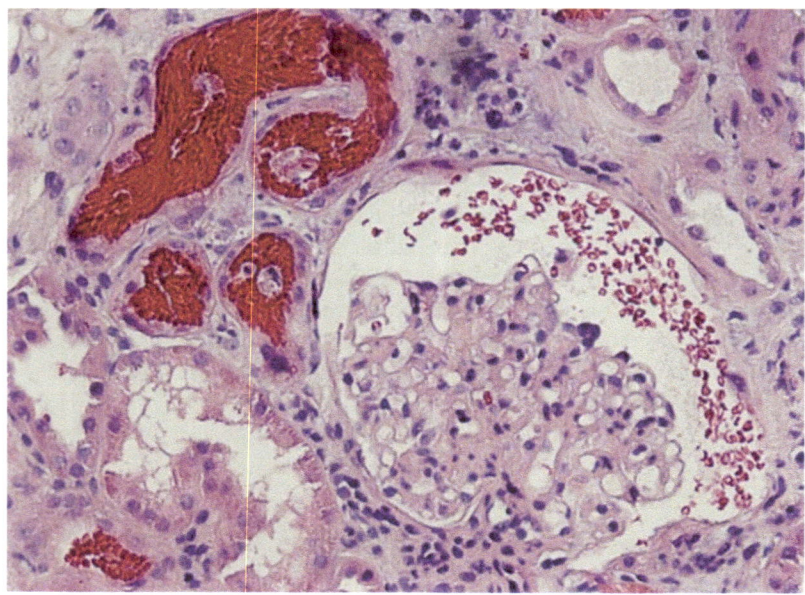

Fig. 9.3 Warfarin-related nephropathy. Note the shrunken glomerulus with bleeding into the Bowman's capsule and adjacent tubules. No inflammatory reaction is noticed. *(Reproduced with permission from Ref.* [75])

ARN is often unrelated to prothrombin concentration (as explained above), and the described glomerular damage may be irreversible.

Anticoagulation *for* Kidney Disease

This section includes kidney diseases that may be prevented or treated by anticoagulants or antiplatelet agents.

Renal Vascular Disorders

Atherosclerotic Renal Artery Stenosis

Inspired by data postcoronary or iliofemoral artery revascularization, the use of antiplatelet agents is often recommended following renal artery stenting for the management of certain types of renovascular hypertension. However, there are no high-quality studies to confirm unequivocal benefit.

Data from respective animal models show that platelet activation occurs in this setting and may be responsible for causing downstream glomerular injury [79]. This provides rationale for the clinical use of antiplatelet agents while awaiting solid clinical evidence. Low-dose aspirin is currently used almost routinely; yet the use of thienopyridines or GPIIb/IIIa inhibitors remains controversial.

Thrombotic Microangiopathy (TMA)

Renal involvement is often a part of systemic TMA, yet there are several occasions where it is isolated without extrarenal criteria. The latter can be only diagnosed by kidney biopsy [80] (Fig. 9.4).

The most common renal TMAs are those associated with the hemolytic uremic syndrome, thrombotic thrombocytopenic purpura (TTP), ANCA-associated vasculitis, and class IV lupus nephritis particularly when associated with antiphospholipid antibodies. Renal transplant TMA may be induced directly by antibody-mediated rejection (ABMR) or indirectly by calcineurin inhibitors used for immunosuppression.

Renal TMA usually presents as acute kidney injury, with rapidly declining function. However, it may be a chronic process ongoing in the background of a systemic disease as systemic lupus.

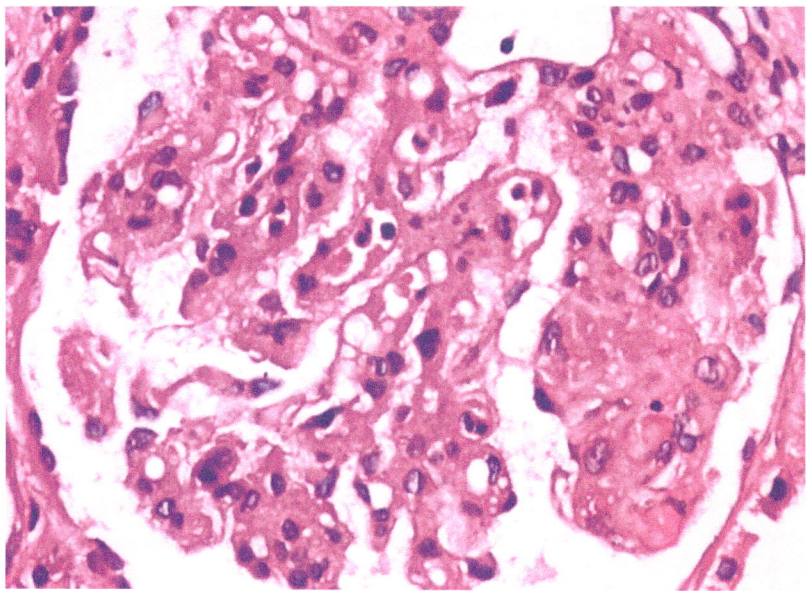

Fig. 9.4 Thrombotic microangiopathy. Note the endothelial swelling, capillary thrombi, and areas of basement membrane duplication. *(From the Cairo Kidney Center histopatholgy Archives, Courtesy Professor Wesam Ismail)*

Since increased platelet aggregation is a major pathogenic factor in TMA, the use of antiplatelet agents is an important therapeutic adjuvant [81]. Low-dose aspirin is standard treatment; the benefit of dual antiplatelet therapy is unclear. Aspirin should be used in conjunction with specific therapeutic lines as plasma exchange, corticosteroids, rituximab, or eculizumab in relevant conditions.

Scleroderma

Renal involvement occurs in 60–80% of patients with scleroderma [82]. The most dramatic scenario is the "renal crisis" (SRC), which accounts for up to 20% of the diffuse cutaneous form [83]. This is characterized by intimal proliferation with subsequent narrowing of the arcuate and interlobular arteries. Associated endothelial injury leads to secondary TMA [84] (Fig. 9.5).

Circulating platelet aggregates and beta-thromboglobulin have been well documented in patients with scleroderma [85] even without renal crisis, thereby providing rationale for antiplatelet therapy. Low-dose aspirin is the usual choice; newer antiplatelet agents have not been tested. The value of antiplatelet therapy is amplified in SRC in view of the associated TMA.

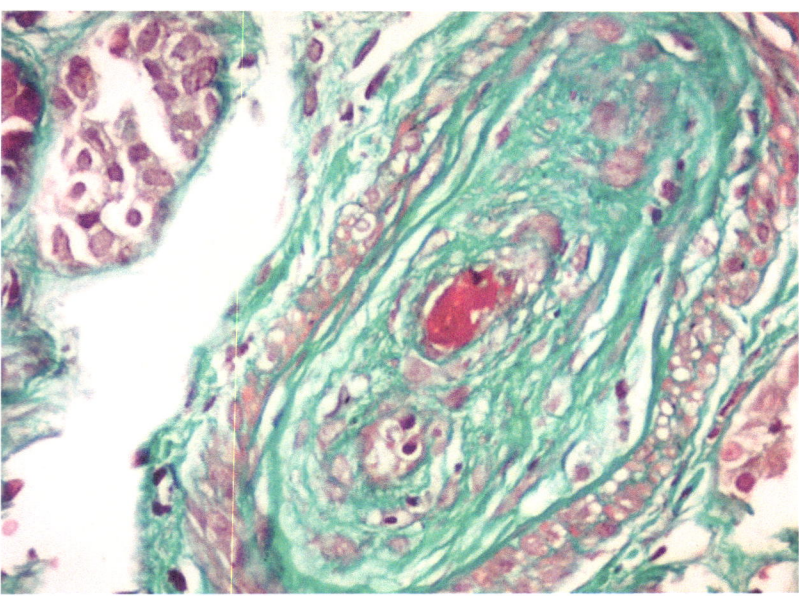

Fig. 9.5 Scleroderma. Arcuate artery showing intimal thickening with an onion skin appearance, luminal narrowing with endothelial activation and thrombus formation. (*From the Cairo Kidney Center histopatholgy Archives, Courtesy Professor Wesam Ismail*)

Cholesterol Crystal Embolism

Showering of cholesterol emboli may occur from atheromatous plaques upon interventional manipulation by intravascular aortic, coronary, or renal arterial catheters. These lodge in the narrow peripheral arteries, measuring 100 to 200 μm [86]. The kidney is the most vulnerable target owing to its anatomical position and circulatory dynamics [87]. Renal affection may be asymptomatic, or manifest with hematuria or acute kidney injury, typically occurring during the 2 weeks following the procedure.

Cholesterol crystal embolization is often induced by anticoagulants. This is explained by bleeding into the atheromatous plaques upon disruption of their fibrous caps, which leads to their rupture, releasing low-density lipoprotein-derived cholesterol crystals [88].

The treatment is mainly supportive by steroids, statins and discontinuation of anticoagulants. Anticoagulation should be minimized if dialysis is required for acute kidney injury.

Renal Vein Thrombosis (RVT)

RVT is rare in normal population. However, it constitutes a significant risk in a) patients with renal malignancy especially renal cell carcinoma and b) those with severe nephrotic syndrome [89].

The reported incidence of RVT is widely variable owing to its silent clinical presentation in most cases, being estimated between 5% and 60% in patients with the nephrotic syndrome [90]. Membranous nephropathy is the most common etiology, with an incidence around 37%, followed in frequency by membranoproliferative glomerulonephritis, minimal change disease, and focal and segmental glomerulosclerosis [90].

The spectrum of clinical presentation varies from silent chronic thrombosis to clinically overt acute kidney disease, manifesting with hematuria, loin pain, and deteriorating GFR, especially in bilateral RVT.

The goals of treatment of RVT are (a) primary prophylaxis in patients at risk, (b) management of established RVT, and (c) management of thromboembolic events such as PE and DVT.

Primary Prophylaxis

The decision of primary prophylaxis should be carefully balanced between the risks of RVT on one hand and anticoagulant-induced bleeding on the other. In membranous nephropathy, hypoalbuminemia is the most significant risk factor. The danger is increased as the serum albumin drops below 2.8 gm/dl and doubles with every further gram/dl decrement [91]. With other causes of the nephrotic syndrome, the risk of RVT is more closely associated with adjuvant comorbidities, such as major surgery and immobilization, severe heart failure, or atrial fibrillation. The counterbalancing bleeding risk can be stratified according to one of the available scores (see above).

Aspirin 75 mg /day is the standard prophylaxis if serum albumin is between 2 to 3 gm/dl. Anticoagulation with low-molecular-weight heparin, enoxaparin, is indicated if serum albumin is lower than 2 gm/dl. The standard dose is 20 mg/day for 3 months to be switched to warfarin with target INR from 1.5 to 2.5, if the serum albumin persisted below 2 gm/dl [92].

Management of Established RVT

Established RVT is suspected with the recent onset of hematuria or rapid deterioration of kidney function, and confirmed by ultrasonic, spiral CT or MRI imaging or occasionally by kidney biopsy. On the other hand, RVT may be silent, being accidentally discovered by imaging for the evaluation of a suspected renal neoplasm or another extrarenal condition. In either case, anticoagulation is mandatory with due consideration to the contemporary kidney function and potential risks.

Local thrombolytic therapy with or without thrombus extraction by catheter is safer than systemic thrombolytic therapy which carries a higher risk of bleeding. It leads to rapid recovery of kidney function in patients with acute renal vein thrombosis [93].

Management of RVT with Thromboembolic Events

RVT with thromboembolic events should be treated with anticoagulation, initially with unfractionated or low-molecular-weight heparin in the same manner as in treatment of PE (Chap. 2) or DVT (Chap. 2). Treatment should be continued for 6–12 month or longer if the nephrotic syndrome persists [94]. If anticoagulation is contraindicated for a reason or another, a suprarenal inferior vena caval filter may be used [95].

Glomerulonephritis

Following the historic attempts to ameliorate the course of glomerulonephritis, the scope of their use regressed to the more severe forms, typically associated with crescent formation. These included anti-glomerular basement membrane disease and ANCA-associated vasculitides. Nevertheless, owing to the current advances in the management of these conditions, anticoagulants are no longer recommended in any of the recent guidelines.

Anticoagulants for Extracorporeal Treatment

Extracorporeal membranes, used for hemodialysis, hemodiafiltration, plasmapheresis, and related treatment modalities, are thrombogenic and procoagulant. They attract blood cells and activate Hageman factor (FXII). FXIIa has a central role in triggering the intrinsic coagulation pathway and also in activating the classical complement, fibrinolytic, and kinin pathways. The negative charge on the membrane also activates the alternative complement pathway, yet C3a and C5a are adsorbed by the membrane, which limits their pathogenicity (Fig. 9.6).

Anticoagulation, therefore, is an essential component of any extracorporeal treatment. Antiplatelet aggregation agents may also be used, though a rapid blood flow through the extracorporeal circuit is usually necessary to prevent thrombosis.

There are different anticoagulation strategies in extracorporeal treatment, targeting different levels of the coagulation cascade (Fig. 9.7).

Unfractionated Heparin (UFH)

UFH is the most widely used in extracorporeal treatments, being efficient, easy to use and monitor, economical, and fairly safe. The main risks are those of anticoagulation at large, hence the issues with old age, recent intracranial events or local bleeding in the gastrointestinal tract or other deep sites, and systemic coagulopathies.

No other condition in medicine mimics regular dialysis in exposing patient to heparin three times weekly for many years. This amplifies the importance of adverse reactions unrelated to its anticoagulant activity, including osteoporosis, hypertriglyceridemia, and hyperkalemia (due to aldosterone inhibition), and "burning feet syndrome." In 3–5% of patients on regular hemodialysis, heparin leads to immune-mediated thrombocytopenia (HIT) (See Chap. 2) in which case an alternative anticoagulant (Table 9.4), most commonly recombinant hirudin, is used instead.

In all the extracorporeal circuits, the "filter" is initially washed with saline and 2000–5000 i.u. of heparin, and the washing solution is discarded before blood is let in. Following this, heparin may be administered in five different protocols, depending on the patient's condition and the center's experience and equipment.

Continuous Heparin Infusion

An initial bolus of 25–50 IU/Kg is injected into the inlet tubing, followed by an infusion of 800–1500 IU/hour through a machine-integrated syringe pump, until 30–60 minutes before termination of the procedure. The wide range of recommended doses reflects the inter-patient variability that has to be taken seriously. This method does not require any monitoring except in patients at risk of bleeding, or those who have issues like repeated clotting of the filter or prolonged bleeding at the puncture sites. In these cases, the rate of infusion is modified to achieve an extracorporeal aPTT target of 200–250 seconds.

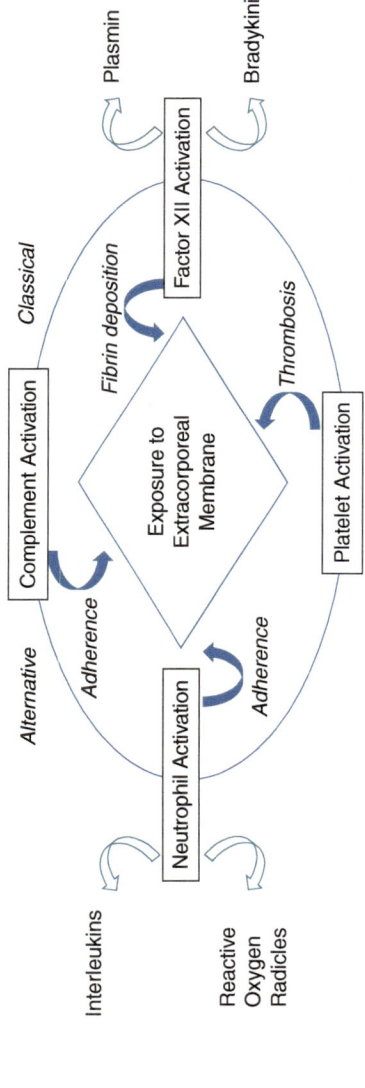

Fig. 9.6 Thrombophilic mechanisms induced by extracorporeal circulation

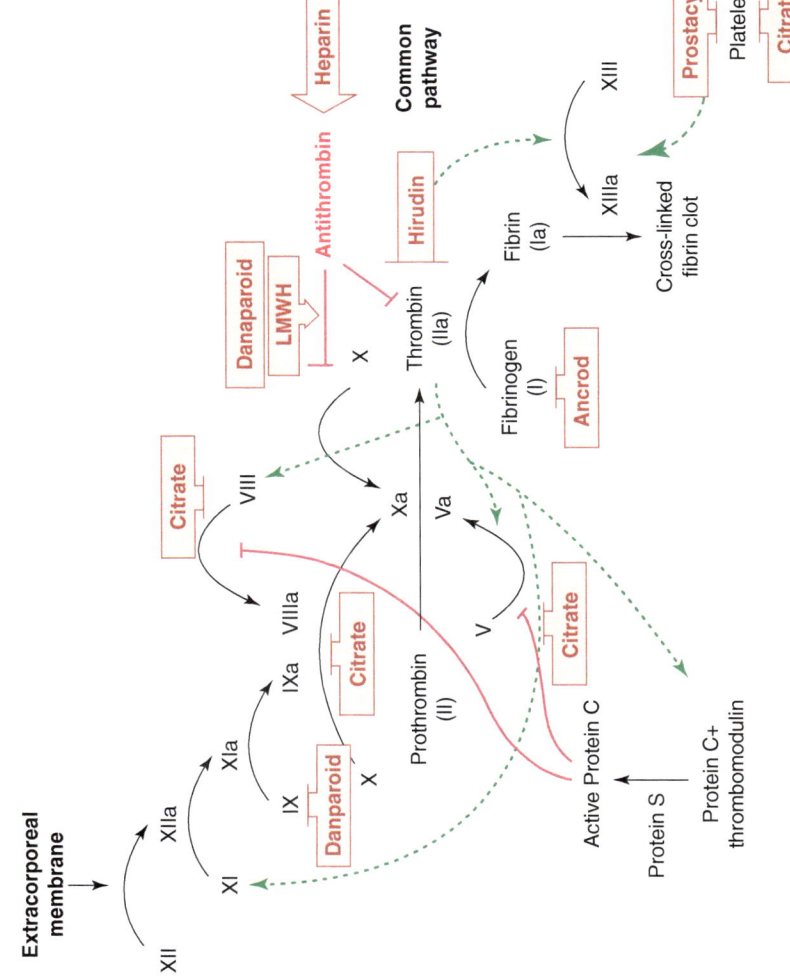

Fig. 9.7 Sites of action of anticoagulants used in the extracorporeal circulation

Table 9.4 Alternative anticoagulation for hemodialysis patients with heparin-induced thrombocytopenia

	Dose for HD		Dose for CVVHD	Dose for catheter lock	Monitoring		Remarks
	Bolus	MD			Test	Target	
Direct thrombin inhibitors	First HD: 0.1 mg/kg	—	Initiate at 0.005–0.01 mg/kg/h	5 mg/ml per port[a]	aPTT	HD: 2–2.5[b] CVVHD: 1.5–2[b]	High risk of bleeding complications due to markedly prolonged half-life in dialysis patients
Hirudin, Lepirudin (recombinant hirudin)	Subsequent HD: 0.05–0.1 mg/kg depending on pre-HD aPTT						Dialysis should be performed with high-flux dialyzers
							Dosing may be as infrequent as every 6–12 days depending on the degree of residual renal function and the pre-HD aPTT
							No antidote is available
Argatroban	250 µg/kg	1.7 to 3.3 µg/kg × min (in normal liver function)	Initiate at 0.5–1.0 µg/kg/min and dose adjustment to aPTT	Not available	aPTT	HD: 1.5–3[b] CVVHD: 1.5–2[b]	Initial assessment of liver function is a must (the dose should be readjusted in hepatic impairment)

Anti factorXa						Anti-factor Xa level	HD: 0–0.4 CVVHD: 0.5–1	Half-life is prolonged in HD patients, so pre-HD anti-factor Xa levels should be carefully monitored and kept below the maximal allowed level
Danaparoid	Rinse system with 750 IU	–	2500 anti-factor Xa U bolus	750 U in 50 ml saline, then 5–10 ml per port				
	Bolus according to BW (IU):							
		<55Kg	>55Kg					
	1st HD	2500	3750	Then 600 U/hr·4 hr,				
	2nd HD	2000	3750	Then 400 U/hr·4 hr,				
				Then 200–600 U/hr				
	From third HD according to anti-Xa:			Based on levels[c]				
	<0.3:	2000	3000					
	0.3 to 0.35	2000	2500					
	>0.35	1500	2000					

Table derived from References [96, 97]

[a]Must be aspirated prior to HD=Hemodialysis

[b]times the mean of the normal range (Target results for the aPTTs are based on individual coagulation laboratory mean values. Do not exceed 100 seconds

[c]Use lower bolus dosing if weight is less than 50 kg

Intermittent Heparin Injection

An initial bolus of 25-50 IU/Kg is injected into the inlet tubing, followed by a bolus of 400–800 iu/30 minutes. This method carries some risk of alternating over- and under-anticoagulation. Like with continuous infusion, no monitoring is required except in the mentioned situations.

Regional Heparinization

Heparin is infused in the inlet tubing by continuous infusion as above and a corresponding dose (1:100) of protamine sulfate in the outlet tubing [98]. This is supposed to provide enough anticoagulation of the extracorporeal circuit while sparing the patient's systemic circulation. The dose of protamine sulfate may be fine-tuned by a protamine-titration test prior to the procedure. The patient's systemic aPTT should be checked every 30 minutes to ensure efficacy of heparin neutralization. Unfortunately, the heparin-protamine complex formed during this procedure may dissociate a few hours later leading to severe bleeding. Owing to this risk, as well as the technical complexity of the procedure, regional heparinization is seldom used nowadays.

Low-Dose Heparin

No initial high-dose bolus is administered. Anticoagulation is achieved by direct injection of 500 units of heparin every 30 minutes, the last dose being administered 60 minutes before the end of the procedure.

No-Heparin

Apart from the initial rinsing, the procedure is performed without any more heparin. The system has to be flushed by 100–200 ml of N-saline every 15–60 minutes to wash any fibrin clots into the clot trap. While this method is successful in many patients, there is always the risk of "filter" clotting on one hand, and thrombocytopenia due to the loss of platelets which adhere to the membranes and tubing. Fluid overload is a frequent complication owing to failure of ultrafiltration caused by occlusion of a significant proportion of the dialyzer capillaries.

Low-Molecular-Weight Heparin

There are several advantages to using LMWH rather than heparin (see Chap. 1). However, owing to its exclusive excretion by the kidneys, it tends to accumulate in patients with renal impairment in general. And since it is not dialyzable, it may further accumulate in patients on regular dialysis. Monitoring its anti-coagulant activity is only possible by measuring Factor Xa, which is not accessible to many routine laboratories. aPTT is unreliable for monitoring LMWH activity [99]. LMWH is incompletely neutralized by protamine sulfate, even with very high doses (>40 µg to 1 IU/ml), and can lead to protamine toxicity [100].

For these reasons, LMWH is not FDA-approved for use in regular dialysis, although it is widely used in Western Europe and off-label in some centers in North America [101, 102]. A single dose (20–40 mg based on body weight) is administered at the beginning of dialysis without monitoring.

Hirudin

While natural hirudin is a highly effective anticoagulant, its clinical use is limited by unavailability being extracted in a small yield from leaches. Its role has been revisited upon the discovery of recombinant hirudin. This has been successfully used as a single bolus of 0.15 mg/kg at the onset of dialysis [103]. Even this small dose can lead to over-anticoagulation owing to the drug's long half-life which may exceed the duration of the dialysis session. It is more expensive than heparin; hence, its use is limited to patients with HIT.

Danaparoid

This anticoagulant inhibits thrombin generation by antithrombin-dependent inactivation of factor Xa and inhibition factor IX, which is an important feedback loop for thrombin generation. It is administered as a single pre-dialysis intravenous bolus of 1500 to 3750 units depending on body weight and dialysis frequency. For CRRT, an initial bolus of 2500 units is followed by 600 units/hour for 4 hours and then 200–600 units/hour for the rest of treatment. Plasma anti-factor Xa level should be monitored, aiming at 500–1000 units/L [104].

Argatroban

Argatroban is a direct thrombin inhibitor that has been successfully used in standard hemodialysis, including patients with HIT. It is partly cleared by dialysis, but this does not significantly affect its anticoagulant effect following a single dose before dialysis. Argatroban is successfully used in catheter lock solutions [105].

Melagatran

Melagatran is a thrombin inhibitor with predictable pharmacokinetics and pharmacodynamics for parenteral use. It is eliminated by HD, so it could be a suitable alternative in HIT especially in patients with high risk of bleeding. However, a fixed dosing protocol needs to be investigated [106].

Ancrod

This interesting anticoagulant is a natural poison extracted from Malaysian snakes. It has a strong anticoagulant activity for which it was used in extracorporeal dialysis during the early 1970s [107]. It has been seldom used ever since, owing to its unknown pharmacokinetics and mechanism of action, though it is of proven fibrinolytic activity, enough to sustain a safe anticoagulation throughout a dialysis session.

Citrate

With long extracorporeal treatments as CRRT, the use of heparin would expose the patient to a much higher dose than what can be cleared by the impaired catabolic capacity. Citrate is a safe anticoagulant that works by binding serum calcium to a pre-dialyzer level of 1 to 1.4 mg/dl, which leads to impairment of blood coagulation by (a) induction of conformational changes in factors V and VIII, (b) downregulation of several convertase enzymes in the intrinsic pathway, and (c) interfering with platelet biochemistry and aggregation (Fig. 9.6). Calcium is infused into the blood return tubing to limit anticoagulation to the extracorporeal circuit and to maintain a physiological intracorporeal serum level [108].

There are two ways of using citrate anticoagulation in CRRT, namely, citrate dialysate and extracorporeal circuit regional anticoagulation. Citrate is also used as a catheter lock anticoagulant with lower incidence of infection compared to heparin [109].

Citrate Dialysate

Dialysate citrate may be used as the sole anticoagulation modality or combined with low-dose heparin or heparin-impregnated dialysis membranes. When used alone, sodium citrate is added to the dialysate at the expense of sodium chloride to achieve a final concentration of 15 mg/dl, without changing the target sodium concentration. Calcium is eliminated from the dialysate. Intravenous calcium replacement is calculated by a special formula based on online ionic dialysance and the desired serum concentration [110–112].

Extracorporeal Circuit Anticoagulation

Sodium citrate is infused at a constant rate of 600 mg citrate/L blood flow (i.e., 12gm/h at a blood flow of 350 mL/min to reach a target activated clotting time (ACT) of 200 to 250 s in the venous line. Calcium chloride is infused into the outlet to target >1 mmol/L ionized calcium (Ca^{++} in arterial line. Early concerns about the effect of conversion of citrate into bicarbonate with consequent blood pH changes have been eliminated [113].

Prostacyclin

Prostacyclin is a vasodilator and an inhibitor of platelet aggregation. Prostacyclin regional dialysis can be achieved by infusion of 4 ng/kg/min into the dialyzer circuit. The use of this method is limited by the hypotensive effect of prostacyclin [114].

Extracorporeal Anticoagulation in Patients on Oral Anticoagulant Treatment

Since hemodialysis adds a transient procoagulant burden to the balanced anticoagulated milieu, additional short-acting anticoagulant should be a logical requirement. However, heparin-free dialysis was often successfully performed, thereby obviating the risk of bleeding. In a small study including 10 patients, the clotting scores were 1.49 and 1.53 with and without enoxaparin, respectively ($P = 0.97$) [115]. There is no uniform agreement on this issue, which awaits large scale clinical trials. In our unit, we adopt a low-dose heparin policy, with individual patient dose adjustment by frequent monitoring of the aPTT.

Summary and Conclusions

Chronic kidney disease is a procoagulant state that accelerates atherosclerosis and constitutes a risk to cardiovascular disease and strokes, hence the frequent need for using antiplatelets and anticoagulants. The latter may also be needed for the treatment of certain intrinsic kidney disease that are often associated with impaired function.

There should be no problem in using these drugs like in the general population so long as the kidney function is only mildly or moderately impaired (creatinine clearance >30 ml/min), and the drug doses are modified accordingly.

However, the art of prescription of these agents in advanced chronic or acute renal insufficiency is confounded by many factors including:

- The risk of bleeding, introduced into the scenario as a result of platelet dysfunction. This can be quantitated by balancing the thrombosis versus bleeding risk by specific scores that were validated in patients with kidney impairment.
- Drug pharmacokinetics, with particular emphasis on the route of elimination.
- Drug dializability when prescribed for patients receiving dialysis treatment.
- Drug-drug interactions particularly at the level of hepatic degradation by the cytochrome system.
- The frequent need for therapeutic drug monitoring.

While there is still some room for using warfarin with frequent INR monitoring and dose adjustment, a lot of non-vitamin K-dependent oral anticoagulants (NOACs) are now available, many of which can be used in adjusted doses. Many cardiovascular comorbidities associated with kidney disease may need antiplatelet drugs with or without anticoagulants, which requires very careful consideration of doses, pharmacokinetics, and drug-drug interactions.

Patients receiving dialysis treatment require regular anticoagulation to avoid blood clotting upon contact with cellophane membranes in the extracorporeal circulation. While heparin is the standard drug of choice, it must be avoided with the development of HIT and preferably replaced by another anticoagulant for prolonged dialysis as in CRRT. Fortunately there are many available options as citrate, direct thrombin inhibitors, prostacyclin, and others.

References

1. Abel JJ, Rowntree LG, Turner BB. The removal of diffusible substances from the circulating blood by means of vividiffusion. Trans Assoc Amer Phys. 1914;58:51–4.
2. Haas G. Ueber Versuche der Blutauswaschung am Lebenden mit Hilfe der Dialyse. Archiv Exp Path Pharmakol. 1926;106:158–72.
3. Sartorius H, Moench A, Fellmer KE. Effect of heparin on the course of experimental nephritis-nephrosis. Z Gesamte Exp Med. 1955;125(6):572–86.
4. Halpern BN, Lagrue G, Milliez P, Morard JC, Fray A. Remarkable inhibition by heparin of experimental heteroimmune nephropathy. C R Seances Soc Biol Fil. 1964;158:2297–302.
5. Halpern B, Milliez P, Lagrue G, Fray A, Morard JC. Protective action of heparin in experimental immune nephritis. Nature. 1965;16(205):257–9.
6. Halpern B, Lagrue G, Bariéty J, Morard JC, Fray A. Studies on experimental hetero-immune nephritis. II. Prevention by immunosuppressive agents and certain anticoagulants. Pathol Biol. 1967;15(7):373–7.
7. Humair LM. Prevention and treatment of experimental glomerulonephritis in mice by urokinase. Curr Probl Clin Biochem. 1968;2:260–1.
8. Kincaid-Smith P, Laver MC, Fairley KF. Dipyridamole and anticoagulants in renal disease due to glomerular and vascular lesions. A new approach to therapy. Med J Aust. 1970;1(4):145–51.
9. Kincaid-Smith P. Anticoagulants in renal disease. Am Heart J. 1969;44(6):840–1.

10. Ishikawa Y, Kitamura M. Inhibition of glomerular cell apoptosis by heparin. Kidney Int. 1999;56:954–63.
11. Floege J, Eng E, Young B, Couser WG, Johnson RJ. Heparin suppresses mesangial cell proliferation and matrix expansion in experimental mesangioproliferative glomerulonephritis. Kidney Int. 1993;43:369–80.
12. Verzetti G, Busilacchi M, Pisano E, Perpignano G. On the treatment of acute glomeruloinephritis with heparin. Preliminary clinical results. Minerva Nefrol. 1966;13(4):136–40.
13. Kincaid-Smith P, Saker BM, Fairley KF. Anticoagulants in "irreversible" acute renal failure. Lancet. 1968;2(7583):1360–3.
14. Herdman RC, Edson R, Pickering RJ, Fish AJ, Marker S, Good RA. Anticoagulants in renal disease in children. Am J Dis Child. 1970;119(1):27–35.
15. Freedman P, Meister HP, De la Paz A, Ronaghy H. The clinical, functional, and histologic response to heparin in chronic renal disease. Investig Urol. 1970;7(5):398–409.
16. Thijs A, Nanayakkara PW, Ter Wee PM, Huijgens PC, van Guldener C, Stehouwer CD. Mild-to-moderate renal impairment is associated with platelet activation: a cross sectional study. Clin Nephrol. 2008;70(4):325–31.
17. Lutz J, Menke J, Sollinger D, Schinzel H, Thurmel K. Haemostasis in chronic kidney disease. Nephrol Dial Transplant. 2014;29:29–40.
18. Shlipak MG, Fried LF, Crump C, Bleyer AJ, Manolio TA, Tracy RP, Furberg CD, Psaty BM. Elevations of inflammatory and procoagulant biomarkers in elderly persons with renal insufficiency. Circulation. 2003;107(1):87–92.
19. Huang MJ, Wei RB, Wang Y, Su TY, Di P, Li QP, Yang X, Li P, Chen XM. Blood coagulation system in patients with chronic kidney disease: a prospective observational study. BMJ Open. 2017;7(5):e014294.
20. Tomura S, Nakamura Y, Deguchi F, Ando R, Chida Y, Marumo F. Coagulation and fibrinolysis in patients with chronic renal failure undergoing conservative treatment. Thromb Res. 1991;64:81–90.
21. Cetin O, Bekpinar S, Unlucerci Y, Turkmen A, Bayram C, Ulutin T. Hyperhomocysteinemia in chronic renal failure patients: relation to tissue factor and platelet aggregation. Clin Nephrol. 2006;65:97–102.
22. Chu AJ. Tissue factor mediates inflammation. Arch Biochem Biophys. 2005;440:123–32.
23. Pawlak K, Tankiewicz J, Mysliwiec M, Pawlak D. Tissue factor/its pathway inhibitor system and kynurenines in chronic kidney disease patients on conservative treatment. Blood Coagul Fibrinolysis. 2009;20(7):590–4.
24. Ganguly P, Alam SF. Role of homocysteine in the development of cardiovascular disease. Nutr J. 2015;14:6.
25. Bostom AG, Athrop L. Hyperhomocysteinemia in end-stage renal disease: prevalence, etiology, and potential relationship to arteriosclerotic outcomes. Kidney Int. 1997;52:10–20.
26. Tay KH, Lip GY. What "drives" the link between the renin-angiotensin-aldosterone system and the prothrombotic state in hypertension? Am J Hypertens. 2008;21(12):1278–9.
27. Sechi LA, Novello M, Colussi G, Di Fabio A, Chiuch A, Nadalini E, Casanova-Borca A, Uzzau A, Catena C. Relationship of plasma renin with a prothrombotic state in hypertension: relevance for organ damage. Am J Hypertens. 2008;21(12):1347–53.
28. Hertig A, Rondeau E. Role of the coagulation/fibrinolysis system in fibrin-associated glomerular injury. J Am Soc Nephrol. 2004;15:844–53.
29. Rabelink TJ, Zwaginga JJ, Koomans HA, Sixma JJ. Thrombosis and hemostasis in renal disease. Kidney Int. 1994;46(2):287–96.
30. Escolar G, Díaz-Ricart M, Cases A. Uremic platelet dysfunction: past and present. Curr Hematol Rep. 2005;4(5):359–67.
31. Hedges SJ, Dehoney SB, Hooper JS, Amanzadeh J, Busti AJ. Evidence-based treatment recommendations for uremic bleeding. Nat Clin Pract Nephrol. 2007;3(3):138–53.
32. Escolar G, Diaz-Ricart M, Cases A, Calls J, López-Pedret J, Carretero M, Castillo R, Ordinas A, Escolar G. Abnormal cytoskeletal assembly in platelets from uremic patients. Am J Pathol. 1993;143:823–31.

33. Lambert MP. Platelets in liver and renal disease. Hematology Am Soc Hematol Educ Program. 2016;1:251–5.
34. Sohal AS, Gangji AS, Crowther MA, Treleaven D. Uremic bleeding: pathophysiology and clinical risk factors. Thromb Res. 2006;118(3):417–22.
35. Remuzzi G, Cavenaghi AE, Mecca G, Donati MB, de Gaetano G. Prostacyclin-like activity and bleeding in renal failure. Lancet. 1977;2:1195–7.
36. Vlachoytis J, Schoeppe W. Adenylate cyclase activity and cAMP content of human platelets in uraemia. Eur J Clin Investig. 1982;12:379–81.
37. Lutz J, Menke J, Sollinger D, Schinzel H, Thurmel K. Haemostasis in chronic kidney disease. Nephrol Dial Transplant. 2014;29:29–40.
38. Pawlak K, Pawlak D, Mysliwiec M. Oxidative stress effects fibrinolytic system in dialysis uraemic patients. Thromb Res. 2006;117(5):517–22.
39. Turpie AGG, Purdham D, Ciaccia A. Nonvitamin K antagonist oral anticoagulant use in patients with renal impairment. Ther Adv Cardiovasc Dis. 2017;11(9):243–56.
40. Harder S. Anticoagulant dosing in renal impairment. Phlebologie. 2015;44(06):316–9.
41. Dager WE, Kiser TH. Systemic anticoagulation considerations in chronic kidney disease. Adv Chronic Kidney Dis. 2010;17(5):420–7.
42. Hughes S, Szeki I, Nash MJ, Thachil J. Anticoagulation in chronic kidney disease patients—the practical aspects. Clin Kidney J. 2014;7(5):442–9.
43. Di Lullo L, Ronco C, Cozzolino M, Russo D, Russo L, Di Iorio B, De Pascalis A, Barbera V, Galliani M, Vitaliano E, Campana C, Santoboni F, Bellasi A. Nonvitamin K-dependent oral anticoagulants (NOACs) in chronic kidney disease patients with atrial fibrillation. Thromb Res. 2017;155:38–4.
44. Walters KJ, Meador A, Galdo JA, Ciarrocca K. A pharmacotherapy review of the novel, oral antithrombotics. Spec Care Dentist. 2017;37(2):62–70.
45. Ibrahim H, Rao SV. Oral antiplatelet drugs in patients with chronic kidney disease (CKD): a review. J Thromb Thrombolysis. 2017;43:519–27.
46. Basra SS, Tsai P, Lakkis NM. Safety and efficacy of antiplatelet and antithrombotic therapy in acute coronary syndrome patients with chronic kidney disease. J Am Coll Cardiol. 2011;58(22):2263–9.
47. Summaria F, Giannico MB, Talarico GP, Patrizi R. Antiplatelet therapy in hemodialysis patients undergoing percutaneous coronary interventions. Nephrourol Mon. 2015;7(4):e28099.
48. Friberg L, Rosenqvist M, Lip GY. Evaluation of risk stratification schemes for ischaemic stroke and bleeding in 182 678 patients with atrial fibrillation: the Swedish Atrial Fibrillation cohort study. Eur Heart J. 2012;33:1500.
49. Pisters R, Lane DA, Nieuwlaat R, de Vos CB, Crijns HJ, Lip GY. A novel user-friendly score (HAS-BLED) to assess one-year risk of major bleeding in atrial fibrillation patients: the Euro Heart Survey. Chest. 2010;138(5):1093–100.
50. Senoo K, Proietti M, Lane DA, Lip GYH. Evaluation of the HAS-BLED, ATRIA, and ORBIT bleeding risk scores in patients with atrial fibrillation taking warfarin. Am J Med. 2016;129:600–7.
51. Hylek EM, Evans-Molina C, Shea C, Henault LE, Regan S. Major hemorrhage and tolerability of warfarin in the first year of therapy among elderly patients with atrial fibrillation. Circulation. 2007;115(21):2689.
52. Siontis KC, Zhang X, Eckard A, Bhave N, Schaubel DE, He K, Tilea A, Stack AG, Balkrishnan R, Yao X, Noseworthy PA, Shah N, Saran R, Nallamothu BK. Outcomes associated with Apixaban use in end-stage kidney disease patients with atrial fibrillation in the United States. Circulation. 2018;138(15):1519–29. https://doi.org/10.1161/CIRCULATIONAHA.118.035418.
53. Liao JN, Chao TF, Liu CJ, et al. Incidence and risk factors for new-onset atrial fibrillation among patients with end-stage renal disease undergoing renal replacement therapy. Kidney Int. 2015;87:1209–15.
54. Marinigh R, Lane DA, Lip GY. Severe renal impairment and stroke prevention in atrial fibrillation: implications for thromboprophylaxis and bleeding risk. J Am Coll Cardiol. 2011;57(12):1339.

55. Vázquez E, Sánchez-Perales C, Borrego F, Garcia-Cortés MJ, Lozano C, Guzmán M, Gil JM, Borrego MJ, Pérez V. Influence of atrial fibrillation on the morbido-mortality of patients on hemodialysis. Am Heart J. 2000;140(6):886.
56. Guo Y, Wang H, Zhao X, Zhang Y, Zhang D, Ma J, Wang Y, Lip GY. Sequential changes in renal function and the risk of stroke and death in patients with atrial fibrillation. Int J Cardiol. 2013;168:4678–84.
57. Vazquez E, Sanchez-Perales C, Garcia-Garcia F, Castellano P, Garcia-Cortes MJ, Liebana A, Lozano C. Atrial fibrillation in incident dialysis patients. Kidney Int. 2009;76:324.
58. Genovesi S, Vincenti A, Rossi E, Pogliani D, Acquistapace I, Stella A, Valsecchi MG. Atrial fibrillation and morbidity and mortality in a cohort of long-term hemodialysis patients. Am J Kidney Dis. 2008;51:255.
59. Vázquez E, Sánchez-Perales C, Lozano C, García-Cortés MJ, Borrego F, Guzmán M, Pérez P, Pagola C, Borrego MJ, Pérez V. Comparison of prognostic value of atrial fibrillation versus sinus rhythm in patients on long-term hemodialysis. Am J Cardiol. 2003;92:868.
60. Olesen JB, Lip GY, Kamper AL, Hommel K, Køber L, Lane DA, Lindhardsen J, Gislason GH, Torp-Pedersen C. Stroke and bleeding in atrial fibrillation with chronic kidney disease. N Engl J Med. 2012;367:625.
61. Bonde AN, Lip GY, Kamper AL, Hansen PR, Lamberts M, Hommel K, Hansen ML, Gislason GH, Torp-Pedersen C, Olesen JB. Net clinical benefit of antithrombotic therapy in patients with atrial fibrillation and chronic kidney disease: a nationwide observational cohort study. J Am Coll Cardiol. 2014;64:2471–82.
62. Shin J, Secora A, Alexander GC, Inker LA, Coresh J, Chang AR, Grams ME. Risks and benefits of direct oral anticoagulants across the spectrum of GFR among incident and prevalent patients with atrial fibrillation. Clin J Am Soc Nephrol. 2018;13(8):1144–52.
63. Goldenberg I, Subirana I, Boyko V, Vila J, Elosua R, Permanyer-Miralda G, Ferreira-González I, Benderly M, Guetta V, Behar S, Marrugat J. Relation between renal function and outcomes in patients with non-ST segment elevation acute coronary syndrome: real-world data from the European Public Health Outcome Research and Indicators Collection Project. Arch Intern Med. 2010;170:888–95.
64. Franczyk-Skóra B, Gluba A, Banach M, Kozłowski D, Małyszko J, Rysz J. Prevention of sudden cardiac death in patients with chronic kidney disease. BMC Nephrol. 2012;13:162.
65. Van Domburg RT, Hoeks SE, Welten GMJM, Chonchol M, Elhendy A, Poldermans D. Renal insufficiency and mortality in patients with known or suspected coronary artery disease. J Am Soc Neph. 2008;19:158–63.
66. Coats WC, Baig SZ, Alpert MA, Aggarwal K. Management of coronary artery disease in patients with chronic kidney disease. Adv Perit Dial. 2009;25:125–8.
67. Park SH, Kim W, Park CS, Kang WY, Hwang SH, Kim W. A comparison of clopidogrel responsiveness in patients with versus without chronic renal failure. Am J Cardiol. 2009;104:1292–5.
68. James S, Budaj A, Aylward P, Buck KK, Cannon CP, Cornel JH, Harrington RA, Horrow J, Katus H, Keltai M, Lewis BS, Parikh K, Storey RF, Szummer K, Wojdyla D, Wallentin L. Ticagrelor versus clopidogrel in acute coronary syndromes in relation to renal function: results from the Platelet Inhibition and Patient Outcomes (PLATO) trial. Circulation. 2010;122:1056–67.
69. Fifth Organization to Assess Strategies in Acute Ischemic Syndromes Investigators, Yusuf S, Mehta SR, Chrolavicius S, Afzal R, Pogue J, Granger CB, Budaj A, Peters RJ, Bassand JP, Wallentin L, Joyner C, Fox KA. Comparison of fondaparinux and enoxaparin in acute coronary syndromes. N Engl J Med. 2006;354(14):1464–76.
70. Franczyk-Skóra B, Gluba A, Banach M, Rozentryt P, Polonski L, Rysz J. Acute coronary syndromes in patients with chronic kidney disease. Curr Vasc Pharmacol. 2013;11:758–67.
71. Chertow GM, Normand SL, Silva LR, McNeil BJ. Survival after acute myocardial infarction in patients with end-stage renal disease: results from the cooperative cardiovascular project. Am J Kidney Dis. 2000;35:1044–105.

72. Chew DP, Bhatt DL, Kimball W, Henry TD, Berger P, McCullough PA, Feit F, Bittl JA, Lincoff AM. Bivalirudin provides increasing benefit with decreasing renal function: a meta-analysis of randomized trials. Am J Cardiol. 2003;92:919–23.
73. Brodsky SV, Nadasdy T, Rovin BH, Satoskar AA, Nadasdy GM, Wu HM, Bhatt UY, Hebert LA. Warfarin-related nephropathy occurs in patients with and without chronic kidney disease and is associated with an increased mortality rate. Kidney Int. 2011;80:181–9.
74. Reilly EB, Perry A, Fujita K, Nakamura RM. Haematuria and anticoagulants. Lancet. 1964;1:554–6.
75. Brodsky SV, Satoskar A, Chen J, Nadasdy G, Eagen JW, Hamirani M, Hebert L, Calomeni E, Nadasdy T. Acute kidney injury during warfarin therapy associated with obstructive tubular red blood cell casts: a report of 9 cases. Am J Kidney Dis. 2009;54:1121–6.
76. Brodsky SV, Collins M, Park E, Rovin BH, Satoskar AA, Nadasdy G, Wu H, Bhatt U, Nadasdy T, Hebert LA. Warfarin therapy that results in an international normalization ratio above the therapeutic range is associated with accelerated progression of chronic kidney disease. Nephron Clin Pract. 2010;115:c142–6.
77. Coughlin SR. Thrombin signalling and protease-activated receptors. Nature. 2000;407:258–64.
78. Ryan M, Ware K, Qamri Z, Satoskar A, Wu H, Nadasdy G, Rovin B, Hebert L, Nadasdy T, Brodsky SV. Warfarin-related nephropathy is the tip of the iceberg: direct thrombin inhibitor dabigatran induces glomerular hemorrhage with acute kidney injury in rats. Nephrol Dial Transplant. 2013;29:2228–34.
79. Safian RD, Textor SC. Renal-artery stenosis. N Engl J Med. 2001;344(6):431–42.
80. Brocklebank V, Wood KM, Kavanagh D. Thrombotic microangiopathy and the kidney. Clin J Am Soc Nephrol. 2018;13:300–17. https://doi.org/10.2215/CJN.00620117.
81. Ruggenenti P, Noris M, Remuzzi G. Thrombotic microangiopathy, hemolytic uremic syndrome, and thrombotic thrombocytopenic purpura. Kidney Int. 2001;60(3):831–46.
82. Traub YM, Shapiro AP, Rodnan GP, Medsger TA, McDonald RH Jr, Steen VD, Osial TA Jr, Tolchin SF. Hypertension and renal failure (scleroderma renal crisis) in progressive systemic sclerosis. Review of a 25-year experience with 68 cases. Medicine (Baltimore). 1983;62(6):335.
83. Denton CP, Lapadula G, Mouthon L, Müller-Ladner U. Renal complications and scleroderma renal crisis. Rheumatology (Oxford). 2009;48(Suppl 3):iii32–5.
84. Donohoe JF. Scleroderma and the kidney. Kidney Int. 1992;41(2):462.
85. Kahaleh MB, Osborn I, Leroy EC. Elevated levels of circulating platelet aggregates and beta-thromboglobulin in scleroderma. Ann Intern Med. 1982;96(5):610–3.
86. Venturelli C, Jeannin G, Sottini L, Dallera N, Scolari F. Cholesterol crystal embolism (atheroembolism). Heart Int. 2006;2:155.
87. Li X, Bayliss G, Zhuang S. Cholesterol crystal embolism and chronic kidney disease. Int J Mol Sci. 2017;18(6):1120.
88. Scolari F, Ravani P. Atheroembolic renal disease. Lancet. 2010;375:1650–60.
89. Wysokinski WE, Gosk-Bierska I, Greene EL, Grill D, Wiste H, McBane RD 2nd. Clinical characteristics and long-term follow-up of patients with renal vein thrombosis. Am J Kidney Dis. 2008;51(2):224.
90. Singhal R, Brimble KS. Thromboembolic complications in the nephrotic syndrome: pathophysiology and clinical management. Thromb Res. 2006;118(3):397.
91. Lionaki S, Derebail VK, Hogan SL, Barbour S, Lee T, Hladunewich M, Greenwald A, Hu Y, Jennette CE, Jennette JC, Falk RJ, Cattran DC, Nachman PH, Reich HN. Venous thromboembolism in patients with membranous nephropathy. Clin J Am Soc Nephrol. 2012;7(1):43.
92. Medjeral-Thomas N, Ziaj S, Condon M, Galliford J, Levy J, Cairns T, Griffith M. Retrospective analysis of a novel regimen for the prevention of venous thromboembolism in nephrotic syndrome. Clin J Am Soc Nephrol. 2014;9(3):478–83.

93. Kim HS, Fine DM, Atta MG. Catheter-directed thrombectomy and thrombolysis for acute renal vein thrombosis. J Vasc Interv Radiol. 2006;17(5):815.
94. Wu CH, Ko SF, Lee CH, Cheng BC, Hsu KT, Chen JB, Chien YS, Yang CC, Huang MC, Chuang FR. Successful outpatient treatment of renal vein thrombosis by low-molecular weight heparins in 3 patients with nephrotic syndrome. Clin Nephrol. 2006;65(6):433.
95. Greenfield LJ, Cho KJ, Proctor MC, Sobel M, Shah S, Wingo J. Late results of suprarenal Greenfield vena cava filter placement. Arch Surg. 1992;127(8):969.
96. Fischer KG. Essentials of anticoagulation in hemodialysis. Hemodial Int. 2007;11(2):178–89.
97. O'Shea SI, Ortel TL, Kovalik EC. Alternative methods of anticoagulation for dialysis-dependent patients with heparin-induced thrombocytopenia. Semin Dial. 2003;16(1):61–7.
98. Maher JF, Lapierre L, Schreiner GE, Geiger M, Westervelt FB Jr. Regional heparinization for hemodialysis — technic and clinical experiences. N Engl J Med. 1963;268:451–6.
99. Ip BK, Thomson AR, Moriarty HT. A comparison of the sensitivity of APTT reagents to the effects of enoxaparin, a low-molecular weight heparin. Pathology. 2001;33(3):347–52.
100. Schroeder M, Hogwood J, Gray E, Mulloy B, Hackett AM, Johansen KB. Protamine neutralisation of low molecular weight heparins and their oligosaccharide components. Anal Bioanal Chem. 2011;399(2):763–71.
101. Schrader J, Rieger J, Müschen M, Stibbe W, Köstering H, Kramer P, Schele F. Anwendung von niedermolekularem Heparin bei Hämodialysepatienten. Klin Wochenschr. 1985;63(2):49–55.
102. Pon TK, Dager WE, Roberts AJ, White RH. Subcutaneous enoxaparin for therapeutic anticoagulation in hemodialysis patients. Thromb Res. 2014;133(6):1023–8.
103. Ulbricht K, Bucha E, Pöschel KA, Stein G, Wolf G, Nowak G. The use of PEG-Hirudin in chronic hemodialysis monitored by the Ecarin Clotting Time: influence on clotting of the extracorporeal system and hemostatic parameters. Clin Nephrol. 2006;65(3):180–90.
104. Lindhoff-Last E, Betz C, Bauersachs R. Use of a low-molecular-weight heparinoid (danaparoid sodium) for continuous renal replacement therapy in intensive care patients. Clin Appl Thromb Hemost. 2001;7(4):300–4.
105. Murray PT, Reddy BV, Grossman EJ, Hammes MS, Trevino S, Ferrell J, Tang I, Hursting MJ, Shamp TR, Swan SK. A prospective comparison of three argatroban treatment regimens during hemodialysis in end-stage renal disease. Kidney Int. 2004;66(6):2446–53.
106. Attman P-O, Ottosson P, Samuelsson O, Eriksson UG, Eriksson-Lepkowska M, Fager G. Prevention of clot formation during haemodialysis using the direct thrombin inhibitor melagatran in patients with chronic uraemia. Nephrol Dial Transplant. 2005;20(9):1889–97.
107. Hall GH, Holman HM, Webster ADB. Anticoagulation by Ancrod for haemodialysis. Br Med J. 1970;4:591–3.
108. Fischer KG. Essentials of anticoagulation in hemodialysis. Hemodial Int. 2007;11(2):178–89.
109. Grudzinski A, Agarwal A, Bhatnagar N, Nesrallah G. Benefits and harms of citrate locking solutions for hemodialysis catheters: a systematic review and meta-analysis. Can J Kidney Health Dis. 2015;2:13.
110. Tai DJ, Leung K, Ravani P, Quinn RR, Scott-Douglas N, MacRae JM, Alberta Kidney Disease Network. The effect of citrate dialysate on intradialytic heparin dose in haemodialysis patients: study design of a randomised controlled trial. BMC Nephrol. 2015;16:147.
111. François K, Wissing KM, Jacobs R, Boone D, Jacobs K, Tielemans C. Avoidance of systemic anticoagulation during intermittent haemodialysis with heparin-grafted polyacrilonitrile membrane and citrate-enriched dialysate: a retrospective cohort study. BMC Nephrol. 2014;15:104.
112. Faguer S, Saint-Cricq M, Nogier MB, Labadens I, Lavayssiere L, Kamar N, Cointault O. Heparin-free prolonged intermittent hemodialysis using calcium-free citrate dialysate in critically ill patients. Crit Care Med. 2017;45(11):1887–92.

113. Mariano F, Bergamo D, Gangemi EN, Hollo Z, Stella M, Triolo G. Citrate anticoagulation for continuous renal replacement therapy in critically ill patients: success and limits. Int J Nephrol. 2011;2011:748320.
114. Deep A, Zoha M, Dutta KP. Prostacyclin as an anticoagulant for continuous renal replacement therapy in children. Blood Purif. 2017;43:279–89.
115. Krummel T, Scheidt E, Borni-Duval C, Bazin D, Lefebvre F, Nguyen P, Hannedouche T. Haemodialysis in patients treated with oral anticoagulant: should we heparinize? Nephrol Dial Transplant. 2014;29:906–13.

Chapter 10
VTE Prophylaxis in General and Orthopedic Surgery

Ahmed Abdulgawad, Vinita Sundaram, Ibraheem Othman, and Hadi Goubran

Abbreviations

ACCP	American College of Chest Physicians
BMI	Body mass index
DOACs	Direct oral anticoagulants
ES	Elastic stockings
GCS	Graduated compression stockings
IPC	Intermittent pneumatic compression devices
LDUH	Low-dose unfractionated heparin
LMWH	Low-molecular-weight heparin
NOACs	Non-vitamin K antagonist oral anticoagulants
THR	Total hip replacement
TKR	Total knee replacement

A. Abdulgawad (✉)
Hematology Department, Faculty of Medicine, Cairo University, Giza, Egypt
e-mail: aahameed@kasralainy.edu.eg

V. Sundaram
Saskatoon Cancer Centre, Saskatoon, SK, Canada
e-mail: Vinita.Sundaram@saskcancer.ca

I. Othman
Alain Blair Cancer Centre and College of Medicine, University of Saskatchewan, Regina, SK, Canada
e-mail: Ibraheem.Othman@saskcancer.ca

H. Goubran
Saskatoon Cancer Centre, College of Medicine, University of Saskatchewan, Saskatoon, SK, Canada
e-mail: Hadi.goubranmessiha@saskcancer.ca

© Springer Nature Switzerland AG 2020
H. Goubran et al. (eds.), *Precision Anticoagulation Medicine*,
https://doi.org/10.1007/978-3-030-25782-8_10

239

VFP	Venous foot pump
VKA	Vitamin K antagonist
VTE	Venous thromboembolism

Introduction

Venous thromboembolism (VTE) in surgical patients is the most common preventable cause of death. The use of low-dose unfractionated heparin (LDUH) in 1975 in an International Multicenter Trial heralded a new era of postoperative management [1]. The incidence of venographically confirmed DVT in general surgery patients not receiving prophylaxis is about 20%, while major orthopedic surgery has one of the highest incidences of VTE ranging between 40% and 60% [2]. VTE prophylaxis has since become a routine practice for most centers [3–5]. There still remains ambiguity about the optimal anticoagulant utilized and the duration of therapy. Preference of anticoagulant depends on individual's predisposing factors, surgical procedure, and risk of bleeding [6]. Most evidence-based clinical guidelines advocate for the use of low-molecular-weight heparins (LMWH) compared to low-dose unfractionated heparin (LDUH) or vitamin K antagonist. The new anticoagulants such as direct oral anticoagulants (DOACs) are being considered for VTE prophylaxis and clinical trials are ongoing.

Risk Stratification

Risk stratification for VTE is based on the patient-specific risk factors and the procedure-specific risks. These factors are intrinsic components guiding the clinician in determining the level of thromboembolism risk and are highlighted in Fig 10.1.

Very low risk	Most outpatient and day surgeries
Low risk	Minor surgery in mobile patients
	Medical patients who are fully mobile
Moderate risk	Most general, open gynecologic, or urologic surgery patients
High risk	Hip or knee arthroplasty Major trauma, spinal cord injury Abdominal–pelvic surgery for cancer Bariatric surgery Pneumonectomy Craniotomy

Fig. 10.1 Levels of thromboembolism risk [7, 8]

Risk factors for VTE include the following [2]:

- Surgery
- Trauma (major trauma or lower-extremity injury)
- Reduced mobility, lower-extremity paresis, stroke
- Cancer
- Cancer therapy (chemotherapy, hormonal, angiogenesis inhibitors, radiotherapy)
- Previous VTE
- Positive family history of VTE
- Increasing age
- Pregnancy and the postpartum period
- Estrogen-containing oral contraceptives or hormone replacement therapy
- Selective estrogen receptor modulators
- Erythropoiesis-stimulating agents
- Acute medical illness
- Inflammatory bowel disease
- Nephrotic syndrome
- Myeloproliferative disorders
- Venous compression (tumor, enlarged lymph nodes, hematoma)
- Obesity
- Central venous catheterization
- Inherited or acquired thrombophilia

Risk stratification models have limitations. Caprini introduced a risk assessment model which has been validated for numerous surgical interventions [9, 10]. Though the study was validated for general, vascular, and urologic surgery populations and outcomes reported 30 days postoperatively, it remains a useful guide for VTE prophylaxis [10]. It is relatively simple to use and is adopted by the American College of Chest Physicians' (ACCP) practice guidelines for the prevention of VTE, 9th edition [7]. Fig 10.2 illustrates the modified Caprini's risk assessment model.

To safely determine the choice of VTE prophylaxis requires assessment of high-risk bleeding. The risks of bleeding are clustered into procedure-related (those identified as having a >1% risk of bleeding) and intrinsic, patient-related ones and are highlighted in Fig 10.3.

The choice of thromboprophylaxis strategy therefore rests on the balance between the thrombotic risks and the bleeding risks of individual patients.

1 point	2 points	3 points	5 points
Age 41–60 years	Age 61–74 years	Age ≥75 years	Stroke (<1 month)
Minor surgery	Arthroscopic surgery	History of VTE	Elective arthroplasty
BMI >25 kg/m2	Major open surgery (>45 minutes)	Family history of VTE	Hip, pelvis, or leg fracture
Swollen legs	Laparoscopic surgery (>45 minutes)	Factor V Leiden	Acute spinal cord injury (<1 month)
Varicose veins	Malignancy	Prothrombin 20210A	
Pregnancy or postpartum	Confined to bed (>72 hours)	Lupus anticoagulant	
History of unexplained or recurrent spontaneous abortion	Immobilizing plaster cast	Anticardiolipin antibodies	
Oral contraceptives or hormone replacement	Central venous access	Elevated serum homocysteine	
Sepsis (<1 month)		Heparin-induced thrombocytopenia	
Serious lung disease, including pneumonia (<1 month)		Other congenital or acquired thrombophilia	
Abnormal pulmonary function			
Acute myocardial infarction			
Congestive heart failure (<1 month)			
History of inflammatory bowel disease			
Interpretation			
Surgical risk category	Score	Estimated VTE risk in the absence of pharmacologic or mechanical prophylaxis (percent)	
Very low	0	<0.5	
Low	1–2	1.5	
Moderate	3–4	3	
High	≥5	6	

Fig. 10.2 Modified Caprini risk assessment model [7]

Procedure-related risks of bleeding	
Cardiac surgery	5%
Vascular surgery	0.3–1.8%
Major trauma	3.4–4.7%
Plastic/reconstructive surgery	0.5–1.8%
Craniotomy	0.5–1.8%
Patient's related bleeding risks	
Bleeding disorders (marked thrombocytopenia and/or coagulopathy)	
Massive bleeding as an indication for surgery (aneurysm, bleeding peptic ulcer, or major trauma)	

Fig. 10.3 Bleeding risk in various surgeries [8]

Strategies to Prevent VTE in the Surgical and Orthopedic Context

Early Ambulation

This should be encouraged as soon as possible with all surgical interventions. Frequent ambulation alone or along with other measures is believed to reduce VTE risk as suggested from indirect evidence from various studies. This might be all what is needed in very low-risk procedures in rather fit patients.

Mechanical Methods

These are generally used with

- Low-risk patients, for example, laparoscopic cholecystectomy
- As an adjunct to pharmacologic agents in high-risk situation
- When pharmacologic agents are contraindicated because of high bleeding risk [11]

Mechanical methods include intermittent pneumatic compression (IPC) devices, elastic stockings (ES), and venous foot pump (VFP). Although ACCP recommends IPC over other methods [8, 12], other authors advise both IPC and ES [13].

(i) *Intermittent Pneumatic Compression (IPC) Devices*

They are thought to be the most effective mechanical method in VTE prophylaxis by ACCP [2]. A large meta-analysis confirmed the efficacy of IPC when used alone or in combination with pharmacologic agents [14, 15].

However, efficacy is linked to proper application and compliance which were challenged in various studies [16, 17].

Portable, battery-powered devices allow better tolerability. Devices are applied for 18/24 hours especially while the patient is sitting or lying in bed. Device can be disconnected while the patient is ambulant.

IPC devices are thought to act as peripheral pumps which reduce peripheral stagnation of blood and thrombus formation. Early application is demonstrated by a study [18], while late application (>72 hours) is thought to impose a risk of dislodging micro-thrombi and cause PE showers.

IPC devices are contraindicated in patients with peripheral arterial disease and patients with extensive skin allergy or skin lesions. IPC cannot be applied in case of amputation operations.

(ii) *Elastic Stockings (ES)/Graduated Compression Stockings (GCS)*

ES are not preferred by ACCP [8] and are inferior to IPC as shown in a large meta-analysis [13–15]. However, being available, relatively tolerable, and safe, ES are of wide clinical use either alone or in conjunction with pharmacologic agents.

(iii) *Venous Foot Pump (VFP)*

This is similar in theory to IPC devices although high-quality evidence to support its use is still lacking.

Pharmacological Agents

These are the principal method (along with early ambulation with or without mechanical methods) in moderate- and high-risk patients.

A local policy should be followed in timing/agent and doses whenever possible.

Timing of initiation of thromboprophylaxis is crucial to its efficacy. There is no consensus regarding the exact timing to commence thromboprophylaxis. Generally, the sooner the better. Early anticoagulation was shown to reduce VTE with no added bleeding risk in neurosurgical patients with head trauma [19].

In all procedures with moderate to high risk of bleeding, pharmacological thromboprophylaxis will not be initiated until hemostasis is established. This usually is 12 hours postoperatively if there are no complications [8, 20]. In elective surgeries with high risk of VTE, the patient may be initiated on pharmacological thromboprophylaxis with LMWH which will be held approximately 12 hours prior to the surgery [21].

The individual risk factors for bleeding are coagulopathy, thrombocytopenia, and massive bleeding due to aneurysm, bleeding peptic ulcer, or major trauma. The risk of bleeding is detrimental in the outcome of plastic surgery; caution must be taken to initiate anticoagulation only after hemostasis is established. Life-threatening bleeding in the brain and those with previous history of bleeding from multiple gastrointestinal telangiectasias are contraindications to pharmacological anticoagulation. If neuraxial anesthesia is scheduled, the patient should not receive anticoagulation till the epidural catheter is removed [9].

(i) *Low-Dose Unfractionated Heparins (LDUH)*

It is preferable in patients with severe renal impairment. However, it carries a higher risk of heparin-induced thrombocytopenia (HIT), and platelet count should be monitored at least at baseline and 4 days later.

A dose of 5000 U BD is widely used. A higher dose of 5000 U three times daily is recommended in high-risk cancer patients [22].

Similarly, no agreement exists on optimal dosing in obese individuals. Data from various studies are contradictory with some showing no benefit [23], others showing harm [24], and a third showing no difference both in efficacy and safety [24].

LDUH – 5000 IU SC BID OR three times daily

(ii) *Low-Molecular-Weight Heparins (LMWH)* (For full dose and description, please refer to Chap. 1)

These are the standard pharmacologic agents to be used unless contraindicated (renal impairment or HIT) [8]. Various preparations exist with no clear difference in efficacy or safety.

Enoxaparin [25]
The most commonly used preparation worldwide and the most extensively studied.

One suggested dosing regimen is 40 mg (4000 u) SC daily, starting 2–72 hours postoperatively, provided that secure hemostasis has been achieved and that no risk of excessive bleeding exists. An approach with 30 mg SC q 12 hours is also implemented in certain countries.

Similar schedule can be used in cancer operation with a 6–12-hour postoperative starting point.

Dalteparin [26]
A common preparation. To be started preoperatively or as soon as hemostasis is warranted, 5000 u SC daily.

Tinzaparin [27]
At a daily SC dose of 4500 U, weight-adjusted dosage (75 IU/kg) has also been suggested for high-risk patients.

Other less commonly used preparations as *bemiparin, certoparin, nadroparin* [28], *parnaparin*, and *reviparin* are similarly effective and safe.

No consensus is present with obese patients. Local policies should be followed. This might be through increasing the dose with 30% or twice daily dosing.

Fig 10.4 illustrates the dosage and administration of various LMWHs in various indications (modified from [29]).

Indication	Preparation/dosage
Abdominal surgery	*Bemiparin:* 2500–3500 IU SC q 24 hours *Certoparin:* 3000 IU SC q 24 hours × 7–10 days *Dalteparin:* 2500 IU preoperative then 2500 IU SC q 24 hours × 7–10 days *Enoxaparin:* 40 mg SC q day; initiate 2 hours preoperatively × 7–10 days With renal impairment: prophylaxis in abdominal surgery: 30 mg SC q day *Nadroparin:* 2850 IU SC q 24 High risk 38 IU/kg SC q 24 × 3 days then 57 IU/kg SC q 24 hours *Parnaparin:* 3200 IU SC 2 hours pre-op, then 3200 u SC q 24 hours × 7 *Reviparin:*1750 SC 12 hours pre-op then every 24 hours *Tinzaparin:* 3500 IU SC q 24 hours
Total hip replacement [THR] **Total knee replacement [TKR]**	*Bemiparin:* 2500–3500 IU SC q 24 hours *Dalteparin:* 2500 IU preoperative or immediate postoperative then 5000 IU SC q 24 *Enoxaparin:* 30 mg SC q 12 hours; initiate therapy 12–24 hours postoperatively and continued for 10 days or up to 35 days postoperatively or until the risk of DVT has been significantly reduced or patient is on anticoagulant therapy *For hip replacement surgery,* consider administering 40 mg SC q day, initiated 9–15 hours preoperatively, and continue for 10 days or up to 35 days postoperatively or until the risk of DVT has been significantly reduced or the patient is on anticoagulant therapy With renal impairment: co-administered with warfarin: maximum 1 mg/kg SC q day *Nadroparin:* High risk 38 IU/kg SC q 24 × 3 days then 57 IU/kg SC q 24 hours from day +4 post-op) *Parnaparin:* 4250 IU SC 12 hours pre-op, then 4250 IU SC 12 hours post-op and then q 24 hours × 10 days *Reviparin:* 4200 IU SC 12 hours prior then q 24 *Tinzaparin:* Hip 50 IU/kg SC q 24 hours. Knee 75 IU/kg SC q 24 hours
Hip fracture	*Dalteparin* pre-op: 2500 U SC once daily post-op: 5000 U SC once daily *Enoxaparin* pre-op: 30 mg SC once daily post-op: 40 mg SC once daily *Nadroparin* 38 U/kg SC once daily (days 1–3 post-op), followed by 57 U/kg SC once daily (day 4+ post-op) *Tinzaparin* pre-op: 3500 U SC once daily post-op: 4500 U SC once daily
Major orthopedic trauma	when hemostasis is evident *Dalteparin* 5000 U SC once daily *Enoxaparin* 30 mg SC twice daily *Tinzaparin* 4500 U SC once daily *Mechanical method* if high risk for bleeding with switch to LMWH when bleeding risk decreases

Fig. 10.4 LMWH dosage and administration in various surgical and orthopedic indications

Indication	Preparation/dosage
Spine surgery: (a) Uncomplicated (b) Complicated (cancer, leg weakness, prior VTE, combined anterior/posterior approach)	(a) Mobilization alone (b) *LMWH* once daily starting the day after surgery
Knee arthroscopy: (a) Low risk (b) Higher risk (major knee reconstruction, prior VTE, other VTE risk factors)	(a) None (b) *LMWH* once daily 5–30 days

Fig 10.4   (continued)

(iii) *Fondaparinux*

This would be an ideal alternative in patients with history of HIT who are unable to receive heparins.

In patients undergoing abdominal surgery, the recommended dose of fondaparinux is 2.5 mg administered by subcutaneous injection once daily after hemostasis has been established. Administer the initial dose no earlier than 6–8 hours after surgery. Administration of fondaparinux earlier than 6 hours after surgery increases the risk of major bleeding.

The usual duration of administration is 5–9 days, and up to 10 days of fondaparinux was administered in clinical trials [30]; Thrombosis Canada suggests 14–35 days of therapy [29].

Fondaparinux 2.5 mg SC 6–8 hours prior to surgery and then reinitiated 6–8 hours post-surgery for 5–9 days

(iv) *Injectable Direct Thrombin Inhibitors/Hirudin*

The recombinant hirudins, desirudin or rb-hirudin [31, 32], are direct thrombin inhibitors with a renal route of elimination that are approved in certain countries, at a subcutaneous dose of 2 × 15 mg per day, for primary VTE prevention after elective hip or knee arthroplasty. They represent a suitable option, if available, for patients with HIT.

Recombinant hirudin at a dose of 15 mg SC twice daily is a prophylaxis in orthopedic patients

(v) *Direct Oral Anticoagulants (DOACs)/Non-Vitamin K Antagonist Oral Anticoagulants (NOACs)* (For detailed description, please refer to Chap. 1)

Many anti-Xa and anti-II orally active, directly acting, biophysically predictable pharmacologic agents have been introduced over the past few years.

Trials showed similar efficacy and safety of many DOACs as compared to LMWHs in VTE prophylaxis especially in orthopedic procedures, namely total hip arthroplasty and total knee arthroplasty, but not in the context of general surgery [33, 34].

There is no direct head-to-head comparison among various DOACs. The anti-IIa dabigatran and the 2 anti-Xa rivaroxaban and apixaban have the bigger share in various trials.

They are contraindicated in patients with marked renal impairment. Their use when LMWHs are contraindicated in HIT is not well evidenced (as fondaparinux, for instance).

Patient preference according to adverse effect profile (e.g., marked gut upset with dabigatran) or drug administration (once daily in rivaroxaban versus twice daily in dabigatran and apixaban) carries the higher impact in choosing one agent against the others [8, 35].

DOACs/NOACs are recommended for knee and hip arthroplasty in the dosage and duration shown in Fig 10.5 [29].

(vi) *Warfarin and Other Vitamin K Antagonists (VKAs)*

Warfarin was compared to aspirin prior to the emergence of newer agents, namely LMWHs, pentasaccharide, and DOACs.

Warfarin and other vitamin K antagonists (VKAs) are still mentioned among pharmacologic options within the most recent guidelines [8, 35].

Fig. 10.5 Recommended dosage and duration of DOACs/NOACs for thromboprophylaxis in orthopedic patients

Agent	Dose	Duration
Rivaroxaban[a]	10 mg PO once daily	14–35 [a]
Apixaban	2.5 mg PO once daily	14–35 days
Dabigatran	220 mg PO once daily	14–35 days
Edoxaban[b]	30 mg PO once daily	–

[a]For patients not at high risk of VTE, consideration can be given to rivaroxaban 10 mg orally per day until postoperative day 5, followed by ASA 81 mg daily for an additional 9 days following total knee arthroplasty or for 30 days after total hip arthroplasty [29]
[b]Data published but not part of current recommendation or product monograph [36]

However, the extensive drug-to-drug interactions and food-to-drug interaction which necessitates continuous INR monitoring and dose adjustments made warfarin a less appealing option as a sub-therapeutic INR confers higher VTE risks [37].

However, warfarin is still the safest in case of severe renal failure along with UFH and as a long-term option in patients with history of HIT.

(vii) *Aspirin*

It has a debatable role in VTE prophylaxis [38]. ACCP lists aspirin as an alternative to heparins when contraindicated. However, this role is not uniformly accepted among ACCP panel members [8].

A recent study, however, has shown comparable efficacy and safety for hybrid use of rivaroxaban for 5 days and then ASA 81 mg for the rest of the VTE prophylaxis course (9 more days in therapeutic knee arthroplasty (TKA) and 30 days in therapeutic hip arthroplasty (THA)) to rivaroxaban use for the total standard duration [39]. This approach can be adopted only for low-risk cases with unilateral procedures, no intervention within 3 months before and after the procedure.

Choice of Pharmacological Agents in the Presence of HIT
Heparin-induced thrombocytopenia (HIT) is a contraindication to LMWH and LDUH. This can occur in 0.2–3% of patients exposed to heparin [15]. The catastrophic thrombosis resulting from the immune-mediated hypercoagulable state is treated with direct thrombin inhibitors. Danaparoid, argatroban, and bivalirudin are used in the treatment; however, fondaparinux is being used off-label [40]. Thrombosis Canada has published in their guideline that in prior history of HIT, patients who require VTE prophylaxis will be initiated on treatment with fondaparinux 2.5 mg OD subcutaneously [41]. This will continue until the patient has recovered a platelet count of $>120 \times 10^9/L$.

Inferior Vena Cava Filters (IVC Filters)

ACCP advises against IVC filter placement to prevent VTE in the context of surgical interventions [8, 35]. Short-term placement of IVC filters is often considered in complicated patients; however, it has been seen that many times these filters may not be retrieved.

IVC filter placement is not recommended to prevent VTE in the context of surgical interventions.

Doppler Monitoring for DVT Prior to Discharge

Evidence-based VTE prophylaxis has reduced the risk of postoperative mortality and morbidity by 50%. This has a major impact on the cost-effectiveness and outcome of hospitalized patients. It is imperative that the guidelines must be incorporated in the hospital systems. However, the clinician must be vigilant to assess for VTE despite the prophylaxis. The recent ACCP guidelines do not recommend the routine Doppler to assess for deep vein thrombus prior to discharge post hip arthroplasty [21].

Duration of Prophylaxis

For general surgeries, most centers advocate for thromboprophylaxis for an average of 7–10 days or till patient is discharged from hospital. This concept is being revised and extended duration prophylaxis is beneficial in those with moderate to high risk of VTE.

Extended duration prophylaxis is vital in patients with cancer as they are at high risk for VTE and also have a worse prognosis after developing VTE postoperatively [38].

Thrombosis Canada recommends that patients admitted for general and abdominal–pelvic cancer surgery at high risk for VTE (6%, Caprini score: >4) and not at high risk for bleeding receive LMWH for 30 days [40].

For orthopedic procedure, the recommended duration of anticoagulation for THR and TKR as well as for hip fracture surgery is 14–35 days, whereas it is usually administered till discharge in most of the other indications [29].

The risk of VTE is now seen to extend to more than 30 days in major trauma, hip fracture, and arthroplasty. A recent multicenter double-blinded randomized controlled trial of 3424 patients undergoing hip and knee arthroplasty compared the use of rivaroxaban 10 mg for 5 days followed by randomized allocation to continue rivaroxaban or aspirin 81 mg for 30 days for hip arthroplasty and 9 days for knee arthroplasty [39]. The results revealed aspirin was comparable to rivaroxaban (after the initial 5 days of rivaroxaban) in the prevention of VTE in a high-risk surgery of hip or knee arthroplasty. This study showed similar efficacy of aspirin as the Extended Prophylaxis Comparing Low-Molecular-Weight Heparin to Aspirin in Total Hip Arthroplasty (EPCAT 1) trial [38].

NOACs are undergoing clinical trials to assess their efficacy in various patient groups, and we expect more high-quality evidence on outcomes in surgical patients. In the future, the randomized clinical trials on extensively validated risk assessment models in well-defined models will provide the necessary adjustments to the present guidelines on VTE prophylaxis. Fig 10.6 illustrates the recommended thromboprophylaxis in different surgical situations based on current published data.

Patient Group	Risk: Caprini score/remarks	Recommendation (grade)
Major General Surgery, thoracic or urological Surgery	Low risk: 0	Early ambulation
	Low risk: 1-2	IPC (2C)
	Moderate Risk: 3-4	LMWH, LDUH (2C)[a]
	if high risk of bleeding	IPC (2C)
	High risk: 5	LMWH, LDUH (1B)
Cancer surgery	High risk: 5	LMWH, LDUH Extended 30 days
Neurosurgery	High risk for Craniotomy and spinal surgery	IPC until adequate hemostasis Add LMWH ,LDUH
Bariatric Surgery	High Risk	LMWH, LDUH
Vascular Surgery	Low risk	Early ambulation
	High risk	LMWH, LDUH, fondaparinux
Laparoscopic Surgery	Low risk	Early ambulation
	High risk	LMWH, LDUH, fondaparinux +/- IPC
Hip fracture surgery	No contraindication to anticoagulation (if surgery delayed start pre-op)	LMWH, LDUH, fondaparinux
	Contraindication to anticoagulation	IPC and reassess daily
THR, TKR	Continue anticoagulation 14–35 days possibly post discharge	LMWH, apixaban, rivaroxaban, dabigatran[a]
	Lower risk patients THR/TKR	Rivaroxaban + ASA 5+30/ 5+9
	Contraindication to anticoagulation	IPC
Upper Limb surgery	Under local or regional anesthesia	none
	General Anesthesia >90 min	Consider VTE prophylaxis
Major trauma or Spinal cord injury	High risk	IPC and LMWH after hemostasis achieved

[a]Dose of medications explained in details in Chapter 1

Fig. 10.6 Recommended prophylaxis and its duration based on surgical and patient's characteristics [8, 10, 42]

Conclusions

Thromboprophylaxis is efficient and well established in the context of general and orthopedic surgery. It has evolved significantly and is becoming more standardized, thanks to the large studies conducted on the novel and existing anticoagulants and thanks to the work of large scientific bodies generating guidelines.

References

1. Kakkar VV, Corrigan TP, Fossard DP. Prevention of fatal postoperative pulmonary embolism by low doses of heparin. Lancet. 1975;2:45–51.
2. Geerts WH, Pineo GF, Heit JA, et al. Prevention of venous thromboembolism: the seventh ACCP conference on antithrombotic and thrombolytic therapy. Chest. 2004;126(suppl):338S–400S.
3. Farfan M, Bautista M, Bonilla G, Rojas J, Llinás A, Navas J. Worldwide adherence to ACCP guidelines for thromboprophylaxis after major orthopedic surgery: a systematic review of the literature and meta-analysis. Thromb Res. 2016;141:163–70.
4. Kalyani BS, Roberts CS. Low molecular weight heparin: current evidence for its application in orthopaedic surgery. Curr Vasc Pharmacol. 2011;9(1):19–23.
5. Yoshida Rde A, Yoshida WB, Maffei FH, El Dib R, Nunes R, Rollo HA. Systematic review of randomized controlled trials of new anticoagulants for venous thromboembolism prophylaxis in major orthopedic surgeries, compared with enoxaparin. Ann Vasc Surg. 2013;27(3):355–69.
6. Muntz J, Michota FA. Prevention and management of venous thromboembolism in the surgical patient: options by surgery type and individual patient risk factors. Am J Surg. 2010;199(1, Supplement):S11–20.
7. Falck-Ytter Y, Francis CW, Johanson NA, et al. Prevention of VTE in orthopedic surgery patients: antithrombotic therapy and prevention of thrombosis, 9th ed: American College of chest physicians evidence-based clinical practice guidelines. Chest. 2012;141(2):e278S–325S.
8. Gould MK, Garcia DA, Wren SM, et al. Prevention of VTE in nonorthopedic surgical patients. Antithrombotic therapy and prevention of thrombosis, 9th ed: American College of chest physicians evidence-based clinical practice guidelines. Chest. 2012;141(2):e227S–77S.
9. Geerts WH, Bergqvist D, Pineo GF, et al. Prevention of venous thromboembolism: American College of Chest Physicians evidence-based clinical practice guidelines (8th edition). Chest. 2008;133:381S–453S.
10. Obi AT, Pannucci CJ, Nackashi A, et al. Validation of the Caprini venous thromboembolism risk assessment model in critically ill surgical patients. JAMA Surg. 2015;150(10):941–8. https://doi.org/10.1001/jamasurg.2015.1841.
11. Kakkos SK, Caprini JA, Geroulakos G, Nicolaides AN, Stansby GP, Reddy DJ. Combined intermittent pneumatic leg compression and pharmacological prophylaxis for prevention of venous thromboembolism in high-risk patients. Kakkos SK, editor. Cochrane database Syst Rev [Internet]. 2008 Oct 8 [cited 2018 Jun 10];(4):CD005258. Available from: http://doi.wiley.com/10.1002/14651858.CD005258.pub2.
12. Gould MK, Jones JP. Thromboprophylaxis in the real world: strengths and limitations of comparative effectiveness research. Chest. 2011;140(6):1401–4.
13. Morris RJ, Woodcock JP. Intermittent pneumatic compression or graduated compression stockings for deep vein thrombosis prophylaxis? A systematic review of direct clinical comparisons. Ann Surg [Internet]. 2010 [cited 2018 Jun 10];251(3):393–6. Available from: https://insights.ovid.com/crossref?an=00000658-201003000-00001.
14. Sachdeva A, Dalton M, Lees T. Graduated compression stockings for prevention of deep vein thrombosis. Cochrane Database Syst Rev. 2018;11:CD001484. https://doi.org/10.1002/14651858.
15. Ho KM, Tan JA. Stratified meta-analysis of intermittent pneumatic compression of the lower limbs to prevent venous thromboembolism in hospitalized patients. Circulation [Internet]. 2013[cited 2018 Jun 10];128(9):1003–20. Available from: http://circ.ahajournals.org/cgi/doi/10.1161/CIRCULATIONAHA.113.002690.
16. Elpern E, Killeen K, Patel G, Senecal PA. The application of intermittent pneumatic compression devices for thromboprophylaxis: AN observational study found frequent errors in the application of these mechanical devices in ICUs. Am J Nurs [Internet]. 2013 [cited 2018 Jun 10];113(4):30–6; quiz 37. Available from: https://insights.ovid.com/crossref?an=00000446-201304000-00027.

17. Cornwell EE, Chang D, Velmahos G, Jindal A, Baker D, Phillips J, et al. Compliance with sequential compression device prophylaxis in at-risk trauma patients: a prospective analysis. Am Surg [Internet]. 2002 [cited 2018 Jun 10];68(5):470–3. Available from: http://www.ncbi.nlm.nih.gov/pubmed/12017149.
18. Clements RH, Yellumahanthi K, Ballem N, Wesley M, Bland KI. Pharmacologic prophylaxis against venous thromboembolic complications is not mandatory for all laparoscopic Roux-en-Y gastric bypass procedures. J Am Coll Surg [Internet]. 2009 [cited 2018 Jun 10];208(5):917–21; discussion 921–3. Available from: http://linkinghub.elsevier.com/retrieve/pii/S1072751509001239.
19. Byrne JP, Mason SA, Gomez D, Hoeft C, Subacius H, Xiong W, et al. Timing of pharmacologic venous thromboembolism prophylaxis in severe traumatic brain injury: a propensity-matched Cohort study. J Am Coll Surg [Internet]. 2016 [cited 2018 Jun 10];223(4):621–631.e5. Available from: http://linkinghub.elsevier.com/retrieve/pii/S1072751516306512.
20. Bilgi K, Muthusamy A, Subair M, Srinivasan S, Kumar A, Ravi R, Kumar R, Sureshkumar S, Mahalakshmy T, Kundra P, Kate V. Assessing the risk for development of Venous Thromboembolism (VTE) in surgical patients using adapted Caprini scoring system. Int J Surg. 2016;30:68–73.
21. Guyatt G, Akl EA, Crowther M, et al. Executive summary : antithrombotic therapy and prevention of thrombosis 9th ed: American College of chest physicians evidence based practice guidelines. Chest. 2012;141:7S–47S. https://doi.org/10.1378/chest.1412S3.
22. Lyman GH, Khorana AA, Kuderer NM, Lee AY, Arcelus JI, Balaban EP, et al. Venous thromboembolism prophylaxis and treatment in patients with cancer: American Society of Clinical Oncology clinical practice guideline update. J Clin Oncol [Internet]. 2013 [cited 2018 Jun 13];31(17):2189–204. Available from: http://ascopubs.org/doi/10.1200/JCO.2013.49.1118.
23. Samuel S, Iluonakhamhe EK, Adair E, Macdonald N, Lee K, Allison TA, et al. High dose subcutaneous unfractionated heparin for prevention of venous thromboembolism in overweight neurocritical care patients. J Thromb Thrombolysis [Internet]. 2015[cited 2018 Jun 13];40(3):302–7. Available from: http://link.springer.com/10.1007/s11239-015-1202-x.
24. Joy M, Tharp E, Hartman H, Schepcoff S, Cortes J, Sieg A, et al. Safety and efficacy of high-dose unfractionated Heparin for prevention of venous Thromboembolism in overweight and obese patients. Pharmacotherapy [Internet]. 2016 Jul [cited 2018 Jun 13];36(7):740–8. Available from: http://doi.wiley.com/10.1002/phar.1775.
25. PRODUCT MONOGRAPH PrLOVENOX®(Enoxaparin sodium solution for injection, manufacturer's standard) ATC Code: B01AB05 Anticoagulant/Antithrombotic Agent sanofi-aventis Canada Inc. 2905 Place Louis-R.-Renaud Laval, Quebec H7V 0A3 Date of Approval: September 11, 2018.
26. Pr FRAGMIN® Monograph. Dalteparin Sodium Injection Solution Anticoagulant/Antithrombotic Agent © Pfizer Canada Inc. 2018 Date of Initial Approval: September 30, 1994 Date of Revision:October 18, 2018.
27. PRODUCT MONOGRAPH Prinnohep® tinzaparin sodium Sterile solution for SC injection. Anticoagulant / Antithrombotic LEO Pharma Inc Thornhill, ON L3T 7W8 www.leo-pharma.com/canada Date of Revision: Date of Approval: May 26, 2017.
28. PRODUCT MONOGRAPH PrFRAXIPARINE® nadroparin calcium injection (9,500 anti-Xa IU/mL) 0.2 mL, 0.3 mL, 0.4 mL, 0.6 mL and 1.0 mL prefilled syringe. Aspen Pharmacare Canada Inc 111 Queen Street East, Suite 450, Toronto, Ontario, M5C 1S2 Submission Control No: 195973 Date of Revision: July 11, 2017.
29. Thromboprophylaxis in orthopedic surgery, Thrombosis Canada guidelines, http://thrombosis-canada.ca/wp-content/uploads/2018/03/Thromboprophylaxis-Orthopedic-2018Feb21-Final.pdf
30. PRODUCT MONOGRAPH PrARIXTRA® fondaparinux sodium injection 2.5 mg/0.5 mL 5.0 mg/0.4 mL 7.5 mg/0.6 mL 10.0 mg/0.8 mL ATC Classification: B01AX05 Synthetic Antithrombotic Aspen Pharma Trading Limited 3016 Lake Drive Citywest Business Campus Dublin 24 Ireland Date of Preparation: 12 March 2015.

31. Eriksson BI, Ekman S, Lindbratt S, Baur M, Bach D, Torholm C, Kälebo P, Close P. Prevention of thromboembolism with use of recombinant hirudin. Results of a double-blind, multicenter trial comparing the efficacy of desirudin (Revasc) with that of unfractionated heparin in patients having a total hip replacement. J Bone Joint Surg Am. 1997;79(3):326–33.

32. Goubran HA, Hanna AAZ, Sholkamy S, Efficacy and Safety of a novel Hansenula polymorpha-derived recombinant RB-variant Hirudin for thromboprophylaxis in orthopaedic patients, ISTH Geneva, 2007. J Thromb Haemost (5) Suppl.2, July, 2007 P-M-667.

33. Nieto JA, Espada NG, Merino RG, González TC. Dabigatran, rivaroxaban and apixaban versus enoxaparin for thromboprophylaxis after total knee or hip arthroplasty: pool-analysis of phase III randomized clinical trials. Thromb Res [Internet]. 2012[cited 2018 Jun 24];130(2):183–91. Available from: http://linkinghub.elsevier.com/retrieve/pii/S004938481200059X.

34. Huisman M V, Quinlan DJ, Dahl OE, Schulman S. Enoxaparin versus dabigatran or rivaroxaban for thromboprophylaxis after hip or knee arthroplasty: results of separate pooled analyses of phase III multicenter randomized trials. Circ Cardiovasc Qual Outcomes [Internet]. 2010 [cited 2018 Jun 24];3(6):652–60. Available from: http://circoutcomes.ahajournals.org/cgi/doi/10.1161/CIRCOUTCOMES.110.957712.

35. Falck-Ytter Y, Francis CW, Johanson NA, Curley C, Dahl OE, Schulman S, et al. Prevention of VTE in orthopedic surgery patients: Antithrombotic therapy and prevention of thrombosis, 9th ed: American College of chest physicians evidence-based clinical practice guidelines. Chest [Internet]. 2012 Feb [cited 2018 Jun 24];141(2 Suppl):e278S–e325S. Available from: http://linkinghub.elsevier.com/retrieve/pii/S0012369212601263.

36. AlHajri L, Jabbari S, AlEmad H, AlMahri K, AlMahri M, AlKitbi N. The efficacy and safety of Edoxaban for VTE Prophylaxis post-orthopedic surgery: a systematic review. J Cardiovasc Pharmacol Ther. 2017;22(3):230–8.

37. Nordstrom BL, Kachroo S, Fraeman KH, Nutescu EA, Schein JR, Fisher A, Bookhart BK. Warfarin prophylaxis in patients after total knee or hip arthroplasty--international normalized ratio patterns and venous thromboembolism. Curr Med Res Opin. 2011;27(10):1973–85.

38. Anderson DR, Dunbar MJ, Bohm ER, et al. Aspirin versus low-molecular-weight heparin for extended venous thromboembolism prophylaxis after total hip arthroplasty: a randomized trial. Ann Intern Med. 2013;158:800–6.

39. Anderson D, Dunbar M, Murgnagham J, et al. Aspirin or Rivaroxaban for VTE Prophylaxis after hip and knee arthroplasty. N Engl J Med. 2018;378:699–707. https://doi.org/10.1056/NEJMoa1712746.

40. Savi P, Chong BH, Greinacher A, et al. Effect of fondaparinux on platelet activation in the presence of heparin-dependent antibodies: a blinded comparative multicenter study with unfractionated heparin. Blood. 2005;105(1):139–144. 122.

41. https://thrombosiscanada.ca/clinicalguides/thromboprophylaxis; non orthopedic surgery.

42. www.nice.org.uk/guidance/ng98. Venous thromboembolism in over 16s: reducing the risk of hospital-acquired deep vein thrombosis of pulmonary embolism.

Chapter 11
Thromboprophylaxis for Hospitalized Medical Patients

Hany Guirguis, Mark Bosch, Kelsey Brose, and Hadi Goubran

Abbreviations

ACCP	American College of Chest Physicians
CrCl	Creatinine clearance
DVT	Deep vein thrombosis
ECS	Elastic compression stockings
LDUH	Low-dose unfractionated heparin
LMWH	Low-molecular-weight heparin
MTHFR	Methylene tetrahydrofolate reductase
PE	Pulmonary embolism
UFH	Unfractionated heparin
VTE	Venous thromboembolism

H. Guirguis (✉)
Scarborough Health Network, Toronto, ON, Canada
e-mail: hguirguis@shn.ca

M. Bosch · K. Brose · H. Goubran
Saskatoon Cancer Centre, College of Medicine, University of Saskatchewan, Saskatoon, SK, Canada
e-mail: Mark.bosch@saskcancer.ca; Kelsey.brose@saskcancer.ca; Hadi.goubranmessiha@saskcancer.ca

© Springer Nature Switzerland AG 2020
H. Goubran et al. (eds.), *Precision Anticoagulation Medicine*,
https://doi.org/10.1007/978-3-030-25782-8_11

Introduction

By the end of the twentieth century, venous thromboembolism was recognized as a common autopsy finding in medical patients who died in hospital [1, 2]. At that time, the frequency of venous thromboembolism in this patient population was unknown, but was estimated to be at least as high as in surgical patients. Furthermore, medical patients who receive treatment for VTE have a higher incidence of major hemorrhage, fatal hemorrhage, and fatal PE when compared to surgical patients [3]. As a result, research has since focused on risk stratification and prevention of VTE in this population [4, 5].

Risk Stratification

As a cohort, hospitalized medical patients have an incidence of VTE of approximately 14.9% [6], but it is recognized that patients' individual risk is influenced by their comorbidities. Multiple risk factors have been identified, including age >70 years, previous VTE, immobility $\geq$3 days, stroke, active cancer (see Chap. 5 that covers specifically this topic), acute inflammatory and infectious conditions and sepsis, known thrombophilia, trauma <1 month, recent surgery <1 month, obesity (body mass index >30), hormone therapy, and cardiac and respiratory failure [7].

At least eight risk assessment models (RAMs) have been developed, including the 4-Element RAM, Caprini RAM, Geneva Risk Score, a full logistic model, Kucher Model, IMPROVE-RAM, a "Multivariable Model," and Padua Prediction Score. All of them, however, are difficult to apply, and none have fulfilled the criteria of an ideal model [8]. The Padua Score and Geneva Score, however, are commonly used.

(a) *The Padua Score*

Risk factor	Absent	Present
Active cancer	0	3
Previous VTE	0	3
Reduced mobility	0	3
Known thrombophilia	0	3
Recent (= < 1 month) trauma/surgery	0	2
Elderly > = 70 years	0	1
Heart or respiratory failure	0	1
Acute MI/ischemic stroke	0	1
Acute infection/rheumatic disease	0	1
Obesity BMI > =30	0	1
Ongoing hormonal treatment	0	1

- Padua Score < 4: low risk of VTE

Thromboprophylaxis should be considered on a case-by-case basis.

- Padua Score ≥ 4: high risk of VTE

Thromboprophylaxis (i.e., heparin/enoxaparin) is recommended for nonpregnant patients without contraindications (major bleeding, low platelets, or creatinine clearance <30 mL/min) who are >18 years.

(b) *The Geneva Score* (score of 3 necessitating thromboprophylaxis)

Cardiac failure	2
Respiratory failure	2
Recent stroke <3 months ago	2
Recent myocardial minfarction <4 weeks ago	2
Acute infectious disease including sepsis	2
Acute rheumatic disease	2
Active malignancy	2
Myeloproliferative syndrome	2
Nephrotic syndrome	2
Any prior VTE	2
Known hypercoagulable state	2
Immobilization for ≥ 3 days <30 min of walking per day	1
Recent travel for >6 h	1
Age > 60 years	1
Obesity BMI >30	1
Chronic venous insufficiency	1
Pregnancy	1
Hormonal therapy contraceptive or replacement therapy	1
Dehydration	1

Efficacy and Application

In the first prophylaxis study for acutely ill medical patients, prophylaxis with enoxaparin 40 mg reduced the incidence of VTE to 5.5%. This benefit was maintained at 3 months, and there was no significant difference in the frequency of adverse events [5]. Such reported data prompted the American College of Chest Physicians (ACCP) to include these patients in their guidelines, sixth edition [9]. The International Union of Angiology also quickly recommended thromboprophylaxis with either LMWH or UFH in medical patients at risk of VTE [10].

Unfortunately, the application of these guidelines was found to be inconsistent and, in some cases, inappropriate [11]. For example, the ENDORSE global survey gathered data from 37,356 hospitalized medical patients across 32 countries, and less than 40% of at-risk hospitalized medical patients received ACCP-recommended prophylaxis [12]. Despite previous mandates from international antithrombotic guidelines, such as those of the American College of Chest Physicians (ACCP), for the "universal" use of thromboprophylaxis in hospitalized medical patients, global audits continue to suggest that implementation of thromboprophylaxis is challenging, and this has been attributed to the perceived higher risk of bleeding and lower risk of VTE than that reported in clinical trials [13].

Guidelines for the Application of Thromboprophylaxis in Medically Ill Patients

In an effort to improve outcomes, some guideline groups use simplified recommendations, such as the following:

> Acutely ill hospitalized medical patients at increased risk of VTE who are not bleeding or at high risk of bleeding should receive pharmacological thromboprophylaxis [7].

> Pharmacological thromboprophylaxis should not be extended beyond the hospitalization period.

Pharmacological Thromboprophylaxis

Unfractionated Heparin

Although the ACCP guidelines recommended twice-daily low-dose unfractionated heparin (LDUH) (5000 IU SC q 12 hours), current evidence suggests that twice-daily LDUH may not be sufficiently efficacious in the acutely ill medical inpatient. Although increasing the frequency of LDUH to three times daily may increase the efficacy, it is associated with an increased risk for bleeding [14].

Unlike most other thromboprophylactic agents, LDUH is not renally excreted and should be offered to patients with renal impairment.

> *LDUH:* In the presence of renal impairment or if short-term anticoagulation is needed in anticipation of surgery or invasive procedures, LDUH could be administered at a dose of 5000 IU SC BID or TID.

Low-Molecular-Weight Heparin

Bemiparin

In a prospective trial of 100 critically ill patients at high risk for developing VTE, patients were randomized to receive subcutaneous injections of either of bemiparin sodium 3500 IU anti-factor Xa or enoxaparin 40 mg given once a day. Patients were followed for 60 days after initiation of anticoagulant therapy for the development of VTE as well as complications related to injectable anticoagulants. DVT was observed in two patients (4%) in the bemiparin group compared with 10 patients (20%) in the enoxaparin group ($p < 0.05$), and ecchymosis or hematoma at the injection site was observed in one patient (2%) in the bemiparin group and eight patients (16%) in the enoxaparin group ($p < 0.05$) [15].

Certoparin

In a study of 3239 older patients (>70 years) comparing certoparin with UFH, the incidence of the VTE was 3.94% in the certoparin group and 4.52% in the UFH group ($p < 0.0001$ for noninferiority), with an OR of 0.87 (95% CI 0.60–1.26; $p = 0.0001$ for noninferiority). Major bleeding occurred in 0.43% of certoparin-treated patients and 0.62% of UFH-treated patients (OR 0.69; 95% CI 0.26–1.83). Any bleeding occurred at 3.20% in certoparin-treated patients versus 4.58% in UFH-treated patients (OR 0.69; 95% CI 0.48–0.99; $p < 0.05$). All-cause mortality was 1.27% in certoparin-treated patients and 1.36% in UFH-treated patients.

In acutely ill, nonsurgical elderly patients, thromboprophylaxis with certoparin (3000 U of anti-FXa once daily) was, therefore, noninferior to 5000 IU of UFH TID, with a favorable safety profile [16].

Dalteparin

A fixed low dose of dalteparin sodium of 5000 U/d is effective and safe in preventing VTE in obese and elderly hospitalized medical patients [17]. There is no dose adjustment of dalteparin if CrCl < 30 mL/min [7].

Enoxaparin

The MEDENOX study randomized 866 critically ill patients to receive enoxaparin 20 mg, 40 mg, or placebo once daily for 6–14 days [6, 10]. The incidence of VTE was significantly lower in the group that received 40 mg of enoxaparin (5.5%)

compared with the group that received placebo (14.9%) (RR, 0.37; 97.6% CI, 0.22 to 0.63; $p < 0.001$) or the group that received 20 mg. The benefit observed with 40 mg of enoxaparin was maintained at 3 months [10] and extended to include all subgroups of patients [18].

Dose reduction should be considered for patients with weight <40 kg; dose increase should be considered for patients with weight > 100 kg. For patients weighing over 120 kg, even higher doses should be considered. In morbidly obese, medically ill patients, use of weight-based enoxaparin dosed at 0.5 mg/kg once daily resulted in peak anti-Xa levels within or near recommended range for thromboprophylaxis, without any evidence of excessive anti-Xa activity, and therefore, a weight-adjusted dose could be offered [19].

In patients with renal impairment (CrCl < 30 mL/min), administration of UFH or a dose reduction of enoxaparin to 30 mg SC once daily should be considered [7].

Nadroparin

In nonsurgical populations at risk of VTE, nadroparin administered at a dose of 2850 anti-Xa IU SC q 24 hours reduced VTE by about one half compared with placebo or no treatment and appeared similarly effective and safe as other prophylactic anticoagulants [20].

Tinzaparin

In many centers, tinzaparin is the commonly used agent for thromboprophylaxis in the medical setting. It is usually administered at a dose of 4500 IU SC q 24 hours. In a pharmacodynamic study performed in elderly patients with impaired renal function, no statistically significant accumulation effect was observed after 8 days of prophylactic treatment with tinzaparin [21].

There is no dose adjustment of tinzaparin if CrCl < 30 mL/min [7].

All LMWH

A systematic review and mixed treatment comparison (MTC) meta-analysis to compare the efficacy and safety of LMWHs for VTE prophylaxis in hospitalized medically ill patients showed that enoxaparin, dalteparin, nadroparin, and certoparin are similar in relative efficacy for the prevention of mortality and VTE and also carry a similar risk of bleeding complications. It also showed that enoxaparin, nadroparin, and certoparin are similar in relative efficacy for the prevention of PE and DVT in hospitalized medical patients [22].

Prophylactic dosages of tinzaparin and dalteparin are likely to be safe in patients with renal insufficiency and do not need dose reduction based on the absence of accumulation. However, prophylactic dosages of enoxaparin, bemiparin, and certoparin did show accumulation in patients with a creatinine clearance (CrCl) below 30 ml/min, and therefore, dose reduction is required [23].

In general, thromboprophylaxis with LMWH does not require any monitoring. Monitoring with anti-Xa activity may only be needed in renal impairment or in extremes of body weight with a reasonable anti-Xa target range of 0.2–0.5 IU/mL [24].

LMWH prophylaxis in medically ill patients

Bemiparin:	3500 IU SC q 24 hours
Certoparin:	3000 IU SC q 24 hours
Dalteparin:	5000 IU SC q 24 hours
Enoxaparin:	40 mg SC q 24 hours (weight-adjusted dose in extreme body weights)
Nadroparin:	2850 IU SC q 24 hours
Tinzaparin:	4500 IU SC q 24 hours

Guidelines recommend the use of these parenteral anticoagulants for 6–14 days but advise against extended-duration thromboprophylaxis after hospital discharge because no compelling scientific evidence has been provided for pharmacological prophylaxis beyond hospital stay. Five large randomized clinical trials, one with low-molecular-weight heparin and four with DOACs, have failed to show significant clinically relevant benefit in this indication [25].

Fondaparinux

Fondaparinux is effective in the prevention of asymptomatic and symptomatic venous thromboembolic events in older acute medical patients with a relative risk reduction of 46.7% [26]. It may also be a very suitable option for patients with or without a previous history of heparin-induced thrombocytopenia [27].

In a study of 210 elderly patients (median age 81 years) treated with fondaparinux, one episode (0.48%, 95% CI 0.1–2.6%) of major bleeding and six episodes (2.86%, 95% CI 1.3–6.1%) of clinically relevant nonmajor bleeding were recorded. Only one thromboembolic event (0.48%, 95% CI 0.1–2.6%) was documented. Therefore, thromboprophylaxis with fondaparinux 2.5 mg daily is safe and effective in preventing VTE without increasing bleeding risk [28].

Fondaparinux is not associated with increased hemorrhagic complications compared with UFH in patients with ischemic stroke [29].

The addition of moderate to severe renal impairment to patients with traditional risk factors for VTE identified a population of very elderly acutely ill medical patients potentially at high risk of both VTE and bleeding complications. The lower prophylactic dose of fondaparinux of 1.5 mg SC q 24 hours appears to be a safe and relatively effective strategy in these patients [30]. It is still recommended, however, to avoid fondaparinux prophylaxis if CrCl < 30 ml/min [7].

Fondaparinux

A dose of 2.5 mg SC q 24 hours is a suitable thromboprophylaxis option in critically ill patients.

In the elderly and patients with renal insufficiency, a dose of 1.5 mg SC q 24 hours has been tried and is effective.

Extended Prophylaxis with Oral Agents

Since medically ill, hospitalized patients are at increased risk for VTE after discharge, many studies aimed to examine thromboprophylaxis patterns, risk factors, and post-discharge outcomes with the extended use of oral agents.

Warfarin

In a study involving 141,628 patients, 3.9% received anticoagulants (3.6% warfarin) [31]. VTE, rehospitalization, and mortality rates were 1.9%, 17.2%, and 6.2%, respectively. The strongest predictors of post-discharge VTE were history of VTE (HR = 4.0, 95% confidence interval [CI]: 3.3–4.8) and rehospitalization (HR = 3.9, 95% CI: 3.6–4.3). Of 504 medical charts, 209 (41.5%) reported in-patient thromboprophylaxis. There was no statistically significant difference in post-discharge VTE rates between patients who did and did not receive in-patient thromboprophylaxis. All-cause mortality was greater among patients without the use of VTE prophylaxis. The post-discharge use of warfarin, however, remains very limited because of the need for monitoring and complex drug interactions.

Rivaroxaban

In a study of 12,024 medical patients randomized to receive either rivaroxaban or placebo as thromboprophylaxis for 45 days after hospital discharge, VTE occurred in 50 of 6007 patients (0.83%) who were given rivaroxaban and in 66 of 6012 patients (1.10%) who were given placebo (hazard ratio, 0.76; 95% confidence interval [CI], 0.52 to 1.09; $p = 0.14$). Rivaroxaban use was not associated with a significantly lower risk of symptomatic VTE and death-related VTE than placebo. The incidence of major bleeding, however, was low [32].

Apixaban

In medically ill patients, an extended course of thromboprophylaxis with apixaban was not superior to a shorter course with enoxaparin. Apixaban was associated with significantly more major bleeding events than was enoxaparin [33].

Betrixaban

Betrixaban differs from other NOACs by having a longer half-life, minimal CYP450 interactions, and minimal renal clearance [34]. Extended-duration VTE prophylaxis from in-hospital through the post-discharge continuum may theoretically improve the quality of care in patients at risk of VTE.

Extended-duration betrixaban showed a significant reduction in venous thromboembolism in the APEX trial (Acute Medically Ill VTE Prevention with Extended Duration Betrixaban Study) [35].

Among hospitalized medically ill patients, extended-duration betrixaban (35–42 days) demonstrated a ≈ 30% reduction in fatal or irreversible ischemic or bleeding events compared with standard-duration enoxaparin. A total of 65 patients would require treatment with betrixaban to prevent one fatal or irreversible event versus enoxaparin [35].

> Extended thromboprophylaxis is not yet standard, but the use of betrixaban can be considered as cost-effective for nonsurgical patients with acute medical illness at risk of VTE, requiring longer VTE prophylaxis from hospitalization through post-discharge [36].

For thromboprophylaxis for inpatients and ambulatory patients with cancer, please refer to Chap. 5.

Nonpharmacological Thromboprophylaxis

In this situation, properly measured and fitted elastic compression stockings (ECS) could be used [7].

The ACCP guidelines highlighted that mechanical methods of thromboprophylaxis should be used primarily in patients at high risk for bleeding (Grade 1A) or possibly as an adjunct to anticoagulant-based thromboprophylaxis (Grade 2A) and that for patients receiving mechanical methods of thromboprophylaxis, careful attention should be directed toward ensuring their proper use and optimal adherence to these methods (Grade 1A) [37].

Conclusions

Thromboprophylaxis in acutely ill medical patients is well established and part of most hospital policies but remains underutilized. It is, therefore, important to increase awareness and reinforce its implementation using preprinted forms or computer decision support systems [37]. LDUH, LMWH, and fondaparinux remain the cornerstone medications used although betrixaban may offer an oral alternative for extended prophylaxis.

References

1. Lindblad B, Sternby NH, Bergqvist D. Incidence of venous thromboembolism verified by necropsy over 30 years. BMJ. 1991;302:709–11.
2. Sandler DA, Martin JF. Autopsy proven pulmonary embolism in hospital patients: are we detecting enough deep vein thrombosis? J R Soc Med. 1989;82:203–5.
3. Monreal M, Kakkar AK, Caprini JA, Barba R, Uresandi F, Valle R, Suarez C, Otero R, RIETE Investigators. The outcome after treatment of venous thromboembolism is different in surgical and acutely ill medical patients. Findings from the RIETE registry. J Thromb Haemost. 2004;2(11):1892–8.
4. Clagett GP, Anderson FA Jr, Geerts WH, et al. Prevention of venous thromboembolism. Chest. 1998;114(Suppl):531S–60S.
5. Prevention of venous thromboembolism: international consensus statement (guidelines according to scientific evidence). Int Angiol. 1997;16:3–38.
6. Samama MM, Cohen AT, Darmon JY, Desjardins L, Eldor A, Janbon C, Leizorovicz A, Nguyen H, Olsson CG, Turpie AG, Weisslinger N. A comparison of enoxaparin with placebo for the prevention of venous thromboembolism in acutely ill medical patients. Prophylaxis in medical patients with enoxaparin study group. N Engl J Med. 1999;341:793–800.
7. Thrombosis Canada, Thromboprophylaxis in hospitalized medical patients, 2013.
8. Stuck AK, Spirk D, Schaudt J, Kucher N. Risk assessment models for venous thromboembolism in acutely ill medical patients. A systematic review. Thromb Haemost. 2017;117(4):801–8.
9. Hirsh J, Dalen J, Guyatt G, American College of Chest Physicians. The sixth (2000) ACCP guidelines for antithrombotic therapy for prevention and treatment of thrombosis. American College of Chest Physicians. Chest. 2001;119(1 Suppl):1S–2S.
10. Samama MM, Kleber FX. An update on prevention of venous thromboembolism in hospitalized acutely ill medical patients. Thromb J. 2006;4:8.
11. Schulman S. Thromboprophylaxis in medical patients--why not for all? Pathophysiol Haemost Thromb. 2006;35(1–2):141–5.
12. Bergmann JF, Cohen AT, Tapson VF, Goldhaber SZ, Kakkar AK, Deslandes B, Huang W, Anderson FA Jr, ENDORSE Investigators. Venous thromboembolism risk and prophylaxis in hospitalized medically ill patients. The ENDORSE global survey. Thromb Haemost. 2010;103(4):736–48.
13. Spyropoulos AC, Raskob GE. New paradigms in venous thromboprophylaxis of medically ill patients. Thromb Haemost. 2017;117(9):1662–70.
14. Michota FA. Venous thromboembolism prophylaxis in the medically ill patient. Clin Chest Med. 2003;24(1):93–101.
15. Abbas MS. Bemiparin versus Enoxaparin in the prevention of venous thromboembolism among Intensive Care Unit patients, Indian J Crit Care Med. 2017;21(7):419–23.

16. Riess H, Haas S, Tebbe U, Gerlach HE, Abletshauser C, Sieder C, Rossol S, Pfeiffer B, Schellong SM. A randomized, double-blind study of certoparin vs. unfractionated heparin to prevent venous thromboembolic events in acutely ill, non-surgical patients: CERTIFY study. J Thromb Haemost. 2010;8(6):1209–15.
17. Kucher N, Leizorovicz A, Vaitkus PT, Cohen AT, Turpie AG, Olsson CG, Goldhaber SZ. Efficacy and safety of fixed low-dose dalteparin in preventing venous thromboembolism among obese or elderly hospitalized patients: a subgroup analysis of the PREVENT trial. Arch Intern Med. 2005;165(3):341–5.
18. Alikhan R, Cohen AT, Combe S, Samama MM, Desjardins L, Eldor A, Janbon C, Leizorovicz A, Olsson CG, Turpie AG. Prevention of venous thromboembolism in medical patients with enoxaparin: a subgroup analysis of the MEDENOX study. Blood Coagul Fibrinolysis. 2003;14(4):341–6.
19. Rondina MT, Wheeler M, Rodgers GM, Draper L, Pendleton RC. Weight-based dosing of enoxaparin for VTE prophylaxis in morbidly obese, medically-ill patients. Thromb Res. 2010;125(3):220–3.
20. Ageno W, Bosch J, Cucherat M, Eikelboom JW. Nadroparin for the prevention of venous thromboembolism in nonsurgical patients: a systematic review and meta-analysis. J Thromb Thrombolysis. 2016;42(1):90–8.
21. Mahé I, Aghassarian M, Drouet L, Bal Dit-Sollier C, Lacut K, Heilmann JJ, Mottier D, Bergmann JF. Tinzaparin and enoxaparin given at prophylactic dose for eight days in medical elderly patients with impaired renal function: a comparative pharmacokinetic study. Thromb Haemost. 2007;97(4):581–6.
22. Dooley C, Kaur R, Sobieraj DM. Comparison of the efficacy and safety of low molecular weight heparins for venous thromboembolism prophylaxis in medically ill patients. Curr Med Res Opin. 2014;30(3):367–80.
23. Atiq F, van den Bemt PM, Leebeek FW, van Gelder T, Versmissen J. A systematic review on the accumulation of prophylactic dosages of low-molecular-weight heparins (LMWHs) in patients with renal insufficiency. Eur J Clin Pharmacol. 2015;71(8):921–9.
24. Wei MY, Ward SM. The anti-factor Xa range for low molecular weight heparin thromboprophylaxis. Hematol Rep. 2015;7(4):5844.
25. Haas S. The role of low molecular weight heparins for venous thromboembolism prevention in medical patients-what is new in 2019? Hamostaseologie. 2019;39(1):62–6.
26. Cohen AT, Davidson BL, Gallus AS, Lassen MR, Prins MH, Tomkowski W, Turpie AG, Egberts JF, Lensing AW, ARTEMIS Investigators. Efficacy and safety of fondaparinux for the prevention of venous thromboembolism in older acute medical patients: randomised placebo controlled trial. BMJ. 2006;332(7537):325–9.
27. Efird LE, Kockler DR. Fondaparinux for thromboembolic treatment and prophylaxis of heparin-induced thrombocytopenia. Ann Pharmacother. 2006;40(7–8):1383–7.
28. Hackett CT, Ramanathan RS, Malhotra K, Quigley MR, Kelly KM, Tian M, Protetch J, Wong C, Wright DG, Tayal AH. Safety of venous thromboembolism prophylaxis with fondaparinux in ischemic stroke. Thromb Res. 2015;135(2):249–54.
29. Silvestri F, Pasca S, Labombarda A, Barbi A, Desideri M, Guidi P, Rogato A, Zaramella M, Bergamo M, Ageno W, Barillari G. Safety of fondaparinux in the prevention of venous thromboembolism in elderly medical patients: results of a single-center, retrospective study. Minerva Med. 2014;105(3):221–8.
30. Ageno W, Riva N, Noris P, Di Nisio M, La Regina M, Arioli D, Ria L, Monzani V, Cuppini S, Lupia E, Giorgi Pierfranceschi M, Dentali F. FONDAIR study group. Safety and efficacy of low-dose fondaparinux (1.5 mg) for the prevention of venous thromboembolism in acutely ill medical patients with renal impairment: the FONDAIR study. J Thromb Haemost. 2012;10(11):2291–7.
31. Mahan CE, Fisher MD, Mills RM, Fields LE, Stephenson JJ, Fu AC, Spyropoulos AC. Thromboprophylaxis patterns, risk factors, and outcomes of care in the medically ill patient population. Thromb Res. 2013;132(5):520–6.

32. Spyropoulos AC, Ageno W, Albers GW, Elliott CG, Halperin JL, Hiatt WR, Maynard GA, Steg PG, Weitz JI, Suh E, Spiro TE, Barnathan ES, Raskob GE, MARINER Investigators. Rivaroxaban for Thromboprophylaxis after hospitalization for medical illness. N Engl J Med. 2018;379(12):1118–27.
33. Goldhaber SZ, Leizorovicz A, Kakkar AK, Haas SK, Merli G, Knabb RM, Weitz JI, ADOPT Trial Investigators. Apixaban versus enoxaparin for thromboprophylaxis in medically ill patients. N Engl J Med. 2011;365(23):2167–77.
34. Lee K, Cham S, Lam S. Betrixaban: a novel factor Xa inhibitor for the prevention of venous thromboembolism in acutely ill medical patients. Cardiol Rev. 2018;26(6):331–8.
35. Gibson CM, Korjian S, Chi G, Daaboul Y, Jain P, Arbetter D, Goldhaber SZ, Hull R, Hernandez AF, Lopes RD, Gold A, Cohen AT, Harrington RA, APEX Investigators. Comparison of fatal or irreversible events with extended-duration Betrixaban versus standard dose enoxaparin in acutely ill medical patients: an APEX trial substudy. J Am Heart Assoc. 2017;6(7). pii: e006015.
36. Guy H, Laskier V, Fisher M, Neuman WR, Bucior I, Deitelzweig S, Cohen AT. Cost-effectiveness of Betrixaban compared with Enoxaparin for venous thromboembolism prophylaxis in non-surgical patients with acute medical illness in the United States. PharmacoEconomics. 2018; https://doi.org/10.1007/s40273-018-0757-8.
37. Geerts WH, Bergqvist D, Pineo GF, et al. American College of Chest Physicians. Prevention of venous thromboembolism: American College of Chest Physicians Evidence-Based Clinical Practice Guidelines (8th ed). Chest. 2008;133(6 suppl):381S–453S.

Chapter 12
Perioperative Management of Anticoagulation and Antiplatelet Therapy

Cherine El-Dabh, Joshua Nero, and Hadi Goubran

Abbreviations

AC	Anticoagulation
ADP	Adenosine diphosphate
AF	Atrial fibrillation
ASA	Acetylsalicylic acid
CABG	Coronary artery bypass grafting
CCS	Canadian Cardiovascular Society
CHF	Congestive heart failure
CHADS2	Score system for anticoagulation in atrial fibrillation
CHA2DS2-VASc	Score system for anticoagulation in atrial fibrillation
COX-1/2	Cyclooxygenase-1/2
CVA	Cerebrovascular accident
DES	Drug eluting stent
DOACs	Direct oral anticoagulants
DVT	Deep vein thrombosis
HIT	Heparin-induced thrombocytopenia
ICH	Intracranial hemorrhage
ICD	Implantable cardioverter-defibrillator

C. El-Dabh (✉)
Cleveland Clinic and Lerner School of Medicine, Abu Dhabi, UAE

J. Nero
Section of Gastroenterology, Department of Internal Medicine, Max Rady College of Medicine, University of Manitoba, Winnipeg, MB, Canada

H. Goubran
Saskatoon Cancer Centre, College of Medicine, University of Saskatchewan, Saskatoon, SK, Canada
e-mail: hadi.goubranmessiha@saskcancer.ca

© Springer Nature Switzerland AG 2020
H. Goubran et al. (eds.), *Precision Anticoagulation Medicine*,
https://doi.org/10.1007/978-3-030-25782-8_12

267

INR   International normalized ratio
LMWH   Low-molecular-weight heparin
LN   Lymph node
M   Month
PCC   Prothrombin complex concentrate
PE   Pulmonary embolism
PT   Prothrombin time
PTT   Partial thromboplastin time
TIA   Transient ischemic attacks
UFH   Unfractionated heparin
VKA   Vitamin K antagonist
VTE   Venous thromboembolism

Introduction

The purpose of this chapter is to suggest an approach to the perioperative management of anticoagulation and antiplatelet therapy based on the current guidelines and available data.

Anticoagulants

The term *bridging* is often used to refer to the use of short-acting anticoagulant before and after elective surgery to ensure the continuity of anticoagulation and reduce thromboembolic risks.

The two variables that interplay in the decision to continue on anticoagulation, temporarily discontinue anticoagulation, or bridge with short-acting preparations are (1) patients' thromboembolic risk and (2) patients' bleeding risk [1–5].

1. *Patient's thromboembolic risks*: The most common indications for anticoagulation are venous thromboembolism, AF, and mechanical valve and heart failure with sinus rhythm. Patients with recent (embolic) cerebrovascular events (CVA) or transient ischemic attacks (TIA). The thromboembolic risk of each of these indications is stratified in Fig. 12.1.
2. *Patient's bleeding risk* is mainly dependent on the type of procedure and patient's history and bleeding risks and is highlighted in Fig. 12.2.

The approach to anticoagulation (AC) bridging is therefore based on the patients' thrombotic risk and the intrinsic as well as operative risks of bleeding.

1. Wafrarin

Figure 12.3 illustrates the approach to bridging when using warfarin. Bridging is achieved with unfractionated heparin (UFH) or low-molecular-weight heparins (LMWH).

Risk	Indication for anticoagulation			
	VTE	AF	Valvular	CHF-SR
High risk	Recent <3M DVT/PE Recent <3M Prior clot with anticoagulation interruption VTE while on therapeutic anticoagulation Active cancer Severe congenital thrombophilia (S or C deficiency) Antiphospholipid syndrome	CHA2DS2-VASc score > 6 CHADS2 4–6 Previous stroke <3M Previous stroke+3 or more CHF Hypertension >75 years DM	Mechanical mitral valve Tricuspid prosthesis Old aortic valve Bileaflet valve and additional risk Rheumatic valve disease	Current or < 3M mural thrombus <3M stroke or TIA
Intermediate risk	Previous VTE 3–12M	CHAD2DS2-VASc score 5–6 Prior stroke/TIA > 3M	Bileaflet aortic valve with AF Bioprosthetic aortic valve with AF	History of stroke/TIA History of mural thrombus
Low risk	Prior VTE >12M	CHAD2DS2-VASc Score 1–4 CHADS2 0–3 Chronic AF	Bileaflet aortic valve with no AF or other risks	No history of mural thrombus

AF CHF Congestive heart failure, *CHAD2DS2-VASc/CHAD2* Score system for *Atrial fibrillation, anticoagulation in atrial fibrillation, DVT* Deep vein thrombosis, *PE* Pulmonary embolism, *VTE* Venous thromboembolism, *TIA* Transient ischemic attack

Fig. 12.1   Risk stratification based on the indication of anticoagulation

Risk	Surgical/procedure	Patient's factors
High risk	Neuraxial anesthesia Neurosurgery Cardiac surgery (CABG/valve) Vascular surgery Major orthopedic surgery Major pulmonary surgery Major cancer surgery Major intra-abdominal or gynecological surgeries and bowel anastomosis Invasive biopsies	Major bleeding <3M ICH < 3M
Intermediate risk	Laparoscopic maneuvers Other invasive surgeries including breast Non-cataract eye Gastroscopy/colonoscopy with biopsy	Platelet abnormalities and use of antiplatelet agents INR is above the therapeutic range Prior bleeding with bridging

Fig. 12.2   Bleeding risk stratification

(continued)

Risk	Surgical/procedure	Patient's factors

Low risk	Coronary angiography
	Cardiac procedures
	  Pacemaker
	  ICD placement
	Bone marrow and LN biopsies, thoraco-, para-, and arthrocentesis
	Multiple tooth extractions
	Dental, dermatologic, cataract, and minor ENT procedures
	Endoscopies without polyp removal
	Dental extractions (2)	

Very low risk	Root canal and periodontal surgery Skin biopsies Cataract removal	

CABG Coronary artery bypass grafting, DVT Deep vein thrombosis, ICH Intracranial hemorrhage, ICD Implantable cardioverter/defibrillator, LN Lymph node, M Month, PE Pulmonary embolism, VTE Venous thromboembolism, TIA Transient ischemic attack

Fig. 12.2 (continued)

Risk	Bleeding risk			
Thrombotic	High	Intermediate	Low	Very low
High	Plan-A bridging Start AC 48–72 hours after surgery Or low dose AC or resume VKA after 12–24 hours	Plan-B bridging Start AC 24–48 hours after surgery	Plan-C bridging Start AC 12–24 hours after surgery	Continue on anticoagulation
Intermediate[a]	Individualized Plan-A bridging decision Start AC 48–72 hours after surgery Or low dose AC or resume VKA after 12–24 hours OR	Individualized Plan-B bridging decision Start AC 24–48 hours after surgery OR	Individualized Plan-C bridging decision Start AC 12–24 hours after surgery OR	Continue on anticoagulation
	No bridging Temporary discontinuation	No bridging Temporary discontinuation	Continue on anticoagulation	
Low	No bridging Temporary discontinuation	No bridging Temporary discontinuation	Continue on anticoagulation	Continue on anticoagulation

[a]The approach to intermediate bleeding risk patients is left to the discretion of the physician to adopt high-risk or low-risk approach

Fig. 12.3 Approach to anticoagulation management based on thromboembolic and bleeding risks

1. *When warfarin and other vitamin k antagonists (VKA) are used, the following action plans can be implemented* [1–5]:

Plan A – Bridging (High and Intermediate Thrombotic Risks with High Bleeding Risk)

- *Day −5:* Stop VKA.
- *Day −3:* Start UFH or subcutaneous LMWH.
- Day *−1:*
  - INR >1.5 – Administer 1–2 mg of vitamin K orally.
  - Stop LMWH on the morning of surgery (omit evening dose in bid) or reduce daily dose 50% in OD dose.
- *Day 0:* Stop UFH 4 hours prior.
- Day *+1/+3:* Assess postoperative hemostasis and could start low dose LMWH or resume VKA.
- Day *+5/+6:* Ensure that INR is therapeutic.

Plan B – Bridging (High and Intermediate Thrombotic Risks with Intermediate Bleeding Risk)

- *Day −5:* Stop VKA.
- *Day −3:* Start UFH or subcutaneous LMWH.
- *Day −1:*
  - INR >1.5 – Administer 1–2 mg of vitamin K orally.
  - Stop LMWH on the morning of surgery (omit evening dose in bid) or reduce daily dose 50% in OD dose.
- *Day 0:* Stop UFH 4 hours prior.
- *Day +1/+2:* Therapeutic dose UFH/LMWH, start VKA.
- *Day +5/+6:* Stop UFH or LMWH when INR is therapeutic.

Plan C – Bridging (High and Intermediate Thrombotic Risks with Low Bleeding Risk)

- *Day −5:* Stop VKA.
- *Day −3:* Start UFH or subcutaneous LMWH.
- *Day −1:*
  - INR >1.5 – Administer 1–2 mg of vitamin K orally.
  - Stop LMWH on the morning of surgery (omit evening dose in bid) or reduce daily dose 50% in OD dose.

- *Day 0:* Stop UFH 4 hours prior – Resume UFH/LMWH 12 hours postoperative.
- *Day +1:* Resume VKA.
- *Day +5/+6:* Stop UFH or LMWH when INR is therapeutic.

No Bridging (Low Thrombotic Risks with High or Intermediate Bleeding Risk)

- *Day −5*: Stop VKA.
- *Day −1*: INR >1.5 – Administer 1–2 mg of vitamin K orally.
- *Day 0*: Resume VKA on the evening if oral feeding allowed.
- *Day +1/+5*: Resume VKA and ensure that INR is therapeutic.

Emergency and Urgent Surgical Interventions on VKA

- *Day −1/0:*
  - Vitamin K 2.5–5 mg IV
  - If needed four-factor prothrombin complex concentrate at a dose of 25–50 IU/kg (average 30 IU/kg) and check INR.
- *Day +1/+5:* UFH/LMWH and resume VKA as per thrombotic/bleeding risk stratification approach.
- (See chapter on anticoagulation reversal for full details.)

For switching to and from other parenteral or oral agents, please refer to the specific agent.

2. Heparin and LMWH

- Stop UFH 4 hours prior to surgery.
- Stop LMWH on the morning of surgery (omit evening dose in bid) or reduce daily dose 50% in OD dose.
- Resume UFH/LMWH 12 hours postoperatively after ensuring that hemostasis is achieved.

3. Hirudin

- Prior to surgical procedure, the medication can be stopped for 4 hours and resumed 12 hours postoperatively after ensuring that hemostasis is achieved.

Transition to Warfarin [6, 7]
- Warfarin initiated only after substantial recovery from HIT has occurred with lepirudin therapy.
- Reduce dosage gradually until the aPTT ratio is just above 1.5, and then initiate therapy with warfarin avoiding loading dose and with modest doses.
- Overlap lepirudin and warfarin therapy for a minimum of 4–5 days until the target INR is reached.

4. Argatroban

- Prior to surgical procedure, the medication can be stopped for 4 hours and resumed 12 hours postoperatively after ensuring that hemostasis is achieved.

Transition to Warfarin [8–10]
- Warfarin initiated only after substantial recovery from HIT has occurred with argatroban therapy.
- If dose is <2 mcg/kg/min D/C when INR is >4 on combined therapy and remeasure INR in 4–6 hours.
- Restart argatroban if INR is below range and repeat until the desired INR is achieved.
- If dose is >2 mcg/kg/min, decrease rate to 2 mcg/kg/min and measure INR at 4–6 hours and proceed accordingly.
- A formula was developed to calculate INR attributable to warfarin when argatroban is given at 2 mcg/kg/min.

$$INR_{warfarin} = 0.19 + \left(0.57 \times INR_{cotherapy} \right).$$

With the use of direct oral anticoagulants (DOACs), which include the direct thrombin inhibitor, dabigatran, or the anti-Xa inhibitors, bridging takes a different perspective.

5. Dabigatran [11, 12]

In clinical trials (RE-LY), treatment was discontinued in the context of procedures with an incidence of major bleeding ranging between 3.8 percent and 5.1 percent for dabigatran doses of 110 milligrams and 150 milligrams, respectively, with a risk of systemic embolization in the range of 0.5 percent [12].

The following table illustrates the suggested time of discontinuation (in hours) of the medication prior to procedures based on creatinine clearance and suggested restarting does and timing.

Discontinuation			Timing (hours)	Timing (hours)
Creatinine clearance ml/min	Half-life in hours		Low bleeding risk	Moderate and high bleeding risk
> = 80	13		24	48
> = 50–80	15		24–48	48–72
> = 30- <50	18		48–72	96
Restarting	Dose (mg)		Timing (hours)	
Minor procedures	75 escalating to 110		Evening of procedure	
Major procedures	Full dose 110–150		48–72	

Bridging with LMWH was done only in a minority of cases in a clinical trial involving high thrombosis risk patients before DOACs are reintroduced.

NB: Normal prothrombin time (PT) and partial thromboplastin time (PTT) do not exclude a significant concentration of dabigatran in the circulation. A normal thrombin time, however, excludes the presence of dabigatran.

If the anticoagulant effect cannot be ruled out completely, neuraxial or celiac block anesthesia should be avoided.

Emergency Surgery: Dabigatran is minimally protein bound and can be removed by dialysis if a procedure can be delayed enough for this to take place.

Tranexamic acid is likely to reduce bleeding in patients who have a residual anticoagulant effect and can be used.

Idarucizumab (Praxbind), a monoclonal antibody to dabigatran, given at a dose of 5 grams (2 × 2.5 g vials) could be used to dose restore hemostasis (see chapter on reversal for full details) [13].

Conversion to Warfarin

When converting from dabigatran to warfarin, adjust the starting time of warfarin based on creatinine clearance as follows:

- For CrCl ≥50 mL/min, start warfarin 3 days before discontinuing dabigatran.
- For CrCl 30–50 mL/min, start warfarin 2 days before discontinuing dabigatran.
- For CrCl 15–30 mL/min, start warfarin 1 day before discontinuing dabigatran.
- For CrCl <15 mL/min, no recommendations can be made.

Converting from or to Parenteral Anticoagulants

- For patients currently receiving a parenteral anticoagulant, start dabigatran 0–2 hours before the next scheduled dose of the parenteral drug or at the time of discontinuation of a continuously administered parenteral drug.
- For patients currently taking dabigatran, wait 12 hours (CrCl ≥ 30 mL/min) or 24 hours (CrCl < 30 mL/min) after the last dose before initiating treatment with a parenteral anticoagulant.

6. Rivaroxaban (Xarelto) [14]

Data from large clinical trials showed that the discontinuation of rivaroxaban for more than 3 days to allow surgery or invasive procedure did not result in any significant major hemorrhage or embolization.

The manufacturer's recommendation is to discontinue for over 24 hours and 48 hours for low and high bleeding risks, respectively.

There is no fixed protocol for pre-procedure discontinuation.

Discontinuation		Timing (hours)	Timing (hours)
Creatinine clearance ml/min	Half-life in hours	Low bleeding risk	Moderate and high bleeding risk
> = 30	9	24	48
<30		48	72
Restarting	Dose (mg)	Timing (hours)	
Minor procedures	20	6–12	
Major procedures	20	Adequate hemostasis – 48	

In patients with high thrombosis risk, it is appropriate to consider prophylactic doses of anticoagulation with LMWH before reintroducing full therapeutic dose of DOACs.

NB: Normal PT and PTT do not exclude a significant concentration of rivaroxaban in the circulation.

- If the anticoagulant effect cannot be ruled out completely, neuraxial or celiac anesthesia should be avoided.

Emergency Surgery: Few data support the use of PCC in the management of emergency surgery, and it should not be used routinely.

Tranexamic acid is likely to reduce bleeding in patients who have a residual anticoagulant effect and can be used.

Andexanet alfa: No data in patients undergoing surgery but promising data on reversal. When available, it should be used for reversal prior to emergency invasive procedures and surgery where bleeding risks are considered significant (see Chap. 12 for full details) [15].

When neuraxial (epidural/spinal) anesthesia or lumbar puncture is performed, patients treated with antithrombotics for prevention of thromboembolic complications are at risk for developing an epidural or spinal hematoma.

The risk of these events is even further increased by the use of indwelling epidural catheters or the concomitant use of drugs affecting hemostasis. Accordingly, the use of rivaroxaban, at doses greater than 10 mg, is not recommended in patients undergoing anesthesia with postoperative indwelling epidural catheters. The risk may also be increased by traumatic or repeated epidural or lumbar puncture. If traumatic puncture occurs, the administration of rivaroxaban should be delayed for 24 hours.

Switching from Parenteral Anticoagulants to Rivaroxaban
- Rivaroxaban can be started when the infusion of full-dose intravenous heparin is stopped or 0–2 hours before the next scheduled injection of full-dose subcutaneous LMWH or fondaparinux.
- In patients receiving prophylactic heparin, LMWH, or fondaparinux, it can be started 6 or more hours after the last prophylactic dose.

Switching from Rivaroxaban to Parenteral Anticoagulants
- Discontinue rivaroxaban and give the first dose of parenteral anticoagulant at the time that the next rivaroxaban dose was scheduled to be taken.

Switching from Vitamin K Antagonists (VKA) to Rivaroxaban
- Stop the VKA and determine the INR.
- If the INR is ≤2.5, start rivaroxaban at the usual dose.
- If the INR is >2.5, delay the start until the INR is ≤2.5.

Switching from Rivaroxaban to a VKA
- Rivaroxaban should be continued concurrently with the VKA until the INR is ≥2.0.
- For the first 2 days of the conversion period, the VKA can be given in the usual starting doses without INR testing.
- Thereafter, while on concomitant therapy, the INR should be tested just prior to the next dose of rivaroxaban, as appropriate. Xarelto can be discontinued once the INR is >2.0.
- Once it is discontinued, INR testing may be done at least 24 hours after the last dose reflecting the anticoagulant effect of the VKA.

7. *Apixaban (Eliquis)* [16]

Data from large clinical trials pointed to the discontinuation of apixaban for 2–5 days to allow surgery or invasive procedure.

The manufacturer's recommendation is to discontinue for over 24 hours and 48 hours for low and high bleeding risks, respectively.

There is no fixed protocol for pre-procedure discontinuation.

Discontinuation		Timing (hours)	Timing (hours)
Creatinine clearance ml/min	Half-life in hours	Low bleeding risk	Moderate and high bleeding risk
> = 30	8	24	48
<30		48	72
Restarting	Dose (mg)	Timing (hours)	
Minor procedures	2.5–5	6–12	
Major procedures	2.5–5	Adequate hemostasis – 48	

In patients with high thrombosis risk, it is appropriate to consider prophylactic doses of anticoagulation with LMWH before reintroducing full therapeutic dose of DOACs.

NB: Normal PT PTT do not exclude a significant concentration of apixaban in the circulation.

- If the anticoagulant effect cannot be ruled out completely, neuraxial or celiac anesthesia should be avoided.

Emergency Surgery: Few data support the use of PCC in the management of emergency surgery, and it should not be used routinely.

Tranexamic acid is likely to reduce bleeding in patients who have a residual anticoagulant effect and can be used.

Andexanet alfa: No data in patients undergoing surgery but promising data on reversal. When available, it should be used for reversal prior to emergency invasive procedures and surgery where bleeding risks are considered significant (see Chap. 12 for full details) [15].

Switching from or to Parenteral Anticoagulants
- In general, switching treatment from parenteral anticoagulants to apixaban (or vice versa) can be done at the next scheduled dose.

Switching from Vitamin K Antagonists (VKA) to Apixaban
- When switching patients from a VKA, such as warfarin, to apixaban, discontinue warfarin or other VKA therapy.
- Start apixaban when the international normalized ratio (INR) is below 2.0.

Switching from Apixaban to VKA
As with any short-acting anticoagulant, there is a potential for inadequate anticoagulation when transitioning from apixaban to a VKA. It is important to maintain an adequate level of anticoagulation when transitioning patients from one anticoagulant to another.

- Apixaban should be continued concurrently with the VKA until the INR is ≥2.0.
- For the first 2 days of the conversion period, the VKA can be given in the usual starting doses without INR testing.
- Thereafter, while on concomitant therapy, the INR should be tested just prior to the next dose of apixaban, as appropriate.
- The medication can be discontinued once the INR is >2.0.
- Once discontinued, INR testing may be done at least 12 hours after the last dose and should then reliably reflect the anticoagulant effect of the VKA.

8. *Edoxaban (Lixiana)* [17, 18]

Edoxaban is excreted only 50% by the kidney.

The manufacturer's recommendation is to discontinue the medication for at least 24 hours before the procedure.

There is no fixed protocol for pre-procedure discontinuation.

Discontinuation			Timing (hours)	Timing (hours)
Creatinine clearance ml/min	Half-life in hours		Low bleeding risk	Moderate and high bleeding risk
> = 30	10–14		24	48
<30			48	72
Restarting	Dose (mg)		Timing (hours)	
Minor procedures	30–60		Evening of procedure	
Major procedures	30–60		Adequate hemostasis – 24	

The usual restarting dose is 60 mg. Dose reduction to 30 mg is recommended in the presence of kidney impairment, a low body weight of less than 60 kg, or the concomitant intake of P-gp inhibitors.

In patients with high thrombosis risk, it is appropriate to consider prophylactic doses of anticoagulation with LMWH before reintroducing full therapeutic dose of DOACs.

NB: Normal PT PTT do not exclude a significant concentration of apixaban in the circulation.

- If the anticoagulant effect cannot be ruled out completely, neuraxial or celiac anesthesia should be avoided.

Emergency Surgery: Few data support the use of PCC in the management of emergency surgery, and it should not be used routinely.

Tranexamic acid is likely to reduce bleeding in patients who have a residual anticoagulant effect and can be used.

Andexanet alfa: No data on edoxaban and in patients undergoing surgery but promising data on reversal. When available, it should be used for reversal prior to emergency invasive procedures and surgery where bleeding risks are considered significant (see Chap. 13 for full details) [15].

From Unfractionated Heparin
- Stop the infusion and start edoxaban 4 hours later.

Switching from Warfarin to Edoxaban
- Discontinue warfarin and start edoxaban when INR is 2.5 or less.
- From non-warfarin anticoagulant (oral or parenteral, e.g., LMWH, rivaroxaban, dabigatran, apixaban) to edoxaban: start edoxaban at the time the next scheduled dose of the non-warfarin anticoagulant was to be administered.

From Edoxaban to Warfarin
- Start warfarin and administer edoxaban at half the prescribed dose (either 30 mg or 15 mg for those on a reduced dose for one or more of the following: CrCl 15–50 mL/min; <60 kg; use with P-gp inhibitor except amiodarone or verapamil).
- Once INR is 2 or greater, discontinue edoxaban. NOTE: Edoxaban can affect INR; therefore, when starting warfarin, INR may be unreliable. If possible, checking INR just prior to next edoxaban dose may better reflect the anticoagulant effect of warfarin.

From Edoxaban to Non-warfarin Anticoagulants (Oral or Parenteral)
(e.g., LMWH, Apixaban, Rivaroxaban, Dabigatran)
- Discontinue edoxaban and give first dose of non-warfarin anticoagulant at the time the next dose of edoxaban is due.

Antiplatelet Agents [19–23]

Acetylsalicylic Acid (Aspirin) (ASA) [19–23]

Aspirin irreversibly inhibits COX-1 to decrease thromboxane and inhibits platelets for 7–10 days. Slow recovery of overall platelet function occurs at 10% per day due to new platelet formation. The doses required for anti-inflammatory effects through COX-2 inhibition are much higher than the doses required for antiplatelet effects (75–100 mg/day). Aspirin has a half-life of 15–20 minutes.

The only randomized trial in noncardiac surgery to assess perioperative antiplatelet management is the Perioperative Ischemic Evaluation-2 (POISE-2) trial. Data from POISE-2 have demonstrated that continuing ASA perioperatively has no protective effect on MI or all-cause mortality (HR 0.99, 95% CI 0.86–1.15) but does increase the risk of major bleeding (HR 1.23, 95% CI 1.01–1.49). However, patients with recent coronary artery stenting or those undergoing carotid endarterectomy were excluded, and only 4% of patients overall had a coronary stent. Consequently, to minimize bleeding risks, ASA is typically withheld for 3 days preoperatively and restarted after 8–10 days postoperatively.

In patients with recent coronary artery stenting (typically 1 month for bare-metal stents and 3 months for drug-eluting stents), elective surgeries should be delayed as interruption of dual antiplatelet therapy in this setting has a high risk of stent thrombosis. Aspirin should be continued in post-PCI patients having noncardiac surgery, while $P2Y_{12}$ therapy is interrupted.

If the patient is not already on ASA, it should not be initiated for the prevention of perioperative cardiac events.

Discontinuation	Timing
Undergoing carotid endarterectomy	Continue perioperatively
Elective noncardiac surgery with previous BMS or DES coronary artery stents	Continue perioperatively
Elective noncardiac surgery without previous coronary artery stents	3 days[a]
ACS requiring CABG	Continue perioperatively
Restarting	Timing
Major noncardiac surgery	8–10 days[b]

[a]Perioperative ASA continuation may be reasonable to prevent local thrombosis for some surgical interventions (e.g., free flap, acute limb ischemia)
[b]When a patient suffers an MI or thrombotic event postoperatively in the absence of bleeding, there might be a net benefit to restarting ASA sooner after surgery

Emergency Surgery: In emergent surgeries, platelet transfusion can be given to counteract the effect of ASA on thrombocytes, although newer literature suggests this does not reverse the effects of other antiplatelet agents due to their longer half-lives. Platelets should be transfused at least 2 hours after the last dose of ASA. *The indications for restoring platelet function in the setting of bleeding are controversial, and the net benefit is uncertain.* Platelet transfusions can put the patient at risk for stent thrombosis, and a risk–benefit analysis should be performed prior to making this decision.

Intravenous desmopressin has been shown to restore platelet activity in ASA-induced platelet dysfunction, but little clinical data is available.

Clopidogrel (Plavix) [19, 20]

Clopidogrel specifically and irreversibly inhibits the $P2Y_{12}$ subtype of ADP receptor, leading to irreversible platelet inhibition. Clopivdogrel is a prodrug requiring activation by hepatic P450 enzymes, and there exists significant interpatient variability of antiplatelet activity. Clopidogrel is eliminated in both the feces and urine and does not require dose adjustment in hepatic or renal disease. Peak plasma concentration is reached 2 hours after oral ingestion. Clopidogrel has a half-life of 7–9 hours.

Clopidogrel is typically used in addition to ASA after PCI, but may be seen as monotherapy in the setting of cerebrovascular disease.

Discontinuation	Timing
Elective noncardiac surgery with previous BMS coronary artery stent, less than 1 month ago	Delay surgery
Elective noncardiac surgery with previous DES coronary artery stent, less than 3 months ago	Delay surgery
Semi-urgent noncardiac surgery with previous DES coronary artery stent, less than 1 month ago	Delay surgery
Elective noncardiac surgery with previous BMS coronary artery stent, more than 1 month ago	5–7 days
Elective noncardiac surgery with previous DES coronary artery stent, more than 3 months ago	5–7 days
Semi-urgent noncardiac surgery with previous DES coronary artery stent, more than 1 month ago	5–7 days
ACS requiring semi-urgent CABG	Minimum 48–72 hours
ACS requiring elective CABG	5 days
Minor procedures with low risk of bleeding	Continue perioperatively[a]
Restarting	Timing
Noncardiac surgery	Restart maintenance dose after surgery, as soon as it is deemed safe by the surgeon

[a]The risk and consequences of perioperative bleeding will vary considerably depending on the type of surgery performed. Some minor surgical procedures carry a low risk of bleeding, whereas others a very high risk of bleeding. For example, some dental, ophthalmological, and endoscopic procedures carry a low risk of bleeding and can be performed without stopping antiplatelet therapy

Emergency Surgery: In emergent surgeries, platelet transfusion can be given to counteract the effect of clopidogrel on thrombocytes, although newer literature suggests this does not reverse the effects of non-ASA antiplatelet agents due to their longer half-lives. Platelets should be transfused at least 12–24 hours after the last dose of clopidogrel. *The indications for restoring platelet function in the setting of bleeding are controversial.* Platelet transfusions can put the patient at risk for stent thrombosis, and a risk–benefit analysis should be performed prior to making this decision.

Bridging with unfractionated or low-molecular-weight heparin has relatively minor effects on platelets and is not recommended. Bridging with short-acting glycoprotein IIb/IIIa inhibitors can be considered in the period of ADP receptor antagonist withdrawal, but not mentioned in the latest CCS guidelines.

Ticagrelor (Brilinta) [24]

Unlike clopidogrel and prasugrel, ticagrelor is a reversible noncompetitive antagonist of the $P2Y_{12}$ subtype of ADP receptor, leading to reversible platelet inhibition. It has a more rapid onset of action and is more potent than either clopidogrel or prasugrel. Ticagrelor is eliminated in the feces. Ticagrelor requires dose adjustment in hepatic dysfunction, but not in renal dysfunction. Ticagrelor has a half-life of 7–9 hours.

Discontinuation	Timing
Elective noncardiac surgery with previous BMS coronary artery stent, less than 1 month ago	Delay surgery
Elective noncardiac surgery with previous DES coronary artery stent, less than 3 months ago	Delay surgery
Semi-urgent noncardiac surgery with previous DES coronary artery stent, less than 1 month ago	Delay surgery
Elective noncardiac surgery with previous BMS coronary artery stent, more than 1 month ago	5–7 days
Elective noncardiac surgery with previous DES coronary artery stent, more than 3 months ago	5–7 days
Semi-urgent noncardiac surgery with previous DES coronary artery stent, more than 1 month ago	5–7 days
ACS requiring semi-urgent CABG	Minimum 48–72 hours
ACS requiring elective CABG	5 days
Minor procedures with low risk of bleeding	Continue perioperatively[a]
Restarting	Timing
Noncardiac surgery	Restart maintenance dose after surgery, as soon as it is deemed safe by the surgeon

[a]The risk and consequences of perioperative bleeding will vary considerably depending on the type of surgery performed. Some minor surgical procedures carry a low risk of bleeding, whereas others a very high risk of bleeding. For example, some dental, ophthalmological, and endoscopic procedures carry a low risk of bleeding and can be performed without stopping antiplatelet therapy

Emergency Surgery: In emergent surgeries, platelet transfusion can be given to counteract the effect of ASA and clopidogrel on thrombocytes, although newer literature suggests this does not reverse the effects of non-ASA antiplatelet agents due to their longer half-lives. Platelets should be transfused at least 12–24 hours after the last dose of ticagrelor. *The indications for restoring platelet function in the setting of bleeding are controversial.* Platelet transfusions can put the patient at risk for stent thrombosis, and a risk–benefit analysis should be performed prior to making this decision.

Bridging with unfractionated or low-molecular-weight heparin has relatively minor effects on platelets and is not recommended. Bridging with short-acting glycoprotein IIb/IIIa inhibitors can be considered in the period of ADP receptor antagonist withdrawal, but not mentioned in the latest CCS guidelines [19].

Prasugrel (Effient) [25]

Prasugrel specifically and irreversibly inhibits the $P2Y_{12}$ subtype of ADP receptor, leading to irreversible platelet inhibition. No dose adjustment is required for hepatic or renal dysfunction. Peak plasma concentration is reached 30 minutes after oral ingestion. Prasugrel is faster and more effective in achieving platelet inhibition than clopidogrel. The FDA recommends lower doses of prasugrel be used in patients ≥75 years of age, weighing <60 kg, or with a previous history of TIAs. Prasugrel has a half-life of 7 hours.

Discontinuation	Timing
Elective noncardiac surgery with previous BMS coronary artery stent, less than 1 month ago	Delay surgery
Elective noncardiac surgery with previous DES coronary artery stent, less than 3 months ago	Delay surgery
Semi-urgent noncardiac surgery with previous DES coronary artery stent, less than 1 month ago	Delay surgery
Elective noncardiac surgery with previous BMS coronary artery stent, more than 1 month ago	7–10 days
Elective noncardiac surgery with previous DES coronary artery stent, more than 3 months ago	7–10 days
Semi-urgent noncardiac surgery with previous DES coronary artery stent, more than 1 month ago	7–10 days
ACS requiring semi-urgent CABG	5 days
ACS requiring elective CABG	7 days
Minor procedures with low risk of bleeding	Continue perioperatively[a]
Restarting	Timing
Noncardiac surgery	Restart maintenance dose after surgery, as soon as it is deemed safe by the surgeon

[a]The risk and consequences of perioperative bleeding will vary considerably depending on the type of surgery performed. Some minor surgical procedures carry a low risk of bleeding, whereas others a very high risk of bleeding. For example, some dental, ophthalmological, and endoscopic procedures carry a low risk of bleeding and can be performed without stopping antiplatelet therapy

Emergency Surgery: In emergent surgeries, platelet transfusion can be given to counteract the effect of ASA and clopidogrel on thrombocytes, although newer literature suggests this does not reverse the effects of non-ASA antiplatelet agents due to their longer half-lives. Platelets should be transfused at least 12–24 hours after the last dose of prasugrel. *The indications for restoring platelet function in the setting of bleeding are controversial.* Platelet transfusions can put the patient at risk for stent thrombosis, and a risk–benefit analysis should be performed prior to making this decision.

Bridging with unfractionated or low-molecular-weight heparin has relatively minor effects on platelets and is not recommended. Bridging with short-acting glycoprotein IIb/IIIa inhibitors can be considered in the period of ADP receptor antagonist withdrawal, but not mentioned in the latest CCS guidelines [19].

References

1. Peri-operative management of patients who are receiving warfarin © 2013 Thrombosis Canada, 2013. http://www.thrombosiscanada.ca/guides/pdfs/Warfarin_perioperative_management.pdf.
2. Warfarin: Peri-operative management. © 2016 Thrombosis Canada http://thrombosiscanada.ca/wp-content/uploads/2016/09/14_Warfarin-Peri-Operative_2016Sept15-2.pdf.
3. Guideline for the management of oral anticoagulation before and after elective surgery or procedures. http://anesthesiology.queensu.ca/assets/Clinical_Policies/Guidelines_for_Bridging_Anticoagulation_-_Oct_2013.pdf.
4. Rechenmacher SJ, Fang JC. Bridging anticoagulation: primum non nocere. J Am Coll Cardiol. 2015;66(12):1392–403.
5. Doherty JU, Gluckman TJ, Hucker WJ, Januzzi JL Jr, Ortel TL, Saxonhouse SJ, Spinler SA. A report of the American College of cardiology clinical expert consensus document task force 2017 ACC expert consensus decision pathway for periprocedural management of anticoagulation in patients with nonvalvular atrial fibrillation. J Am Coll Cardiol. 2017;69(7):871–98.
6. Greinacher A, Volpel H, Janssens U, et al. Recombinant hirudin (lepirudin) provides safe and effective anticoagulation in patients with heparin-induced thrombocytopenia. Circulation. 1999;99:73–80. [PubMed 9884382].
7. Messmore HL, Jeske WP, Wehmacher WH, et al. Benefit-risk assessment of treatments for heparin-induced thrombocytopenia. Drug Saf. 2003;26:625–41.
8. Ansara AJ, Arif S, Warhurst RD. Weight based argatroban dosing nomogram for treatment of heparin-induced thrombocytopenia. Ann Pharmacother. 2009;43:9–18.
9. Argatroban package insert, GlaxoSmithKline September, 2009.
10. Argatroban, Pfizer Canada, revision June 25, 2013.
11. PRODUCT MONOGRAPH Pr PRADAXA® Dabigatran Etexilate Capsules 75 mg, 110 mg and 150 mg Dabigatran Etexilate, (as Dabigatran Etexilate Mesilate) Anticoagulant Boehringer

Ingelheim Canada Ltd. 5180 South Service Road Burlington, ON L7L 5H4 BICL 0266 17, 18 and 19 Date of Revision: February 7, 2019.

12. Wallentin L, Yusuf S, Ezekowitz MD, Alings M, Flather M, Franzosi MG, Pais P, Dans A, Eikelboom J, Oldgren J, Pogue J, Reilly PA, Yang S, Connolly SJ, RE-LY investigators. Efficacy and safety of dabigatran compared with warfarin at different levels of international normalised ratio control for stroke prevention in atrial fibrillation: an analysis of the RE-LY trial. Lancet. 2010;376(9745):975–83.

13. Pollack CV Jr, Reilly PA, van Ryn J, Eikelboom JW, Glund S, Bernstein RA, Dubiel R, Huisman MV, Hylek EM, Kam CW, Kamphuisen PW, Kreuzer J, Levy JH, Royle G, Sellke FW, Stangier J, Steiner T, Verhamme P, Wang B, Young L, Weitz JI. Idarucizumab for Dabigatran reversal - full cohort analysis. N Engl J Med. 2017;377(5):431–44.

14. PRODUCT MONOGRAPH PrXARELTO® rivaroxaban tablets 2.5 mg, 10 mg, 15 mg and 20 mg Anticoagulant (ATC Classification: B01AF01) Bayer Inc. 2920 Matheson Boulevard East Mississauga, Ontario L4W 5R6 Canada http://www.bayer.ca Date of Revision: September 18, 2018.

15. Connolly SJ, Crowther M, Eikelboom JW, Gibson CM, Curnutte JT, et al. Full study report of Andexanet Alfa for bleeding associated with factor Xa inhibitors. N Engl J Med. 2019; https://doi.org/10.1056/NEJMoa1814051.

16. PRODUCT MONOGRAPH PrELIQUIS® apixaban tablets 2.5 mg and 5 mg Anticoagulant Pfizer Canada Inc. 17,300 Trans-Canada Highway Kirkland, Quebec H9J 2M5 Bristol-Myers Squibb Canada Co. Montreal, Canada H4S 0A4 www.bmscanada.ca Date of Preparation: 23 October 2018.

17. Lixiana product monograph. (Servier Canada Inc), July 26, 2017.

18. Giugliano RP, Ruff CT, Braunwald E, Murphy SA, Wiviott SD, Halperin JL, Waldo AL, Ezekowitz MD, Weitz JI, Špinar J, Ruzyllo W, Ruda M, Koretsune Y, Betcher J, Shi M, Grip LT, Patel SP, Patel I, Hanyok JJ, Mercuri M, Antman EM, ENGAGE AF-TIMI 48 Investigators. Edoxaban versus warfarin in patients with atrial fibrillation. N Engl J Med. 2013;369(22):2093–104.

19. Levine GN, Bates ER, Bittl JA, Brindis RG, Fihn SD, Fleisher LA, Granger CB, Lange RA, Mack MJ, Mauri L, Mehran R, Mukherjee D, Newby LK, O'Gara PT, Sabatine MS, Smith PK, Smith SC Jr. 2016 ACC/AHA guideline focused update on duration of dual antiplatelet therapy in patients with coronary artery disease: a report of the American College of Cardiology/American Heart Association task force on clinical practice guidelines: an update of the 2011 ACCF/AHA/SCAI guideline for percutaneous coronary intervention, 2011 ACCF/AHA guideline for coronary artery bypass graft surgery, 2012 ACC/AHA/ACP/AATS/PCNA/SCAI/STS guideline for the diagnosis and management of patients with stable Ischemic heart disease, 2013 ACCF/AHA guideline for the management of ST-elevation myocardial infarction, 2014 AHA/ACC guideline for the management of patients with non-ST-elevation acute coronary syndromes, and 2014 ACC/AHA guideline on perioperative cardiovascular evaluation and management of patients undergoing non-cardiac surgery. Circulation. 2016;134(10):e123–55.

20. Oprea AD, Popescu WM. Perioperative management of antiplatelet therapy. Br J Anaesth. 2013;111(Suppl 1):i3–17.

21. British Society of Hematology. Guidelines: Peri-Operative Management of Anticoagulation and Antiplatelet Therapy, October, 2016 https://b-s-h.org.uk/guidelines/guidelines/peri-operative-management-of-anticoagulation-and-antiplatelet-therapy/.

22. Duceppe E, Parlow J, MacDonald P, Lyons K, McMullen M, Srinathan S, Graham M, Tandon V, Styles K, Bessissow A, Sessler DI, Bryson G, Devereaux PJ. Canadian Cardiovascular Society guidelines on perioperative cardiac risk assessment and management for patients who undergo non-cardiac surgery. Can J Cardiol. 2017;33(1):17–32.

23. Mehta SR, Bainey KR, Cantor WJ, Lordkipanidzé M, Marquis-Gravel GRobinson SD, Sibbald M, So DY, Wong GC, Abunassar JG, Ackman ML, Bell AD, Cartier R, Douketis JD, Lawler PR, McMurtry MS, Udell JA, van Diepen S, Verma S, Mancini GBJ, Cairns JA, Tanguay JF, members of the Secondary Panel. 2018 Canadian Cardiovascular Society/Canadian Association of

interventional cardiology focused update of the guidelines for the use of antiplatelet therapy. Can J Cardiol. 2018;34(3):214–33.

24. PRODUCT MONOGRAPH BRILINTA® ticagrelor tablets 60 and 90 mg Platelet Aggregation Inhibitor AstraZeneca Canada Inc. 1004 Middlegate Road Mississauga, Ontario L4Y 1M4 www.astrazeneca.ca Date of Preparation: October 25, 2018.

25. PRODUCT MONOGRAPH PrEFFIENT® prasugrel (as prasugrel hydrochloride) tablets 10 mg Platelet Aggregation Inhibitor © ELI LILLY CANADA INC. 3650 Danforth Avenue Toronto, Ontario M1N 2E8 1–877–545-5972 www.lilly.ca Date of Revision: June 17, 2014.

Chapter 13
Anticoagulation Reversal Guide and Reversal Agents

Waleed Sabry, Caroline Hart, and Hadi Goubran

Abbreviations

3F-PCC	Three-factor prothrombin complex concentrate
4F-PCC	Four-factor prothrombin complex concentrate
aPCC	Activated prothrombin complex concentrate
ASCO	American Society of Clinical Oncology
CAT	Cancer-associated thrombosis
CrCl	Creatinine clearance
CVC	Central venous catheter
DOACs	Direct oral anticoagulants
DVT	Deep vein thrombosis
FEIBA	Factor eight inhibitor bypassing activity
FFP	Fresh frozen plasma
INR	International normalized ratio
IU	International unit
LMWH	Low-molecular-weight heparin
NCCN	National Comprehensive Cancer Network
PCC	Prothrombin complex concentrate
PE	Pulmonary embolism
PTT	Partial thromboplastin time
rFVIIa	Recombinant activated factor VII

W. Sabry (✉)
Saskatoon Cancer Centre and Division of Oncology, College of Medicine,
University of Saskatchewan, Saskatoon, SK, Canada
e-mail: Waleed.Sabry@saskcancer.ca

C. Hart · H. Goubran
Saskatoon Cancer Centre, College of Medicine, University of Saskatchewan,
Saskatoon, SK, Canada
e-mail: caroline.heart@saskcancer.ca; hadi.goubranmessiha@saskcancer.ca

© Springer Nature Switzerland AG 2020
H. Goubran et al. (eds.), *Precision Anticoagulation Medicine*,
https://doi.org/10.1007/978-3-030-25782-8_13

S/D	Solvent and detergent
U	Unit
UFH	Unfractionated heparin
VH	Vapor heat
VTE	Venous thromboembolism
WFI	Water for injection

Introduction

Pharmaceutical anticoagulants disrupt the process of normal hemostasis directly by inhibiting clotting factor activity, indirectly by depleting vitamin K–dependent clotting factors, or by amplifying native anticoagulant pathways through antithrombin [1].

Coagulation Reversal Guide

In the context of active bleeding with or without over-dosage of the anticoagulant medications or when an urgent state of hemostasis is required due to an eminent surgery, anticoagulation reversal becomes a necessity. Figure 13.1 is a practical anticoagulation reversal guide.

Anticoagulant agent	Half-life	Reversal approach
Unfractionated heparin infusion [2].	60–90 minutes	*Non-urgent:* Holding infusion for 4–6 hours results in a near-complete reversal *Emergent/urgent:* *Protamine sulfate* 1 mg/80–100 U UFH if within 15 minutes of UFH infusion 0.5 mg/80–100 U within 60 minutes or 0.25 mg/80–100 U within 2 hours Maximum 50 mg dose
Enoxaparin [2]	~4–8 hours	*Non-urgent:* Time-dependent, ~24 hours *Emergent/urgent*: PCC at 20 U/kg Partial reversal with protamine, but degree unclear If dosed ≤8 hours: 1 mg/1 mg enoxaparin If dosed >8 hours: 0.5 mg/1 mg enoxaparin *Experimental:* Ciraparantag 300 mg IV

Fig. 13.1 The different anticoagulant agents, their half-lives, and their reversal approach

Anticoagulant agent	Half-life	Reversal approach
Nadroparin [3]	3.5 hours	*Non-urgent:* Time-dependent, ~24 hours *Emergent/urgent:* The dose of protamine should be equal to the dose of nadroparin used, on a mg to mg basis. A second infusion of 0.5 mg protamine per 1 mg nadroparin may be administered if the aPTT measured 2–4 hours after the first infusion remains prolonged
Tinzaparin [4]	3–4 hours	*Non-urgent:* Time-dependent, ~24 hours *Emergent/urgent:* Transfusion of FFP may be used 1 mg of protamine sulfate neutralizes the effect of 100 anti-Xa IU tinzaparin (effective in 3 hours)
Fondaparinux [2]	~17–21 hours	*Non-urgent:* Time-dependent, ~24 hours *Emergent/urgent:* 4F-PCC at 20 U/kg Protamine has not been shown to be effective
Argatroban [5]	39–51 minutes	*Non-urgent:* Time-dependent: full reversal in ~4–6 hours *Emergent/urgent:* No effective means of reversal has been established

Warfarin [2, 6]	40 hours	*Non-urgent:* Time: Hold for 5 d, INR normalization variable depending on age, dose, and drug/enzyme interactions
		If not bleeding and INR >10
		  Oral vitamin K (1–5 mg)
		Emergent/urgent:
		Minor bleeding with any INR:
		  IV vitamin K (1 mg–3 mg)
		Major bleeding:
		INR and weight known
		  Vitamin K 5 mg in 50 mL NS IV STAT if INR 1.6–5.0
		  Vitamin K 10 mg in 50 mL NS IV STAT if INR > 5.0 or ongoing major bleeding prothrombin complex concentrate (4F-PCC)

Weight/INR	1.6–1.9	2.0–2.9	3.0–5.0	>5
<100 Kg	500 U	1000 U	2000 U	3000 U maximum
>100 Kg	1000 U	1500 U	2500 U	3000 U maximum

3F-PCC could be used in conjunction with plasma or vitamin K
Repeat INR 15 minutes after PCC infusion is completed
INR and weight not known
Vitamin K 10 mg in 50 mL NS IV STAT
Administer PCC 2000 IU
Repeat INR 15 minutes after PCC infusion is completed
NB:
If 4F-PCC is not available, use plasma 10–15 mL/kg
aPCC not effective

Fig. 13.1 (continued)

Anticoagulant agent	Half-life	Reversal approach
Dabigatran [7]	7–9 hours in young adults 12–14 hours in older adults [8]	*Non-urgent:* Time-dependent, ~24 hours *Emergent/urgent:* Administer 5 g idarucizumab IV (typically provided as two separate vials, each containing 2.5 g/50 mL) If idarucizumab is not available, administer 4F-PCC or aPCC 50 units/kg IV Consider activated charcoal for known recent ingestion (within 2–4 hours) NB: Plasma not effective
Rivaroxaban [7]	5–9 hours in young adults 11–13 hours in older adults [8]	*Non-urgent:* Time-dependent, ~24 hours *Emergent/urgent:* *Last dose >10 mg or unknown* *<8 hours ago or unknown:* High dose of andexanet alfa Initial IV bolus 800 mg at a target rate of 30 mg/min Follow-on IV infusion: 8 mg/min for up to 120 minutes *Last dose <10 mg or <8 hours:* Low dose of andexanet alfa Initial IV bolus: 400 mg at a target rate of 30 mg/min Follow-on IV infusion: 4 mg/min for up to 120 minutes If andexanet alfa is not available, administer 4F-PCC 50 units/kg IV or aPCC 50 units/kg IV Consider activated charcoal for known recent ingestion (within 2–4 hours) NB: Idarucizumab, plasma not effective *Experimental:* Ciraparantag 100–300 mg IV
Apixaban [2, 7]	~12 hours	*Non-urgent:* Time-dependent, ~24 hours *Emergent/urgent:* *Last dose >5 mg or unknown* *<8 hours ago or unknown:* High dose of andexanet alfa Initial IV bolus 800 mg at a target rate of 30 mg/min Follow-on IV infusion: 8 mg/min for up to 120 minutes *Last dose <5 mg or <8 hours:* Low dose of andexanet alfa Initial IV bolus: 400 mg at a target rate of 30 mg/min Follow-on IV infusion: 4 mg/min for up to 120 minutes If andexanet alfa is not available, administer 4F-PCC 50 units/kg IV or aPCC 50 units/kg IV Consider activated charcoal for known recent ingestion (within 2–4 hours) NB: Idarucizumab, plasma not effective *Experimental:* Ciraparantag 100–300 mg IV

Fig. 13.1 (continued)

Anticoagulant agent	Half-life	Reversal approach

Edoxaban [2, 7]	1–3 hours	*Non-urgent:*
		Time-dependent, ~24 hours
		Emergent/urgent:
		  Administer 4F-PCC 25–50 units/kg IV
		  Second line if 4F-PCC is not available, administer aPCC 50 units/kg IV
		  For all patients, consider activated charcoal for known recent ingestion (within 2–4 hours)
		NB:
		  Idarucizumab, plasma, not indicated
		Experimental:
		  Ciraparantag 100–300 mg IV

Multiple agents LMWH, anti-Xa, anti-IIa	Variable	*Experimental:* Ciraparantag 100–300 mg IV

Fig. 13.1 (continued)

Coagulation Reversal Agents

Vitamin K

(a) Mechanism of Action

Vitamin K administration repletes the warfarin-induced depletion of functional vitamin K and promotes the synthesis of clotting factors VII, IX, X, and II.

(b) Indication

Vitamin K administration is suitable for reversal of vitamin k antagonists, warfarin, and Coumadin.

(c) Dose and Administration

For minor bleeds with any elevation of the INR: vitamin K 2.5–5 mg orally; monitor INR; if INR remains elevated at 24 hours, repeat dose of vitamin K may be given [9].

For major bleeds: If INR 1.6–5.0, vitamin K 5 mg (in 50 mL normal saline) IV; if INR > 5.0, vitamin K 10 mg (in 50 mL, normal saline).

In the setting of severe bleeding, administer 4-factor prothrombin complex concentrate and vitamin K 5–10 mg IV [10].

(d) Warnings/Precautions

Severe allergic reactions, including anaphylactic reactions, can occur as a result of intravenous or intramuscular administration of vitamin K.

In severe bleeding, it may be combined with PCC or plasma.

Protamine Sulfate

Since its discovery and FDA approval, protamine sulfate has occupied an important therapeutic niche as perhaps the only viable option for reversing the anticoagulant effect of heparin use for over 77 years [11, 12].

(a) Mechanism of Action

When administered alone, protamine has an anticoagulant effect. However, when it is given in the presence of heparin (which is strongly acidic), a stable salt is formed and the anticoagulant activity of both drugs is lost. Neutralization of heparin occurs within 5 minutes after intravenous administration of an appropriate dose of protamine sulfate.

It is supplied as a solution containing 10 mg of protamine sulfate/ml (50 mg in 5 ml).

(b) Indication

Protamine sulfate can be used to reverse the anticoagulant effect of unfractionated heparin and for incomplete reversal of low-molecular-weight heparin anticoagulant effect.

(c) Adult Dose and Administration

- UFH reversal: protamine sulfate 1–1.5 mg IV per 100 units of heparin

  - Maximum dose: 50 mg/dose; maximum rate: 5 mg/min.
  - Dose based on the amount of heparin remaining in the body; for intravenous heparin infusion, calculate heparin dose based on infusion rate for prior 2 hours.
  - Dose may be adjusted based on time from heparin admin; if 0–30 minutes, give 1–1.5 mg/100 units; if 30–60 minutes, give 0.5–0.75 mg/100 units; if >2 hours, give 0.25–0.375 mg/100 units.

- LMWH reversal

  - Less than 8 hours since the last LMWH dose:

    o Protamine sulfate 1 mg IV per 100 anti-Xa units LMWH; max: 50 mg/dose; rate: 5 mg/min; info: may give additional 0.5 mg IV per 100 anti-Xa units LMWH if bleeding continues; protamine incompletely neutralizes LMWH effects; 1 mg enoxaparin = 100 anti-Xa units

  - Greater than 8 hours since last LMWH dose:

    o Protamine sulfate 0.5 mg IV per 100 anti-Xa units LMWH; max: 50 mg/dose; rate: 5 mg/min; info: may repeat dose x1 if bleeding continues; protamine incompletely neutralizes LMWH effects; 1 mg enoxaparin = 100 anti-Xa units

(d) Warnings and Precautions

Protamine sulfate can cause rare but severe adverse effects that include systemic hypotension, pulmonary hypertension, liver and kidney tissue damage, and anaphylactic reaction [13].

Fresh Frozen Plasma (FFP)

For the reversal of VKA action, if other products are not available, FFP could be administered at a dose of 10–15 ml/kg.

Three-Factor (3F-PCC)/Four-Factor Prothrombin Complex (4F-PCC) and Activated Prothrombin Complex Concentrate (aPCC)

Three- and 4-factor prothrombin complexes are plasma-derived products used to revert the action of warfarin and stop bleeding. They have the potential for inducing allergic reactions. Being plasma-derived and virally inactivated, their potential for transmission of blood-borne infections is minimal. They are, however, potentially thrombogenic.

Three-Factor Prothrombin Complex Concentrates (3F-PCC) (Bebulin VH [14, 15], Profilnine SD [16])

Three-factor prothrombin complex concentrates (Bebulin, Profilnine) have historically been used to control and/or prevent bleeding associated with hemophilia B.

3-F PCC contains plasma-derived factors II, IX, and X, as well as low/nontherapeutic levels of factor VII. For this reason, four-factor PCC is typically preferred for reversal of warfarin effect.

Figure 13.2 illustrates the difference between Bebulin/Immunine VH and Profilnine SD.

(a) Indication

Three-factor prothrombin complex concentrates can be considered for off-label use in the reversal of severe/life-threatening bleeding associated with warfarin. Due to low factor VII content, concomitant administration of fresh frozen plasma or factor VII could be considered.

Name	Bebulin VH/Immunine VH	Profilnine SD
Source	Plasmatic	Plasmatic
Viral inactivation	Vapour heat, Tween 80	Solvent/detergent
Dose based on	Units of factor IX activity	Units of factor IX activity
Prothrombin content	24–38 IU/m	150 IU/100 fIX IU
Factor VII	<5 IU/ml	<35 IU/100 fIX IU
Factor IX	24–38 IU/ml	100 IU
Factor X	24–38 IU/ml	100 IU/100 fIX IU
Heparin	0.15 IU/1 fIX IU	None

Fig. 13.2 Differences between commercial preparations of 3F-PCC

(b) Dose and Administration

An average dose of 25–50 IU/kg is usually administered.

Co-administer vitamin K (phytonadione) 5–10 mg by slow IV infusion [10, 17, 18]; vitamin K may be repeated every 12 hours if INR is persistently elevated.

(c) Warnings and Precautions

Due to viral inactivation, the potential for transmission of blood-borne infections is minimal.

Three-factor prothrombin complex concentrations have thrombogenic potential. Patients should be monitored for thrombotic sequelae following administration of these concentrates.

Allergic reactions have been reported.

Four-Factor Prothrombin Complex Concentrate (4F-PCC)

(a) Mechanism of Action

Four-factor PCC contains coagulation factors II, VII, IX, and X together with the endogenous inhibitor proteins S and C and is indicated for the urgent reversal of acquired coagulation factor deficiency induced by VKA with bleeding or in the urgent perioperative prophylaxis context to revert the action of VKA. Doses are usually individualized based on severity of disorder, extent and location of bleeding, and clinical status of patient. -Four-factor PCC may result in superior efficacy compared to the use of 3F-PCC [18, 19].

Three preparations are available in North America including Kcentra [20]/ Beriplex [21] and Octaplex [22]. Figure 13.3 illustrates the differences between the available formulations.

(b)Indications

Four-factor PCC is indicated for urgent reversal of acquired coagulation factor deficiency induced by vitamin K antagonists in patients who are bleeding or who require invasive procedures on an urgent basis. In this setting, 4F-PCC may result in superior efficacy compared to the use of 3F-PCC [19].

Brand names	Octaplex	Kcentra/Beriplex
Formulation	Freeze-dried	Freeze-dried
Viral inactivation	Solvent and detergent treated	Chromatographic, heat-treated, nano-filtration
Diluent	20 mL/40 mL of WFI	20 mL/40 mL of WFI
Vial size	500 IU	20–31 Factor IX units/mL after reconstitution. The actual potency for 500 unit vial ranges from 400 to 620 units/vial. The actual potency for 1000 unit vial ranges from 800 to 1240 units/vial
Factor II	280–760 IU	380–800 IU
Factor VII	180–480 IU	200–500 IU
Factor IX	280–760 IU	400–620 800–1240
Factor X	360–600 IU	500–1020 IU
Protein C	140–620 IU	420–820 IU
Protein S	140–640 IU	240–680 IU
Others	Heparin	Heparin: 8–40 IU AT 4–30 IU

Fig. 13.3 Differences between the available 4F-PCC formulations [23]

Empiric dosage				
Pretreatment INR	INR <3.0		INR 3.0–5.0	INR >5.0
Dose of prothrombin complex	40 mL (1000 IU)		80 mL (2000 IU)	120 mL (3000 IU)
Weight-adjusted dosage				
Pretreatment INR	INR 2–2.5	INR 2.5–3	INR 3–3.5	INR >3.5
Dose IU/Kg	22.5–32.5 IU/Kg	32.5–40 IU/Kg	40–47.5 IU/Kg	>47.5 IU/Kg maximum dose: 3000 IU (120mL)

For Kcentra® as per FDA approval:

Pretreatment INR	2–<4	4–6	>6
Dose	25 units of F IX/ Kg body weight	35 units of F IX/ Kg body weight	50 units of F IX/ Kg body weight
Maximum dose** (Units of factor IX)/kg body weight	Not to exceed 2500	Not to exceed 3500	Not to exceed 5000

Fig. 13.4 Dose of Octaplex/Beriplex as per Canadian Blood Services recommendation and dose of Kcentra as per FDA approval

(c) Dose and Administration

Dosing of prothrombin complex concentrate should be based on the INR as per Fig. 13.4 with empiric treatment based on INR or a weight-adjusted dosage.

Notes regarding administration:

* 4F-PCC must be administered intravenously; it may be administered by direct IV push, syringe pump, or minibag
* Maximal infusion rates, as per the manufacturer's recommendations:

  – Octaplex: 3 mL/min
  – Beriplex P/N: 8 mL/min

* Reconstituted Kcentra is administered at a rate of 0.12 mL/kg/min (~3 units/kg/min) up to a maximum rate of 8.4 mL/min (~210 units/min) [20]

A 4F-PCC reversal strategy is efficacious in INR reversal and provides lower thromboembolic risk as compared to 3F PCC with rFVIIa [24].

Activated Prothrombin Complex Concentrate (aPCC)

(a) Mechanism of Action

Activated prothrombin complex concentrate (factor eight inhibitor bypassing activity [FEIBA]/Autoplex) contains plasma-derived precursor and activated forms of coagulation factors II, IX, X, and VII [25].

(b) Indications

FEIBA is approved by the FDA to control spontaneous bleeding episodes and to prevent bleeding with surgical interventions in hemophilia A patients with factor VIII inhibitors.

Recent data have also suggested that FEIBA may be used off-label as an anticoagulant reversal agent [26].

(c) Dose and Administration

Dosage and duration of treatment depend on the location and extent of bleeding and clinical condition of the patient.

Determination of the optimal dosing of aPCC for the purpose of anticoagulant reversal has primarily been determined in the setting of intracranial hemorrhage (ICH) associated with non-vitamin K antagonist anticoagulants administered within three to five drug half-lives (off-label use) [27]:

* Oral direct factor Xa inhibitor-mediated bleeding (apixaban, rivaroxaban, edoxaban; if andexanet alfa is not available): 50 units/kg
* Direct thrombin inhibitor-mediated bleeding (argatroban, dabigatran [if idarucizumab is not available], hirudin, rb-hirudin, bivalirudin, desirudin): 50 units/kg
* Pentasaccharide-mediated (fondaparinux – full therapeutic dose only): 20 units/kg

aPCC seems to reverse the anticoagulant effect of Xa inhibitors more effectively than rFVIIa and 3F or 4F-PCC by evaluation with thromboelastometry [28].

(d) Warnings and Precautions

Activated prothrombin complex concentrate administration can lead to increased risk of thromboembolic events. Patients should be monitored for thrombotic sequelae following administration of aPCC.

Recombinant Activated Factor VII (rFVIIa)

Low-dose rFVIIa was initially tested with success as a rapid reversal modality for major bleeding events in the presence of warfarin and an elevated INR in a dose range of 11–25 mcg/kg (1.2 mg) in ICU patients [29]. It was also shown to reverse the anticoagulant effects of argatroban, bivalirudin, fondaparinux, enoxaparin, and heparin as assessed ex vivo by thromboelastography [30].

Due to its cost and its potential thrombotic properties and the availability of more suitable options, its use in the context of anticoagulation reversal is currently limited.

Idarucizumab (Praxbind) [31]

(a) Mechanism of Action

Idarucizumab is a humanized monoclonal antibody fragment that binds to dabigatran, thereby inhibiting the activity of dabigatran as an anticoagulant. Idarucizumab binds to dabigatran and its metabolites with very high affinity, approximately 300-fold more potent than the binding affinity of dabigatran for thrombin.

(b) Indication

Idarucizumab is indicated for adult patients treated with dabigatran when rapid specific reversal of the anticoagulant effect is required for life-threatening bleeding and/or emergent procedures.

(c) Dose and Administration

The recommended dose of idarucizumab is 5 grams (administered as two separate 2.5 g doses no more than 15 minutes apart) [32].

If a second emergency surgery/urgent procedure is required and patient has elevated coagulation parameters (aPTT), consider administration of an additional 5 g, although data to support this approach is limited.

In patients with dabigatran-associated intracranial hemorrhage, if refractory bleeding occurs after the initial idarucizumab dose, consider re-dosing and/or hemodialysis [26].

(d) Warnings and Precautions

Anaphylactic reactions and possible hypersensitivity adverse events including bronchospasm, rash, pyrexia, pruritus, and hyperventilation have been reported in clinical trials [31].

Andexanet Alfa (Andexxa) [33]

(a) Mechanism of Action

Andexanet alfa is a modified recombinant inactive form of human factor Xa developed for reversal of factor Xa inhibitors [33].

(b) Indication

Andexanet alfa is indicated in patients with acute major bleeding associated with the use of a factor Xa inhibitor [33]. Administration in this setting led to effective hemostasis occurring in approximately 80% of patients [34, 35].

(c) Dose and Administration

Dosing is based on the severity of bleeding and the dose of anti-Xa anticoagulant used. Two dosing approaches were suggested based on the timing and strength of the anticoagulant used (please refer to Fig. 13.1).

- Low dose: 400 mg IV bolus administered at a rate of ~30 mg/minute, followed 2 minutes later by 4 mg/minute IV infusion for up to 120 minutes
- High dose: 800 mg IV bolus administered at a rate of ~30 mg/minute, followed 2 minutes later by 8 mg/minute IV infusion for up to 120 minutes

(d) Warnings and Precautions

Arterial and venous thromboembolic events, ischemic events, and cardiac events, including sudden death, have occurred during treatment with andexanet alfa.

Ciraparantag (Aripazine)

Ciraparantag (aripazine) is a drug under investigation, which consists of two L-arginine units connected with a piperazine containing linker chain, as an antidote for a number of anticoagulant drugs, including factor Xa inhibitors (rivaroxaban, apixaban and edoxaban), dabigatran, LMWH, and UH by binding directly to anticoagulants via hydrogen bonds from or guanidine and amide parts of the molecule [36, 37]. At a dose of 300 mg, it reverses the whole blood clotting time induced by enoxaparin in a dose-related manner and produces no procoagulant signal or deleterious adverse events [38].

In a double-blind controlled fashion, escalating, single IV doses (100–300 mg) of ciraparantag were administered alone and following a 60 mg oral dose of edoxaban to healthy volunteers. Fibrin diameter within clots was restored to normal 30 minutes after a single dose of 100–300 mg ciraparantag as determined by scanning electron microscopy and change in fibrin diameter quantified by automated image analysis [39, 40].

Conclusion

When immediate hemostasis is needed in patients receiving therapeutic anticoagulation, reversal of anticoagulation may be achieved with multiple modalities. Protamine sulfate helps reverting the action of heparin and partly reverts the action of LMWHs, whereas vitamin K and plasma-derived products are used to counteract the action of warfarin. Recombinant FVIIa emerged with a limited role in reversal. Idarucizumab binds dabigatran reversing its action, whereas andexanet alfa, a modified recombinant inactive form of human factor Xa, was developed for the reversal of factor Xa inhibitors. A complete palette of reversal agents is therefore now available.

References

1. Ferreira JL, Wipf JE. Pharmacologic therapies in anticoagulation. Med Clin North Am. 2016;100(4):695–718.
2. Holzmacher JL, Sarani B. Indications and methods of anticoagulation reversal. Surg Clin N Am. December 2017;97(6):1291–305.
3. PRODUCT MONOGRAPH PrFRAXIPARINE®Aspen Pharmacare Canada Inc 111 Queen Street East, Suite 450, Toronto, Ontario, M5C 1S2 Submission. Control No: 195973 Date of Revision: July 11, 2017.
4. PRODUCT MONOGRAPH Prinnohep® tinzaparin sodium sterile solution for SC injection. LEO Pharma Inc Thornhill, ON L3T 7W8 www.leo-pharma.com/canada Date of Revision: February 16, 2016.
5. Argatroban prescription information, ARGATROBAN INJECTION in 0.9% Sodium Chloride, for intravenous infusion U.S. Approval: 2000.
6. http://thrombosiscanada.ca/wp-content/uploads/2016/05/Anticoagulant-relatedBleedMgmntOSv.12.pdf.
7. Tomaselli GF, et al. ACC expert consensus decision pathway on management of bleeding in patients on oral anticoagulants. J Am Coll Cardiol. 2017;70:3042.
8. Brighton T. New oral anticoagulant drugs - mechanisms of action. Aust Prescr. 2010;33(2):38–41.
9. Patriquin C, Crowther M. Treatment of Warfarin-associated coagulopathy with vitamin K. Expert Rev Hematol. 2011;4(6):657–67.
10. Guyatt GH, Norris SL, Schulman S, Hirsh J, Eckman MH, Akl EA, Crowther M, Vandvik PO, Eikelboom JW, McDonagh MS, Lewis SZ, Gutterman DD, Cook DJ, Schünemann HJ. Methodology for the development of antithrombotic therapy and prevention of thrombosis

guidelines: antithrombotic therapy and prevention of thrombosis, 9th ed: American College of Chest Physicians Evidence-Based Clinical Practice Guidelines. Chest. 2012 Feb;141(2 Suppl):53S–70S.

11. Sokolowska E, Kalaska B, Miklosz J, Mogielnicki A. The toxicology of heparin reversal with protamine: past, present and future. Expert Opin Drug Metab Toxicol. 2016 Aug;12(8):897–909.

12. Bromfield SM, Wilde E, Smith DK. Heparin sensing and binding - taking supramolecular chemistry towards clinical applications. Chem Soc Rev. 2013 Dec 7;42(23):9184–95.

13. https://dailymed.nlm.nih.gov/dailymed/drugInfo.cfm?setid=e1964129-33f4-4e4e-86e3-8e6a4e65bd83.

14. Bebulin (factor IX complex) [prescribing information]. Westlake Village, CA: Baxter Healthcare; September 2015.

15. PRODUCT MONOGRAPH IMMUNINE VH (Factor IX Concentrate (Human), Vapor Heated, IMMUNO) Freeze-dried powder with diluent for intravenous injection 480–720 IU1 /5 mL, Pharmacopeial Hemostatic Shire Pharma Canada ULC 22 Adelaide Street West, Suite 3800 Toronto Ontario M5H. 4E3 Submission Control No: 214296 Date of Approval: April 23, 2018.

16. Profilnine (factor IX complex) [prescribing information]. Los Angeles, CA: Grifols Biologicals Inc; March 2017.

17. Masotti L, Di Napoli M, Godoy DA, Rafanelli D, Liumbruno G, Koumpouros N, Landini G, Pampana A, Cappelli R, Poli D, Prisco D. The practical management of intracerebral hemorrhage associated with oral anticoagulant therapy. Int J Stroke. 2011 Jun;6(3):228–40.

18. Baker RI, Coughlin PB, Gallus AS, Harper PL, Salem HH, Wood EM, Warfarin Reversal Consensus Group. Warfarin reversal: consensus guidelines, on behalf of the Australasian Society of Thrombosis and Haemostasis. Med J Aust. 2004;181(9):492–7.

19. Herzog E, Kaspereit F, Krege W, Niebl P. Stefan Schulte and Gerhard Dickneite four-factor Prothrombin Complex Concentrate (4F-PCC) is superior to three-factor Prothombin Complex Concentrates (3F-PCC) for reversal of Coumarin anticoagulation blood, vol. 124; 2014. p. 1472.

20. HIGHLIGHTS OF PRESCRIBING INFORMATION. KCENTRA® (Prothrombin Complex Concentrate (Human)) for Intravenous Use, Lyophilized Powder for Reconstitution. Initial U.S. Approval: 2013

21. PRODUCT MONOGRAPH Beriplex® P/N 500 / Beriplex® P/N 1000 Powder and solvent for solution for injection Human Prothrombin Complex. CSL Behring Canada, Inc. 55 Metcalfe Street, Suite 1460 Ottawa, Ontario K1P 6 L5 Date of Revision: September 08, 2017 Date of Approval: September 25, 2017.

22. PRODUCT MONOGRAPH octaplex® Human Prothrombin Complex, freeze dried powder and solvent for solution for injection. Manufactured by: Octapharma Pharmazeutika Produktionsges m.b.H. Oberlaaer Strasse 235 A-1100 Vienna, Austria. Date of Approval: November 3, 2017.

23. PROTHROMBIN COMPLEX CONCENTRATE (PCC) Comparison table, Canadian Blood Services, 2011-06-30 Page 1 .

24. Barton CA, Hom M, Johnson NB, Case J, Ran R, Schreiber M. Protocolized warfarin reversal with 4-factor prothrombin complex concentrate versus 3-factor prothrombin complex concentrate with recombinant factor VIIa. Am J Surg. 2018;215(5):775–9.

25. Abildgaard CF, Penner JA, Watson-Williams EJ. Anti-inhibitor coagulant complex (Autoplex) for treatment of factor VIII inhibitors in hemophilia. Blood. 1980;56:978–84.

26. FEIBA (Anti-Inhibitor Coagulant Complex) for intravenous use, lyophilized powder for solution, vapour heated, prescibing information. Westlake Village: Baxter Healthcare Corporation; 2005.

27. Dibu JR, Weimer JM, Ahrens C, Manno E, Frontera JA. The role of FEIBA in reversing novel oral anticoagulants in intracerebral hemorrhage. Neurocrit Care. 2016;24(3):413–9.

28. Schultz NH, Tran HTT, Bjørnsen S, Henriksson CE, Sandset PM, Holme PA. The reversal effect of prothrombin complex concentrate (PCC), activated PCC and recombinant activated factor VII against anticoagulation of Xa inhibitor. Thromb J. 2017;15:6.

29. Dager WE, King JH, Regalia RC, Williamson D, Gosselin RC, White RH, Tharratt RS, Albertson TE. Reversal of elevated international normalized ratios and bleeding with low-dose recombinant activated factor VII in patients receiving warfarin. Pharmacotherapy. 2006;26(8):1091–8.
30. Young G, Yonekawa KE, Nakagawa P, Blain R, Lovejoy AE, Diane J. Nugent recombinant factor VIIa reverses the anticoagulant effects of Argatroban, Bivalirudin, Fondaparinux, Enoxaparin, and Heparin as assessed Ex Vivo by thromboelastography. Blood. 2004;104:1867.
31. PRODUCT MONOGRAPH INCLUDING PATIENT MEDICATION INFORMATION PrPRAXBIND® Idarucizumab Solution for Infusion or bolus Injection, 5 g/dose Professed Standard Antidote for Pradaxa® Boehringer Ingelheim (Canada) Ltd. 5180 South Service Road Burlington, Ontario L7L 5H4 Date of Approval: June 28, 2018.
32. Pollack CV. Idarucizumab for dabigatran reversal: updated results of the RE-VERSE AD Study. Presented at 2016 American Heart Association Scientific Sessions 2016; New Orleans, LA.
33. ANDEXXA® Product monograph, (coagulation factor Xa (recombinant), inactivated-zhzo) Lyophilized Powder for Solution For Intravenous Injection Initial U.S. Approval: 2018.
34. Connolly SJ, Crowther M, Eikelboom JW, Gibson CM, Curnutte JT, Lawrence JH, Yue P, Bronson MD, Lu G, Conley PB, Verhamme P, Schmidt J, Middeldorp S, Cohen AT, Beyer-Westendorf J, Albaladejo P, Lopez-Sendon J, Demchuk AM, Pallin DJ, Concha M, Goodman S, Leeds J, Souza S, Siegal DM, Zotova E, Meeks B, Ahmad S, Nakamya J, Milling TJ Jr, ANNEXA-4 Investigators. Full study report of Andexanet Alfa for Bleeding associated with factor Xa inhibitors. N Engl J Med. 2019; https://doi.org/10.1056/NEJMoa1814051.
35. Connolly SJ, Milling TJ Jr, Eikelboom JW, Gibson CM, Curnutte JT, Gold A, Bronson MD, Lu G, Conley PB, Verhamme P, Schmidt J, Middeldorp S, Cohen AT, Beyer-Westendorf J, Albaladejo P, Lopez-Sendon J, Goodman S, Leeds J, Wiens BL, Siegal DM, Zotova E, Meeks B, Nakamya J, Lim WT, Crowther M, ANNEXA-4 Investigators. Andexanet Alfa for acute major bleeding associated with factor Xa inhibitors. N Engl J Med. 2016;375(12):1131–41.
36. Schubert-Zsilavecz, M, Wurglics, M, Ciraparantag. Neue Arzneimittel Herbst 2015 (in German).
37. Ansell JE. Universal, class-specific and drug-specific reversal agents for the new oral anticoagulants. J Thromb Thrombolysis. 2016;41(2):248–52.
38. Ansell JE, Laulicht BE, Bakhru SH, Hoffman M, Steiner SS, Costin JC. Ciraparantag safely and completely reverses the anticoagulant effects of low molecular weight heparin. Thromb Res. 2016;146:113–8.
39. Ansell JE, Bakhru SH, Laulicht BE, Steiner SS, Grosso MA, Brown K, Dishy V, Lanz HJ, Mercuri MF, Noveck RJ, Costin JC. Single-dose ciraparantag safely and completely reverses anticoagulant effects of edoxaban. Thromb Haemost. 2017;117(2):238–45.
40. Ansell JE, Bakhru SH, Laulicht BE, Steiner SS, Grosso M, Brown K, Dishy V, Noveck RJ, Costin JC. Use of PER977 to reverse the anticoagulant effect of edoxaban. N Engl J Med. 2014;371(22):2141–2.

Index

© Springer Nature Switzerland AG 2020
H. Goubran et al. (eds.), *Precision Anticoagulation Medicine*,
https://doi.org/10.1007/978-3-030-25782-8